Problem Solving in Respiratory Medicine & Allergy

Edited by

RICHARD LEACH, MD, FRCP
Consultant Physician and Clinical Director of Medicine
Guy's and St Thomas' NHS Foundation Trust
London, UK

CHRISTOPHER KOSKY, MBBS, FRACP
Consultant Physician, Respiratory, General and Sleep Medicine
Guy's and St Thomas' NHS Foundation Trust
Honorary Senior Lecturer
King's College
London, UK

ELIZABETH HADLEY, MBBS Hons, BSc Hons, MRCP London
Consultant Respiratory and General Physician
Department of Respiratory Medicine
Barking, Havering and Redbridge Hospitals University NHS Trust
London, UK

BORIS LAMS, MBBS, MD, FRCP
Consultant Physician, Respiratory, General and Critical Care Medicine
Clinical Lead for Respiratory and Sleep Medicine
Guy's and St Thomas' NHS Foundation Trust
London, UK

CLINICAL PUBLISHING
OXFORD

CLINICAL PUBLISHING
an imprint of Atlas Medical Publishing Ltd
Oxford Centre for Innovation
Mill Street, Oxford OX2 0JX, UK

Tel: +44 1865 811116
Fax: +44 1865 251550

E mail: info@clinicalpublishing.co.uk
Web: www.clinicalpublishing.co.uk

Distributed in USA and Canada by:
Clinical Publishing
30 Amberwood Parkway
Ashland OH 44805 USA
tel: 800-247-6553 (toll free within US and Canada)
fax: 419-281-6883
email: order@bookmasters.com

Distributed in UK and Rest of World by:
Marston Book Services Ltd
PO Box 269
Abingdon
Oxon OX14 4YN UK
tel: +44 1235 465500
fax: +44 1235 465555
email: trade.orders@marston.co.uk

First published 2011

A catalogue record for this book is available from the British Library.

ISBN 13 978 1 904392 86 6
ISBN e-book 978 1 84692 598 6

Project manager: Gavin Smith, GPS Publishing Solutions, Herts, UK
Typeset by Phoenix Photosetting, Chatham, UK
Printed by Marston Book Services, Abingdon, Oxon, UK

Problem Solving in Respiratory Medicine & Allergy

Contents

SECTION 9 Pleural Disease

Contributors

Consultant Respiratory Physicians, Guy's and St Thomas' NHS Foundation Trust, London, UK

Liju Ahmed
Ronan Breen
Anne Collett
Craig Davidson
Christopher Kosky
Boris Lams
Richard Leach
Heather Milburn
John Rees
Charles Twort

Consultant Respiratory and General Physician, Barking, Havering and Redbridge Hospitals University NHS Trust, London, UK

Elizabeth Hadley

Consultant Respiratory Physician, Royal Brompton and Harefield NHS Foundation Trust, London, UK

Nicholas Hopkinson

Consultant Respiratory Physician, Darent Valley Hospital, Dartford and Gravesham NHS Trust, Dartford, Kent, UK

Burhan Khan

Consultant Respiratory Physician, Medway Maritime Hospital, Medway, Kent, UK

Kate Brignall

Specialist Registrars in Respiratory Medicine, Guy's and St Thomas' NHS Foundation Trust, London, UK

Bethia Bradley
Eleanor Giddings
Lynette Linkson
Jimstan Periselneris
Lucy Schomberg

Previous Core Medical Trainees in Respiratory Medicine, Guy's and St Thomas' NHS Foundation Trust, London, UK

Oni Choudhury
Suma Kumar
Amina Aitsi-Selmi

Abbreviations

ABG	arterial blood gas
ABPA	allergic bronchopulmonary aspergillosis
ACCP	American College of Chest Physicians
ACE	angiotensin converting enzyme
ACE-I	angiotensin converting enzyme inhibitor
AECOPD	acute exacerbation of COPD
AEP	acute eosinophilic pneumonia
AF	*Aspergillus fumigatus*
AFB	acid-fast bacilli
AIDS	acquired immune deficiency syndrome
AIP	acute interstitial pneumonia
ALK-1	activin receptor-like kinase 1
ALT	alanine transaminase
ANA	anti-nuclear antibody
ANCA	anti-neutrophil cytoplasmic antibody
ANNA-1 type 1	anti-neuronal nuclear antibody
anti-Ber-EP4	anti-human epithelial antigen
anti-CEA	anti-carcino-embryonic antigen
anti-CK5/6	anti-cytokeratin 5/6
anti-MPO	anti-myeloperoxidase antibody
anti-PR3	anti-proteinase 3 antibody
anti–TTF-1	anti-thyroid transcription factor 1
anti-WT1	anti-Wilms tumour 1
APACHE	Acute Physiology and Chronic Health Evaluation
APAH	associated pulmonary arterial hypertension
ARDS	acute respiratory distress syndrome
ASH	Action on Smoking and Health
AST	aspartate transaminase
ATS	American Thoracic Society
AV	arteriovenous
AVM	arteriovenous malformation
BAL	bronchoalveolar lavage
BCG	Bacillus Calmette-Guérin
BDP	beclomethasone
BHL	bihilar lymphadenopathy
BM	body mass
BMI	body mass index
BMPR2	bone morphogenetic protein receptor 2
BNP	brain natriuretic peptide
BOOP	bronchiolitis obliterans organizing pneumonia
BP	blood pressure
BREATH-1	Bosentan Randomized trial of Endothelin Antagonist Therapy of pulmonary Hypertension Study
BTS	British Thoracic Society
c-ANCA	cytoplasmic anti-neutrophil cytoplasmic antibody
CAP	community-acquired pneumonia
CAVE	cyclophosphamide, doxorubicin, vincristine, etoposide
CCB	calcium channel blocker
CF	cystic fibrosis
cGMP	cyclic guanosine monophosphate
CHART	continuous hyperfractionated accelerated radiotherapy
CHD	congenital heart disease
CI	confidence interval
CK7	cytokeratin 7
CNS	central nervous system
COP	cryptogenic organizing pneumonia
COPD	chronic obstructive pulmonary disease
CPAP	continuous positive airway pressure
CRP	C-reactive protein
CSF	cerebrospinal fluid
CT	computed tomography
CTD	connective tissue disease
CTEPH	chronic thromboembolic pulmonary hypertension
CTPA	computed tomography pulmonary angiogram

CXR	chest radiograph
DAD	diffuse alveolar damage
DIC	disseminated intravascular coagulation
DIP	desquamative interstitial pneumonia
DLCO	carbon monoxide diffusing capacity
DOT	directly observed therapy
DPI	dry powder inhalers
DPLD/ILD	diffuse parenchymal (interstitial) lung disease
DPT	diffuse pleural thickening
DVT	deep vein thrombosis
EBUS	endoscopic bronchial ultrasound
ECG	electrocardiogram
ECV	epirubicin, cyclophosphamide and vincristine
ELISA	enzyme-linked immunosorbent assay
EMA	epithelial membrane antigen
EORTC	European Organisation for Research and Treatment of Cancer
EPAP	expiratory positive airway pressure
EPP	extrapleuropneumonectomy
ERS	European Respiratory Society
ESR	erythrocyte sedimentation rate
ET-1	endothelin-1
ETS	environmental tobacco smoke
F	female
^{18}FDG	18-fluorodeoxyglucose
FEV_1	forced expiratory volume in 1 second
FiO2	inspired oxygen concentration
FRC	functional residual capacity
FU	follow-up
FVC	forced vital capacity
GBM	glomerular basement membrane
GBS	Guillain-Barré syndrome
GGO	ground glass opacification
GI	gastrointestinal
GORD	gastro-oesophageal reflux disease
GP	general practitioner
GSD	glycogen storage disease
HAART	highly active antiretroviral therapy
HAP	hospital-acquired pneumonia
HbSS	homozygous sickle cell disease
HCAP	health-care-associated pneumonia
HCO_3	partial pressure of arterial bicarbonate
HCRF	hypercapnic respiratory failure
HHT	hereditary haemorrhagic telangiectasia
HIV	human immunodeficiency virus
HLA	human leukocyte antigen
HP	hypersensitivity pneumonitis
HPAH	heritable pulmonary arterial hypertension
HRCT	high-resolution computed tomography
HTLV-1	human T cell lymphotrophic virus type 1
IASLC	International Association for the Study of Lung Cancer
ICS	inhaled corticosteroid
ICU	intensive care unit
IDSA	Infectious Diseases Society of America
IgA	immunoglobulin A
IgE	immunoglobulin E
IgG	immunoglobulin G
IIP	idiopathic interstitial pneumonia
IL-1	interleukin-1
IL-5	interleukin-5
ILD	interstitial lung disease
IPAH	idiopathic pulmonary arterial hypertension
IPAP	inspiratory positive airway pressure
IPF	idiopathic pulmonary fibrosis
ISOLDE	Inhaled Steroids in Obstructive Lung Disease in Europe
IU	international unit
Iγ-1b	interferon gamma-1b
KCO	transfer coefficient; carbon monoxide gas transfer corrected for alveolar volume
LABA	long-acting β2 agonist
LAMA	long-acting muscarinic antagonist
LC	Langerhans cell
LCH	Langerhans cell histiocytosis
LDH	lactate dehydrogenase
LFT	liver function test
LIP	lymphocytic interstitial pneumonia
LOS	lower oesophageal sphincter
LRT	lower respiratory tract
LRTI	lower respiratory tract infection
LTOT	long-term oxygen therapy
M	male
MAC	*M. avium* complex
MALT	mucosal-associated lymphoid tissue

MARS	Mesothelioma and Radical Surgery
MDI	metered dose inhalers
MDR	multidrug resistant
MHC	major histocompatibility complex
MND	motor neurone disease
MPA	microscopic polyangiitis
MPO	myeloperoxidase
MRSA	methicillin-resistant *Staphylococcus aureus*
MS	multiple sclerosis
99mTc	technetium-99m
MV	mechanical ventilation
6MW	six-minute walks
NAC	N-acetylcysteine
nAchR	nicotinic acetylcholine receptors
Nd-Yag	neodymium-yttrium aluminium garnet
NHS	National Health Service
NICE	National Institute for Health and Clinical Excellence
NIPPV	non-invasive positive pressure ventilation
NIV	non-invasive ventilation
NRT	nicotine replacement therapy
NSAID	non-steroidal anti-inflammatory drugs
NSCLC	non-small cell lung cancer
NSIP	non-specific interstitial pneumonia
NT	nebulizer therapy
NTM	non-tuberculous mycobacteria
NYHA	New York Heart Association
OC	oral contraceptive
OHS	obesity hypoventilation syndrome
OP	organizing pneumonia
OR	odds ratio
OSA	obstructive sleep apnoea
OT	oxygen therapy
$PaCO_2$	partial pressure of arterial carbon dioxide
PAH	pulmonary arterial hypertension
p-ANCA	perinuclear anti-neutrophil cytoplasmic antibody
PaO_2	partial pressure of arterial oxygen
PAO_2	alveolar oxygen pressure
PAP	pulmonary artery pressure
PAS	para-aminosalicylic acid
PASP	pulmonary artery systolic pressure
PCI	prophylactic cranial irradiation
PCWP	pulmonary capillary wedge pressure
PE	cisplatin and etoposide
PE	pulmonary embolism
PEC	paclitaxel, etoposide, carboplatin
PEEP	positive end-expiratory pressure
PEFR	peak expiratory flow rate
PET	positron emission tomography
PFT	pulmonary function test
PHT	pulmonary hypertension
PiO2	partial pressure of oxygen in airways
PJP	*Pneumocystis jirovecii* pneumonia
PLCH	pulmonary Langerhans cell histiocytosis
pMDI	pressurized metered dose inhaler
PN	pulmonary nodule
PPE	parapneumonic effusion
PPHN	persistent PHT in the newborn
PPV	positive predictive value
PSP	primary spontaneous pneumothorax
QoL	quality of life
RAP	right atrial pressure
RB	respiratory bronchiolitis
RB-ILD	respiratory bronchiolitis-associated interstitial lung disease
RCT	randomized controlled trial
REM	rapid eye movement
RHC	right heart catheterization
RR	respiratory rate
RV	residual volume
RVF	right ventricular failure
RVSP	right ventricular systolic pressure
Rx	treatment
SABA	short-acting β2 agonist
SAMA	short-acting muscarinic antagonist
SaO_2	oxygen saturation of arterial blood
SCC	squamous cell cancer
SCD	sickle cell disease
SCLC	small cell lung cancer
SIADH	syndrome of inappropriate antidiuretic hormone
SIRS	systemic inflammatory response syndrome
SLE	systemic lupus erythematosus
SPP	secondary pneumothorax
SVCO	superior vena cava obstruction
TB	tuberculosis
TBBx	transbronchial biopsy
Td	deadspace
Th1	helper T cell type 1
Th2	helper T cell type 2
TLC	total lung capacity

TLCO	carbon monoxide gas transfer
TNF-a	tumour necrosis factor alpha
TORCH	Towards a Revolution in COPD Health
TPMT	thiopurine methyltransferase
TTE	transthoracic Doppler echocardiography
TTF-1	thyroid transcription factor 1
Tv	tidal volume
UIP	usual interstitial pneumonia
URTI	upper respiratory tract infection
USS	ultrasound scan
V/Q	ventilation-perfusion
VA	alveolar volume
VAP	ventilator-associated pneumonia
VATS	video-assisted thoracoscopy
VC	ital capacity
VCI	inspiratory vital capacity
VO_2	oxygen consumption
WCC	white cell count
WHO	World Health Organization
WHO-FC	World Health Organization functional class
XR	X-ray/radiograph

Infection

PROBLEM

1 Severe Pulmonary Tuberculosis

Oni Choudhury, Heather Milburn

Case History

A 30-year-old, non-English-speaking Estonian man presented with a four-week history of productive cough, haemoptysis, weight loss, fever and night sweats. He had recently arrived in the UK and was working as a casual labourer. He had no past medical history and was on no medication. He had not been treated for, vaccinated against (i.e. Bacillus Calmette-Guérin [BCG]) or had any known tuberculosis (TB) contact. His alcohol intake was excessive but he did not smoke. He lived in a hostel.

On examination he was unwell with fever (39.2°C) and tachypnoea (18 breaths/min) and his oxygen saturation (SaO_2) was 91% on air. There was no lymphadenopathy. Chest examination revealed reduced breath sounds and bronchial breathing in the left lung. His haemoglobin was 10.4 g/dl with a low white cell count (3.9×10^9/l) and lymphocytosis. The C-reactive protein (CRP; 194 mg/l) and erythrocyte sedimentation rate (ESR; 84 mm/h) were raised. Renal function was normal but liver function tests were slightly elevated. The albumin was 21 g/dl. The chest radiograph (CXR) demonstrated dense left-lung consolidation (Figure 1.1) and a left-sided pneumothorax occurred shortly after admission. Acid-fast bacilli were isolated in sputum. Contact tracing revealed that his partner, who was 11 weeks pregnant, had a strongly positive tuberculin skin test and her CXR was consistent with early TB.

What factors would you take into account when you treat this patient?

How would you manage this patient?

What treatment adjustments are required in liver and renal disease?

When would you use steroid therapy in pulmonary tuberculosis?

How would you manage drug resistance in this patient?

How would you manage this patient's pneumothorax?

How would you treat the pregnant partner of this patient?

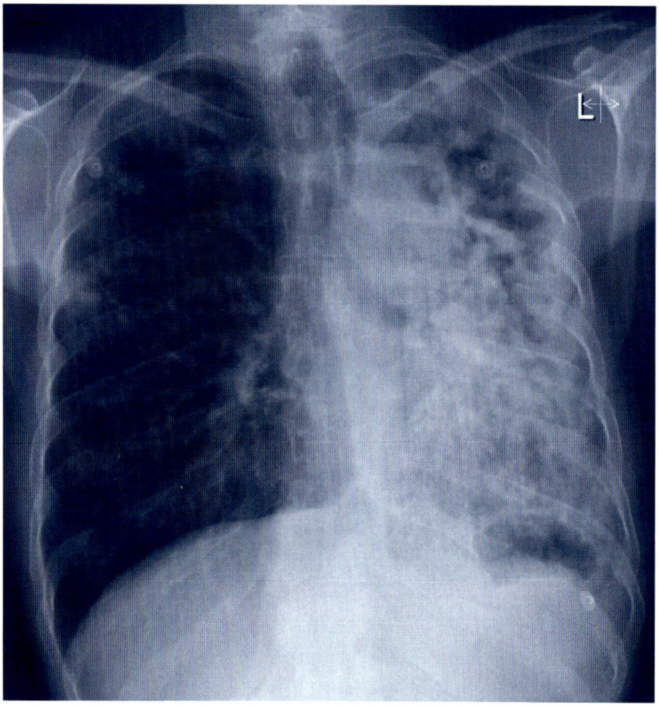

Figure 1.1 Chest radiograph.

Background

Mycobacterium tuberculosis affects 9.4 million people and causes 1.7 million deaths a year worldwide, despite being a curable disease[1] and is one of the commonest causes of infectious mortality. The incidence of tuberculosis (TB) is highest in sub-Saharan Africa but over 50% of cases occur in Asia (i.e. India, China) due to the high population density and incidence is increasing in Eastern Europe and Russia. About 10% of cases globally are multidrug resistant (MDR), and around 10% of TB cases are co-infected with human immunodeficiency virus

(HIV). However, co-infection rates vary geographically, affecting 35%–40% of sub-Saharan African cases, 2.7% of UK cases and 1%–2% of cases in China.

In the UK, 60% of TB occurs in the 15–44-year-old age group, 66% of patients are non-UK born and >70% are from ethnic minority groups.[2] In this case, age, ethnic origin (associated with drug resistance, HIV co-infection), social factors (e.g. isolation, poverty, homelessness) and alcohol consumption (i.e. non-compliance) must be taken into account. The risk factors associated with non-compliance and factors associated with resistant disease are listed in Table 1.1. Although treatment regimens for pulmonary tuberculosis are evidence based,[3,4] the management of complications such as extensive lung damage and pneumothoraces is less clear.

Table 1.1 Risk factors for non-compliance with therapy and resistant disease in TB

a.	**Main risk factors for tuberculosis**
1	Ethnic origin, sex and age
	• Caucasian; >50 years old; M > F
	• Asian/Chinese; <50 years old; M = F
	• African; <40 years old; M = F
2	Medical factors
	• Diabetes; renal and malignant disease
	• Immunosuppression (chemotherapy, steroids)
	• Immunomodulatory drugs (infliximab)
	• Vitamin D deficiency
	• Smoking
3	Poverty, poor nutrition, homelessness, social isolation
4	HIV/AIDS
5	Alcohol addiction
b.	**Risk factors for non-compliance with therapy**
1	Alcohol addiction
2	Homelessness
3	Drug abuse
4	Mental illness
c.	**Factors associated with resistant disease**
1	Contact with resistant disease
2	Treatment failure, inadequate previous anti-TB therapy
3	Adding a single drug to a failing regimen
4	Immigration from area of high resistance

AIDS, acquired immune deficiency syndrome, F, female; M, male.

Management of *Mycobacterium tuberculosis*

Patients with 'open TB' (i.e. sputum smear positive) should be isolated either at home or in a hospital negative-pressure side room (i.e. vented to the outside air) and hospital staff should wear face masks when attending the patient. After two weeks of TB therapy, HIV-negative patients with sensitive organisms are considered non-infectious and although bacilli may be seen in sputum these are usually dead.

The standard TB treatment regimen includes four drugs in the initial two months (rifampicin, isoniazid, pyrazinamide, ethambutol) followed by two drugs for a further four months (rifampicin, isoniazid).[3,4] Initial therapy with four drugs has superseded previous guidelines[5] recommending three drugs because of increasing background isoniazid resistance. In this case, an initial four-drug regimen is essential as isoniazid resistance is greater in immigrants, ethnic minority groups, HIV-positive patients and previously treated patients. A three times weekly directly observed therapy (DOT) regimen for six months is equally effective. Drug doses are calculated according to body weight (Table 1.2). Pyridoxine (vitamin B_6) is given to most patients as their diets are often poor (e.g. alcoholics) or they have diabetes, renal failure or HIV infection.

Central nervous system (CNS) TB requires twelve months' treatment but non-CNS TB usually responds to six months' therapy. Baseline full blood count and renal and liver function tests (LFTs) should be checked and if the patient is not at risk of adverse drug reactions need not be rechecked unless symptoms develop. Steroid therapy may be considered (see below). Essential advice for patients is listed in Table 1.3.

The doctor making the diagnosis has a legal obligation to notify the public health authorities (even if the diagnosis is made after death). This triggers appropriate contact tracing and allows planning of treatment and screening services. As contact tracing is undertaken by the community TB nursing services, they should also be informed about all index cases.

Table 1.2 Standard antituberculous drug doses

Drug	Daily dose	3 × weekly dose
Isoniazid	300 mg	15 mg/kg 3 × weekly (maximum 1 g)
Rifampicin (BM <50 kg)	450 mg	600 mg
Rifampicin (BM >50 kg)	600 mg	900 mg
Pyrazinamide (BM <50 kg)	1.5 g	2.0 g
Pyrazinamide (BM >50 kg)	2.0 g	2.5 g
Ethambutol	15 mg/kg	30 mg/kg

BM, body mass.

Table 1.3 Essential advice for patients starting antituberculous therapy

- Red urine (due to rifampicin)
- Red contact lenses due to rifampicin
- Nausea – usually improves
- Abdominal pain, vomiting or jaundice – stop drugs and contact doctor
- Efficacy of oral contraceptive pill reduced – need alternative contraception
- Potential drug interactions
  - Rifampicin decreases levels of warfarin, phenytoin, digoxin, methadone, sulphonylureas, steroids, theophylline, ciclosporin
  - Isoniazid increases levels of phenytoin, carbamazepine, warfarin, diazepam
- Visual acuity and colour vision loss with ethambutol – stop drugs and contact doctor

Treatment adjustments in liver and renal disease

Liver function tests are often slightly raised in alcoholics or new patients with TB (e.g. hepatic TB). Antituberculous therapy should not be withheld in these patients as LFTs usually improve with therapy or remain stable. Viral hepatitis should be excluded.

In chronic liver disease, baseline LFTs should be followed by regular monitoring (i.e. weekly for two weeks then every two weeks). If aspartate transaminase (AST) and alanine transaminase (ALT) are greater than twice normal, continue to monitor 1–2-weekly;

if greater than five times normal, or if bilirubin rises, stop therapy until liver function recovers. Reintroduce drugs individually, starting with reduced doses of each drug whilst monitoring LFTs and clinical condition. If there is a further reaction, exclude the offending drug and include a second-line alternative (see below). These patients should be managed by a TB expert as antituberculous drug-induced hepatitis can be fatal.

Treatment of TB in renal disease is complicated and should be managed by a TB specialist, and reference should be made to the 2010 British Thoracic Society Guidelines.[6] Generally, isoniazid, rifampicin and pyrazinamide are given in normal doses as they have biliary excretion, although pyrazinamide metabolites may accumulate and cause gout. Ethambutol is renally excreted and the dose should be given less frequently (e.g. three times per week) to avoid optic neuropathy. Peak and trough levels should be measured. Moxifloxacin is a possible alternative to ethambutol. Pyridoxine is required to prevent isoniazid-induced peripheral neuropathy. Drugs are usually given after dialysis in end-stage renal failure.

Corticosteroid therapy in pulmonary tuberculosis

Steroid therapy (30–60 mg daily) is recommended in cerebral, meningeal, pericardial and genitourinary TB to reduce complications due to fibrosis. Steroids also help to prevent hypersensitivity antituberculous drug reactions. Steroids have been used in large tuberculous pleural effusions but their role in pulmonary TB is unclear.

A systematic review of eleven randomized clinical trials of standard chemotherapy with or without steroids (approximately 30 mg/1–3 months) demonstrated early resolution of fever and inflammatory markers, increased weight gain and reduced hospital length of stay with steroids.[7] Unfortunately, most of the trials pre-dated modern anti-TB therapy and only two included rifampicin. Uncontrolled studies show some advantage with steroids in conjunction with rifampicin.[8] Anti-inflammatory effects, cytokine inhibition and suppression of lymphocyte tumour necrosis factor α (TNF-α) release have been proposed as potential mechanisms.

Currently, the American Thoracic Society does not advocate steroid use in pulmonary disease as there is insufficient evidence of benefit.[4] Nevertheless, expert opinion suggests that some patients with severe, cavitating pulmonary TB may benefit. Further well-designed trials are needed. Remember that rifampicin effectively halves the oral dose of steroid.

Management of drug resistance

Numbers of cases of drug resistance are increasing in the UK and in 2009 7.8% of isolates were resistant to at least one first-line drug, 6.9% were resistant to isoniazid, 1.4% to rifampicin and 1.2% were MDR.[2] In this case, after six weeks' culture, the patient's drug sensitivity tests indicated isoniazid mono-resistance. The mono-resistant treatment regimen must include three drugs to which the organism is sensitive:

- **Isoniazid** resistance that is reported before the start of therapy is treated with rifampicin, ethambutol, pyrazinamide and intramuscular streptomycin for two months followed by rifampicin and ethambutol for seven months. If reported after the onset of therapy, stop isoniazid and treat with rifampicin and ethambutol for twelve months with two months of initial pyrazinamide.
- **Pyrazinamide** resistance is uncommon. Use rifampicin and isoniazid for nine months with two months of initial ethambutol.

- **Rifampicin** resistance is rare. It often indicates MDR TB and is treated as such until sensitivities are known. Use isoniazid and ethambutol for 18 months with two months of initial pyrazinamide.
- **Ethambutol** resistance is uncommon. Treat with six months of rifampicin and isoniazid and two months of initial pyrazinamide.

MDR TB is defined as resistance to two or more first-line agents, including isoniazid and rifampicin. Although infectivity is no different from normal TB, treatment is more complex as second-line drugs are more toxic and less effective than first-line agents. Management must involve a specialist experienced in the treatment of MDR TB, isolation in a negative-pressure room, close supervision and monitoring for drug toxicity and compliance. Treatment is with five or more drugs to which the organism is sensitive (including an injectable) until sputum cultures are negative. Treatment is continued with three or four drugs for a total of 18–24 months. Table 1.4 lists available second-line antituberculous therapies.

Table 1.4 Second-line antituberculosis drugs

Drug	Dose	Side effects
Ciprofloxacin	500–750 mg bd	GI upset, headache, drug interaction, connective tissue disorders
Moxifloxacin	400 mg daily	Long QT interval
Ofloxacin	400 mg bd	GI upset, headache
Azithromycin	500 mg od	GI upset
Clarithromycin	500 mg bd	GI upset
Streptomycin	15 mg/kg daily or 3 × per week (maximum total dose 1 g)	Vertigo, tinnitus, ataxia, renal impairment
Amikacin	15 mg/kg	As for streptomycin
Capreomycin	15 mg/kg	As for streptomycin
Kanamycin	15 mg/kg	As for streptomycin
Ethionamide (or prothionamide)	BM <50 kg: 375 mg bd BM >50 kg: 500 mg bd	GI upset, hepatitis; avoid in pregnancy
Aminosalicylic acid (PAS)	4 mg 3 × per day	GI upset, fever, rash, hepatitis
Rifabutin	300–450 mg od	As for rifampicin; uveitis with macrolides

BM, body mass; GI, gastrointestinal.

Contacts of MDR TB should be treated with two drugs (depending on sensitivities in the index case) for six months, although there is no evidence to validate this treatment period. If the resistance is extensive in the index case, no chemoprophylactic regimen may be suitable and these contacts require close follow-up. The British Thoracic Society provide an expert advice panel to assist with the management of MDR TB.[9]

Management of pneumothorax in tuberculosis

Since the advent of effective chemotherapy the occurrence of pneumothorax has decreased and occurs in <1% of hospital TB cases, so there is very little up-to-date evidence for management. Intercostal drainage remains standard therapy although resolution may take up to six weeks.[10] Factors influencing the length of drainage include the extent of underlying parenchymal damage, delay from diagnosis to drainage and the presence of an empyema. There is no evidence to suggest that surgical intervention provides any great benefit over tube drainage.

Tuberculosis treatment in pregnancy

The diagnosis of TB is often delayed in pregnancy as the initial non-specific symptoms are attributed to the pregnancy and chest radiographs are avoided. Tuberculin skin tests are not affected by pregnancy but a negative test should not be followed by BCG, as live vaccines are contraindicated in pregnancy. Diagnosis in the first trimester has a similar outcome to that in non-pregnant women. Diagnosis in the second or third trimester, particularly when associated with inadequate treatment, is associated with pre-eclampsia, small-for-date babies, spontaneous abortion and an increase in pre-term labour and obstetric mortality, particularly in third-world countries.[1]

Rifampicin, isoniazid, pyrazinamide and ethambutol are not teratogenic. Standard therapy using these four drugs for six months is recommended in non-CNS TB. Poor absorption due to morning sickness in early pregnancy is the main problem with treatment and may cause drug resistance. Second-line drugs have variable toxicity and should be used only after specialist advice (e.g. streptomycin causes fetal ototoxicity). Babies of sputum-positive mothers who have been treated for less than two weeks at delivery should be treated with isoniazid and skin-tested at six weeks. If the skin test is negative, the isoniazid is stopped and BCG given one week later (BCG is sensitive to isoniazid). The concentrations of drugs in breast milk are too low to prevent or treat infection in the baby. Consequently breast-feeding is safe.

Conclusion

In this case the patient had 'open TB' (i.e. sputum smear positive) and was homeless (i.e. cannot be isolated at home for two weeks) and consequently was admitted to a hospital negative-pressure side room. He was at high risk of non-compliance because he was alcoholic, homeless and unable to communicate effectively (non-English speaking). To ensure effective therapy his minimum requirements included adequate accommodation, close follow-up including urine examination (i.e. rifampicin stains urine red) and tablet counts by the community TB nursing team. Dosette boxes help people with chaotic lives to remember their medication and ensure correct treatment in those with poor understanding. If there is concern about compliance, sputum should be rechecked and consideration given to DOT, which aims to improve compliance by witnessing the ingestion of medication three times weekly. DOT improves treatment completion, prevents relapses and reduces drug resistance.

Further Reading

1. World Health Organization. Global Health Observatory. Tuberculosis. www.who.int/gho/tb/en (accessed 21 06 11).
2. Health Protection Agency (UK). Tuberculosis. www.hpa.org.uk (accessed 21 06 11).
3. National Institute for Health and Clinical Excellence. Tuberculosis: clinical diagnosis and management of tuberculosis and measures for its prevention and control. Clinical guideline 117. London: NICE, 2006. www.nice.org.uk (accessed 01 06 11).
4. American Thoracic Society, CDC and Infectious Diseases Society of America. Treatment of Tuberculosis. MMWR Recommendations and Reports, 2003; 52 (RR-11): 1–88.

5 Joint Tuberculosis Committee of the British Thoracic Society. Chemotherapy and management of tuberculosis in the United Kingdom: recommendations 1998. *Thorax* 1998; **53**: 536–48.

6 Milburn HJ, Ashman N, Davies P *et al.* Guidelines for the prevention and management of *Mycobacterium tuberculosis* infection and disease in adult patients with chronic kidney disease. British Thoracic Society Guidelines Group on behalf of the BTS Standards of Care Committee and Joint Tuberculosis Committee. *Thorax* 2010; **65**: 557–70.

7 Smego RA, Ahmed N. A systematic review of the adjunctive use of systemic corticosteroids for pulmonary tuberculosis. *Int J Tuberc Lung Dis* 2003; **7**: 208–13.

8 Muthuswamy P, Hu TC, Carasso B, Antonio M, Dandamudi N. Prednisone as an adjunctive therapy in the management of pulmonary tuberculosis. Report of 12 cases and review of the literature. *Chest* 1995; **107**: 1621–30.

9 British Thoracic Society. Tuberculosis. www.brit-thoracic.org.uk/tuberculosis.aspx (accessed 01 06 11).

10 Auerbach O, Lipstein S. Bronchopleural fistulas complicating pulmonary tuberculosis. *J Thorac Surg* 1939; **8**: 384.

PROBLEM

2 Non-tuberculous Mycobacterial Disease

Ronan Breen, Richard Leach

Case History

A 64-year-old man with emphysema (forced expiratory volume in 1 second [FEV_1] 0.9 l, forced vital capacity [FVC] 3.5 l, gas transfer [KCO] 50% predicted), left apical cavitation following previous tuberculosis (TB) and a small aspergilloma presented with a chronic obstructive pulmonary disease (COPD) exacerbation and a small right-sided pneumothorax. Before admission his exercise tolerance had been poor and he had intermittent night sweats.

On examination he was thin with a body mass index (BMI) of 18 kg/m^2. He was breathless and mildly febrile (37.6°C), with a saturation (SaO_2) 89%, reduced right-sided air entry and widespread expiratory wheeze. Sputum microbiology detected a heavy growth of *Moraxella catarrhalis* but sputum was smear negative for acid-fast bacilli (AFB). The C-reactive protein (CRP) was 24 mg/l. Figure 2.1 illustrates his presenting chest radiograph (CXR). The COPD exacerbation was treated with antibiotics, steroids and bronchodilators. Following initial recurrences, the right-sided pneumothorax (arrow in Figure 2.1) was eventually successfully drained.

At follow-up six weeks later the patient was clinically well but sputum mycobacterial culture from the previous admission had isolated a scanty growth of *Mycobacterium kansasii*. Three sputum samples following this appointment were AFB smear negative but at follow-up two months later one of three cultures had again isolated *M. kansasii*. Symptoms were stable apart from 1 kg weight loss, CXR was unchanged and CRP was 32 mg/l. A high-resolution computed tomography (HRCT) scan demonstrated widespread emphysema with apical cavitation but no other abnormality. Three further sputum samples were AFB smear negative but at follow-up two months later, one of the three cultures had again isolated *M. kansasii*. Symptoms and CXR were unchanged apart from a further 1 kg in weight loss and a CRP of 20 mg/l.

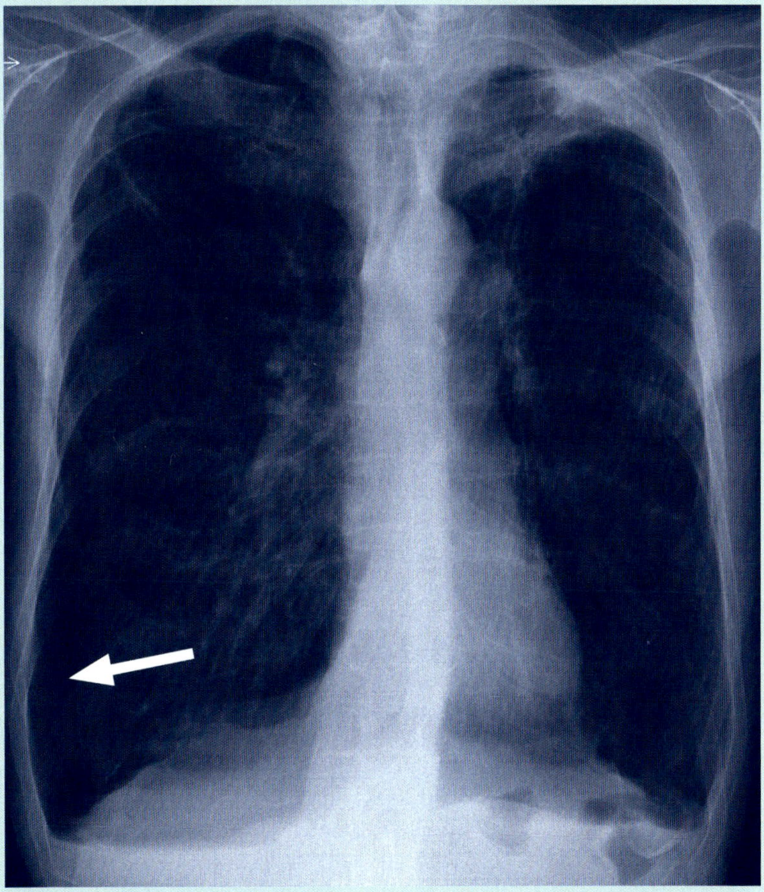

Figure 2.1 Chest radiograph. The right-sided pneumothorax is indicated by the arrow.

What are the criteria to diagnose non-tuberculous mycobacterial (NTM) lung disease?

What are the characteristic clinical features of NTM disease?

How would you manage the *M. kansasii* isolated in this patient?

Should pulmonary NTM infection be notified and contact traced?

Can NTM lung disease affect other sites?

Background

Non-tuberculous mycobacteria (NTM), also called atypical, opportunistic or environmental mycobacteria, are ubiquitous in the environment and are found in water (including tap water), soil, dust, milk, animals and birds. To date, 125 different species have been identified. They are low-grade pathogens and only a few (e.g. *M. avium* complex [MAC], *M. kansasii*, *M. malmoense*, *M. abscessus*, *M. xenopi*) cause significant human illness. Because NTM can be isolated following environmental contamination, more than one culture-positive specimen is often required for diagnostic purposes. Similarly the decision to treat is often dependent on the likelihood of active infection determined from clinical, radiographic and microbiological progression.

The American Thoracic Society (ATS) and the Infectious Diseases Society of America (IDSA) clinical and microbiological criteria for diagnosing NTM lung disease are given in Table 2.1.[1] The 1999 British Thoracic Society guidelines[2] differ slightly and suggest that NTM lung disease is likely if the CXR is suggestive and three or more positive sputum samples are obtained seven days apart with or without symptoms; or if there is one

Table 2.1 Clinical and microbiologic criteria for diagnosing NTM lung disease

Clinical (both required)

1 Pulmonary symptoms, cavitary or nodular opacities on CXR, or a HRCT scan showing multifocal bronchiectasis with multiple small nodules

AND

2 Appropriate exclusion of other diagnoses

Microbiology

1 Positive culture results from at least two separate sputum samples. If the initial sputum results are non-diagnostic consider repeating

OR

2 Positive culture results from at least one bronchial wash or bronchoalveolar lavage (BAL)

OR

3 Transbronchial or other lung biopsy with mycobacterial histopathologic features (granuloma or AFB) and +ve culture for NTM, or biopsy with mycobacterial histopathologic features and 1 or more sputum or BAL samples that are NTM culture +ve

4 Expert advice should be sought when NTM are recovered that are infrequent or usually represent environmental contamination

5 Patients who are suspected of having NTM lung disease but who do not meet the diagnostic criteria should be followed until the diagnosis is firmly established or excluded

6 Making the diagnosis of NTM lung disease does not necessitate the institution of therapy, which is a decision based on the potential risks and benefits of therapy for each case

+ve, positive.

positive culture from a sterile site (e.g. pleural fluid, biopsy); or two positive cultures from bronchoalveolar lavage (BAL) on separate occasions.

Clinical features of non-tuberculous mycobacteria disease

Symptoms and signs of NTM disease are variable and non-specific. Most cases present with a subacute illness, productive cough and weight loss. Fatigue, dyspnoea and fever are common and haemoptysis occasional. Symptoms frequently mimic those seen in TB. The underlying lung disease (e.g. COPD) may complicate evaluation of the symptoms and signs and in these cases the underlying disease progression may be atypical. Occasionally a hypersensitivity-type illness occurs. For example MAC-associated 'hot tub syndrome' resolves when hot-tub exposure stops (± steroids and antibiotics).

- **Radiographic features** in NTM lung disease are either (i) fibrocavitary (often indistinguishable from TB) or (ii) characterized by clusters of small nodules (<5 mm) and multifocal bronchiectasis which is typically located in the mid and lower lung fields. A plain CXR may be sufficient for evaluation of fibrocavitary disease but HRCT scan is often required to confirm nodular/bronchiectatic disease.
- **Mycobacterial culture** and isolation of NTM is essential for the diagnosis of NTM lung disease. Presumptive diagnosis based on clinical and radiographic features is not adequate to initiate therapy. In addition, as a single sputum culture may be due to contamination it is inadequate for diagnosis. Three sputum samples collected on three separate days optimize the predictive value of sputum analysis. A study correlating MAC culture with new radiographic cavitation and infiltration demonstrated that greater than two positive cultures (from three specimens) was associated with radiographic progression in >90% of cases whereas a single positive culture was not.[3] Table 2.1 illustrates the microbiological requirements for NTM diagnosis.

Management of NTM isolation

Chronic pulmonary disease is the most frequent clinical manifestation of NTM. In the USA,[1] the commonest pulmonary pathogens, in order of frequency, are MAC, *M. kansasii* and *M. abscessus* whereas in the UK[2] *M. kansasii*, MAC, *M. malmoense* and *M. xenopi* are the most frequent. Treatment should be in close liaison with the tuberculosis and infectious disease teams.

M. kansasii

M. kansasii is usually acquired from tap water, which is the major reservoir for this NTM. Lung disease due to *M. kansasii* occurs in geographic clusters and is more frequent in south-east England, Wales and central USA. It primarily affects middle-aged to elderly white men or those with pre-existing lung disease, especially those with emphysema, healed TB, alcoholism or immunodeficiency. The clinical course closely parallels that of TB with subacute illness and upper lobe cavitary infiltrates. Untreated, the disease progresses.

Treatment: *M. kansasii* is most sensitive to treatment with rifampicin although isoniazid, ethambutol, clarithromycin and ethionamide are also effective. Drug regimes containing rifampicin report sputum conversion rates of almost 100% with low long-term relapse rates.[1,2] Daily treatment regimes should include rifampicin 10 mg/kg/day (maximum 600 mg), ethambutol 15 mg/kg/day, isoniazid 5 mg/kg/day (maximum 300 mg) and pyridoxine 50 mg/day for a duration that includes twelve months of negative sputum cultures. Patients with rifampicin-resistant *M. kansasii* require a three-drug regime based on *in vitro* susceptibilities including clarithromycin or azithromycin, moxifloxacin, ethambutol, sulfamethoxazole and streptomycin or amikacin. Treatment may be indefinite in non-compliant subjects. Overall response rate is 100%, with >90% five-year cure and <10% relapse.

M. avium *complex*

M. avium complex is most commonly acquired from natural water sources including indoor pools and hot tubs. Lung disease presents as:

- **Apical fibrocavitary disease** in 40–50-year-old male smokers who drink excessive alcohol. If untreated it progresses to severe lung destruction over 1–2 years.
- **Nodular/bronchiectatic disease** in post-menopausal, non-smoking, white females with thin body habitus, scoliosis and pectus excavatum. Consequently it is often referred to as 'Lady Windermere syndrome'. It affects mainly the right middle and lingular lobes. It is characterized by HRCT findings of bronchiectasis and peripheral nodules centred round the bronchovascular bundle with a 'tree-in-bud pattern'. Unlike fibrocavitary disease it progresses slowly.

In human immunodeficiency virus (HIV)-positive patients with a CD4 count <50 cells/μl, MAC is the cause of 90% of NTM infection and is rarely confined to the lungs. Widespread dissemination occurs early. The CXR shows diffuse interstitial, alveolar and nodular infiltrates.

Treatment: the introduction of the macrolides – clarithromycin and azithromycin – to previous regimes using rifampicin or rifabutin, ethambutol and streptomycin represented a major advance in treatment. All untreated MAC strains are macrolide sensitive but as resistance can develop, macrolide monotherapy should be avoided. Drug regimes including a macrolide achieve sputum clearance in 70%–90% of cases with associated negative sputum cultures for twelve months.

Recommendations for initial therapy depend on the type of pulmonary disease and are shown in Table 2.2.[1] The primary microbiological goal is twelve months of negative sputum cultures whilst on therapy. Intermittent drug regimes are not recommended for fibrocavitary disease or those who have been previously treated. Doses may have to be modified for small body mass (<50 kg), age (>70 years) and drug intolerance (i.e. gastrointestinal effects with clarithromycin). Occasionally surgical resection is justified in patients with localized MAC disease.

In HIV-positive cases MAC treatment should be considered lifelong unless immune restoration is achieved with antiretroviral therapy. The risk of drug interactions between rifampicin, macrolides, protease inhibitors and non-nucleoside reverse transcription inhibitors should be considered. MAC prophylaxis is achieved with azithromycin 1200 mg weekly or clarithromycin 500 mg twice daily.

Other NTM

Other NTM causing lung disease (e.g. *M. malmoense*, *M. xenopi*, *M. abscessus*) show varying sensitivity and resistance to treatment and specialist advice should always be sought.

Table 2.2 Therapy for MAC lung disease

Type of pulmonary disease	Initial therapy
• Nodular bronchiectatic disease • Fibrocavitary disease in patients unable to tolerate daily therapy • When disease suppression rather than cure is an appropriate goal	*Three times weekly* regime of: 1 Clarithromycin 1000 mg or azithromycin 500–600 mg 2 Ethambutol 25 mg/kg 3 ± Rifampicin 600 mg
• Fibrocavitary disease • Severe nodular bronchiectatic disease	*Daily* regime of: 1 Clarithromycin 1000 mg/day or azithromycin 250 mg/day 2 Ethambutol 15 mg/kg/day 3 Rifampicin 450–600 mg/day
• Advanced severe fibrocavitary disease • Previously treated disease	*Daily* regime of: 1 Clarithromycin 1000 mg/day or azithromycin 250 mg/day 2 Ethambutol 15 mg/kg/day 3 Rifabutin 150–300 mg/day or rifampicin 450–600 mg/day 4 ± Streptomycin or amikacin

The incidence of *M. malmoense* and *M. xenopi* is similar to *M. kansasii* in parts of the UK. In these areas they often cause NTM lung disease.

- ***M. malmoense***: is best treated with rifampicin and ethambutol (± clarithromycin, ciprofloxacin, isoniazid) for 24 months but up to 10% of patients remain culture positive or relapse after two years' treatment.
- ***M. xenopi***: often colonizes hot water systems as it is an obligate thermophile (i.e. optimal growth at 45°C). It causes fibrocavitary lung disease with an insidious onset and commonly occurs in patients with COPD. Optimal therapeutic regimens include clarithromycin, rifampicin, ethambutol and isoniazid (± streptomycin, ciprofloxacin or moxifloxacin) and are continued until sputum cultures have been negative for twelve months. Although sputum conversion occurs rapidly, relapse rates are high and in one study mortality was 57% at five years, probably reflecting the severe underlying lung disease.[2,4]
- ***M. abscessus***: no treatment has proven efficacy in lung disease. However, multidrug regimens including clarithromycin 1000 mg/day and one or more parenteral agents (e.g. amikacin, imipenem), for several months, may produce symptomatic improvement. The only curative therapy requires surgical resection of localized lung disease combined with multidrug therapy.

Notification of non-tuberculous mycobacteria infection

The risk of cross-infection with NTM lung disease is very low. Notification and contact tracing are not required. If a patient is notified as TB and AFB are subsequently found to be NTM, the patient should be 'de-notified' and medication changed as appropriate.

Non-tuberculous mycobacteria involvement of non-pulmonary tissues

Non-pulmonary NTM is less common but can involve many other sites:

- Lymphadenitis due to NTM (e.g. MAC, *M. malmoense*) occurs mainly in children (1–5 years old) and often presents with non-tender, cervical lymphadenopathy and a normal CXR. Surgical resection of affected nodes is recommended. Antituberculous therapy is reserved for post-operative recurrence.

- Widespread dissemination (e.g. MAC) occurs in the immunocompromised (e.g. HIV positive).
- Skin and soft tissue lesions (e.g. *M. abscessus*, *M. chelonae*, *M. marinum*) may follow local invasion (e.g. injection with a tap water–contaminated needle).

Conclusion

In this patient the isolation of three positive cultures of *M. kansasii* over six months in the absence of progressive clinical or radiological disease suggests 'colonization' but not 'active' disease. Given the slow progression of NTM lung disease, the concept of 'colonization' may not be justified, as slow progression with few initial symptoms may still proceed to severe disease. Nevertheless, as this patient was clinically stable with minimal symptoms (apart from weight loss) and no evidence of radiological progression, expert advice recommended continued microbiological and radiological monitoring without treatment.

Further Reading

1 Griffith DE, Aksamit T, Brown-Elliott BA *et al.* An official ATS/IDSA statement: diagnosis, treatment, and prevention of nontuberculous mycobacterial diseases. *Am J Respir Crit Care Med* 2007; **175**: 367–416.

2 British Thoracic Society. Management of opportunistic mycobacterial infections: Joint Tuberculosis Committee Guidelines 1999. *Thorax* 2000; **55**: 210–8.

3 Tsukamura M. Diagnosis of disease caused by *Mycobacterium avium* complex. *Chest* 1991; **99**: 667–9.

4 Research Committee of the British Thoracic Society. First randomised trial of treatments for pulmonary disease caused by *M avium intracellulare*, *M malmoense*, and *M xenopi* in HIV negative patients: rifampicin, ethambutol and isoniazid versus rifampicin and ethambutol. *Thorax* 2001; **56**: 167–72.

PROBLEM

3 Hospital-acquired Pneumonia

Richard Leach

Case History

A 69-year-old man was admitted to hospital with acute abdominal pain and peritonitis. He had a history of indigestion but no previous cardiorespiratory illness. At surgery a perforated duodenal ulcer was successfully over-sewn. Two days post-operatively he developed low-grade fever (37.8°C), tachycardia (90 beats/min) and tachypnoea (22 breaths/min). The following day he was confused and agitated, with a temperature of 38.5°C, tachycardia (95 beats/min), tachypnoea (26 breaths/min), oxygen saturation (SaO_2) 89% on air and 96% on 40% oxygen, blood pressure (BP) 110/70 mmHg, bilateral crepitations on chest auscultation and falling urine output at 25 ml/hr. Initial investigations demonstrated a raised white cell count of 18×10^9/l, urea of 12 mmol/l and creatinine of 170 μmol/l. Blood gases on air revealed partial pressures of arterial oxygen (PaO_2) of 8.2 kPa and carbon dioxide ($PaCO_2$) of 4.0 kPa, pH 7.3 and bicarbonate 18 mmol/l. A chest radiograph demonstrated bi-basal atelectasis and some minor lower lobe consolidation. A diagnosis of post-operative pneumonia was made and the patient was treated with intravenous amoxicillin by the surgical houseman; the patient appeared to improve over the next 24 hours. The following day the chest team was called to review the patient who had become more confused, tachypnoeic, hypotensive (BP 95/55 mmHg), hypoxaemic (SaO_2 89% on 40% oxygen) and oliguric (urine output <20 ml/hr). A repeat chest radiograph was performed (Figure 3.1).

How is hospital-acquired pneumonia (HAP) defined and the diagnosis established?

What is the pathogenesis and which organisms cause HAP?

What other factors determine the type of causative organism in HAP?

What is the incidence and mortality associated with HAP?

How would you manage this patient?

Background

The pathogenesis, causative organisms and outcome of hospital-acquired pneumonia (HAP) differ from community-acquired pneumonia (CAP).[1–4] Preventative measures and early antibiotic therapy guided by awareness of the role of potential multidrug resistant (MDR) pathogens improves outcome in HAP.[4,5]

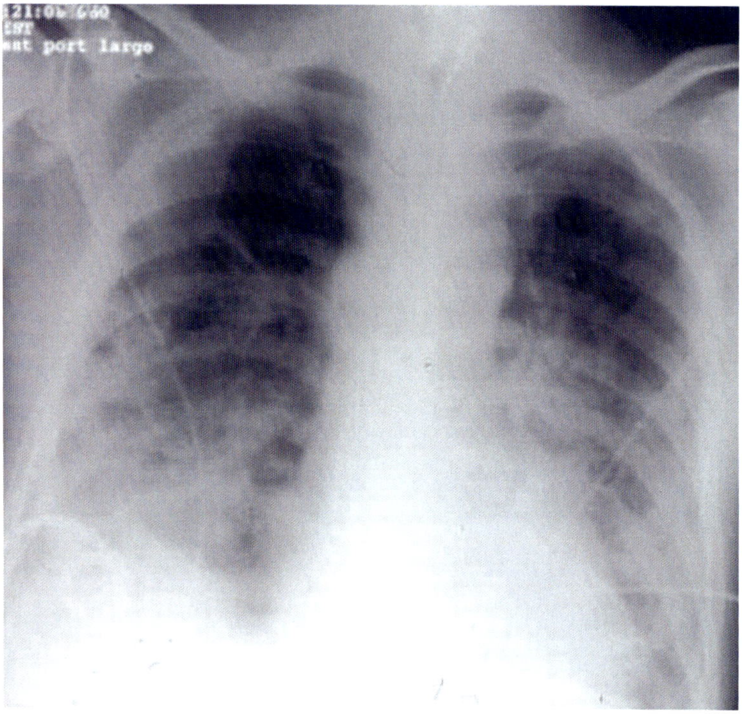

Figure 3.1 Chest radiograph.

HAP is defined as any lower respiratory tract (LRT) infection developing >48 hours after hospital admission that was not incubating at the time of admission. The definition of HAP includes 'ventilator-associated pneumonia' (VAP), which refers to pneumonia developing >48–72 hours after endotracheal intubation. In the USA, health-care-associated pneumonia (HCAP) is described and identifies patients who are at immediate risk of pneumonia caused by 'hospital-acquired' pathogens rather than the expected 'community-acquired' pathogens. HCAP includes any patient admitted to hospital for >2 days within 90 days of the current infection, residing in a nursing home, receiving wound or intravenous therapy within 30 days of the current infection, or who attends a hospital or haemodialysis clinic.[4] Diagnosis of HAP is based on *both clinical and microbiological assessment* but may be difficult as clinical features are often non-specific or confused with concurrent illness (e.g. acute lung injury), and previous antibiotic therapy limits microbiological evaluation. HAP is suspected if a patient develops new radiographic infiltrates, hypoxaemia and at least two of three clinical features suggestive of infection (e.g. temperature >38°C, purulent secretions, leukocytosis or leukopaenia). Diagnostic tests verify infection and determine the causative organism (± antibiotic sensitivity). They include routine blood counts, blood gas analysis, serology, blood cultures, diagnostic thoracentesis of pleural effusions, chest radiography and LRT cultures including endotracheal aspirates and bronchoalveolar lavage in intubated patients. Computed tomography (CT) scanning aids diagnosis and detects complications, which are frequent with cavitation, abscesses, effusions and haemoptysis (Figure 3.2).

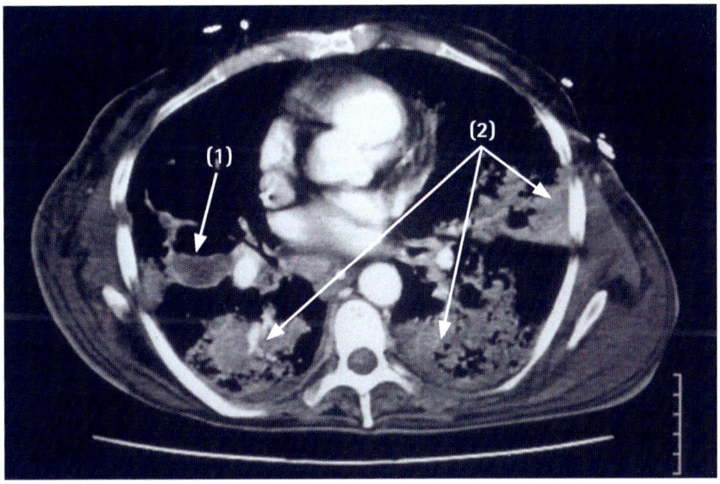

Figure 3.2 Chest CT scan showing abscess formation (1) and consolidation (2).

Incidence and mortality

Hospital-acquired pneumonia is the second commonest nosocomial infection after urinary tract infections and accounts for 15% of hospital-acquired infections in the UK and USA.[4,5] It is the most important in terms of mortality. It affects 0.5%–2% of hospital patients. Incidence varies between 5 and 10 episodes per 1000 discharges and lengthens hospital stay by 3–14 days. Incidence is highest on intensive care units (ICU) and surgical wards. ICU HAP accounts for 37% of all HAP, and VAP for >80% of ICU HAP. The risk of HAP increases 6–20 fold during mechanical ventilation (MV) and it occurs in 9%–27% of intubated patients. In ICU, it accounts for 25% of all infections and approximately 50% of prescribed antibiotic use. The risk of VAP is 3%/day during the first five days of mechanical ventilation, 2%/day during days 5–10 and 1%/day after this.

HAP mortality is 30%–70% but early-onset HAP/VAP (defined as occurring within the first four days of hospitalization) is usually caused by antibiotic-sensitive bacteria and carries a better prognosis than late-onset HAP/VAP, which occurs after five days and is associated with MDR pathogens.[4] However, prior antibiotic therapy or hospitalization predispose to MDR pathogens and are treated as late-onset HAP/VAP even if occurring before five days. Delayed or ineffective antibiotic therapy, bacteraemia (especially with *Pseudomonas aeruginosa* or *Acinetobacter* species), medical rather than surgical illness and VAP increase mortality.[4,5]

Pathogenesis and causative organisms

Oropharyngeal colonization with enteric Gram-negative bacteria occurs in most patients within a few days of hospital admission due to immobility, instrumentation (e.g. nasogastric tubes), inhibition of gastric acid secretion (e.g. proton pump inhibitors) or inadequate attendant hygiene with cross-infection. Subsequent aspiration of nasopharyngeal secretions (± gastric contents) due to supine positioning, reduced consciousness, difficulty swallowing, leakage past endotracheal-tube cuffs or direct inoculation during airways suctioning introduces these organisms into the LRT. Impaired mechanical (e.g. cough), cellular and humoral host defences and inability to clear secretions (e.g. lung disease, sedation, MV, post-operative pain) promote ensuing infection.[4] Haematogenous spread from distant infected sites may also cause HAP.

Accurate microbiological data of the causative organisms in HAP are limited.[4,5] Aerobic Gram-negative bacilli including *Klebsiella pneumoniae*, *Pseudomonas aeruginosa*, *Escherichia coli* or *Acinetobacter* species cause 45%–70% of HAP and Gram-positive bacteria including *Streptococcus pneumoniae* and *Staphylococcus aureus* approximately 10%–40%. *S. pneumoniae* and *Haemophilus influenzae* may be isolated in early-onset HAP/VAP (less than four days in hospital). Polymicrobial infection is increasing (~50%) and isolated anaerobic infections occur in 25% of cases. Viral and fungal infections are rare in immunocompetent hosts.

Factors that determine the type of causative organism

The potential pathogens causing HAP depends on (i) severity of illness, (ii) time of onset (i.e. early/late onset) and (iii) the presence of risk factors for HAP and infection with MDR organisms (Table 3.1, Figure 3.3).[4] Risk factors for developing HAP may be host related (e.g. malnutrition, age, comorbid disease, alcohol dependency, smoking, obesity), epidemiological (e.g. occupation, environment), therapy related (e.g. immunosuppressive therapy, posture, intravenous lines, sedation, MV, pain relief) or associated with infection control (e.g. isolation, hand washing).

Table 3.1 Risk factors for multidrug-resistant pathogens causing hospital-acquired pneumonia

- Antimicrobial therapy in the previous 90 days
- Current hospitalization of >5 days
- High frequency of local antibiotic resistance
- Presence of risk factors for HCAP
  - Hospitalization for >2 days in the previous 90 days
  - Residence in a nursing home
  - Home wound care or intravenous therapy
  - Chronic dialysis within 30 days
  - Family member with MDR pathogen
- Immunosuppressive disease and/or therapy

Critical risk factors for developing HAP include prolonged (>48 hours) mechanical ventilation, duration of hospital or ICU stay, severity of illness (Acute Physiology and Chronic Health Evaluation [APACHE] score), presence of acute respiratory distress syndrome (ARDS) and medical comorbidity. In ventilated patients, prior use of antibiotics appears protective, whereas continuous sedation, cardiopulmonary resuscitation, high ventilatory pressures, upper airway colonization and duration of ventilation were independent risk factors.

Management

Constant vigilance in hospital patients with early diagnosis and treatment of HAP improves morbidity and mortality. Antibiotic therapy must not be delayed whilst awaiting diagnostic tests and microbiological results.

- **Supportive therapy** includes supplemental oxygen to maintain PaO_2 >8 kPa (saturation <90%) and intravenous fluids (± inotropes) to maintain a mean blood pressure >65 mmHg and urine output 0.5–1.0 ml/kg/min. Physiotherapy and analgesia aid

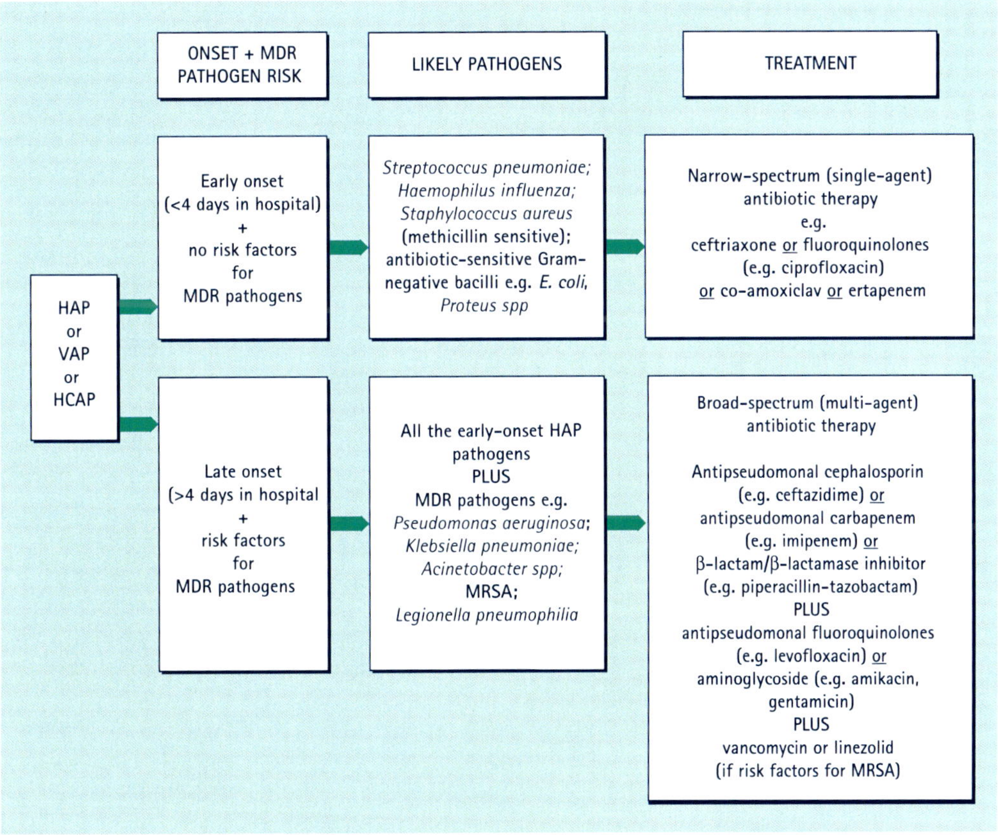

Figure 3.3 Likely pathogens and empirical antibiotic treatment of hospital-acquired pneumonias. MRSA, methicillin-resistant *Staphylococcus aureus*.

sputum clearance post-operatively and in immobile patients. Avoid heavy sedation and paralytic agents that may depress cough. Semi-recumbent nursing of bed-bound patients with elevation of the bed head to 30° reduces aspiration risk.

- **Ventilatory support** including non-invasive (e.g. continuous positive airway pressure [CPAP], non-invasive positive pressure ventilation [NIPPV]) or mechanical ventilation may be required in respiratory failure. Subglottic aspiration using specially designed endotracheal tubes may reduce early-onset VAP but frequency of ventilator circuit changes does not affect VAP incidence.
- **Blood sugar control (4.0–6.5 mmol/l)** with intensive insulin therapy may reduce morbidity and mortality.
- **Stress ulcer prophylaxis** with sucralfate may reduce VAP risk in MV patients.

Antibiotic therapy is initially empirical. The key decisions are (i) does the patient have early- or late-onset HAP and (ii) are there risk factors for MDR organisms (Table 3.1), which determines the need for broad-spectrum antibiotic therapy. Initial empiric antibiotic therapy requires modification in 50% of cases because of failure to respond or microbiological detection of resistant organisms. Nevertheless getting 'the treatment regimen correct the first time' is important, as effective initial therapy is associated with better outcomes. Therefore local patterns of bacterial antibiotic resistance should be used to modify therapeutic guidelines. Figure 3.3 illustrates the American Thoracic Society (ATS) guidelines for initial, empiric, intravenous antibiotic therapy.[4] It should also be recognized that antibiotic regimens in the UK tend to be less aggressive (i.e. use of two broad-spectrum antibiotics to cover Gram-negative organisms in late-onset HAP would be unusual).

- In **early-onset HAP/VAP** (<4 days in hospital) with no risk factors for MDR organisms, antibiotic ***monotherapy*** is advised with either a β-lactam/β-lactamase inhibitor (e.g. piperacillin-tazobactam 4.5 g qds IV) ***or*** a third-generation cephalosporin (e.g. ceftazidime 2 g tds IV) ***or*** a fluoroquinolone (e.g. ciprofloxacin 400 mg tds IV).
- In **late-onset HAP/VAP** (>4 days in hospital) or with risk factors for MDR pathogens (Table 3.1) and most VAP or HCAP, ***combination therapy***, with at least two broad-spectrum antibiotics to cover MDR Gram-negative bacilli and one antibiotic to treat methicillin-resistant *Staphylococcus aureus* (MRSA), is recommended by the ATS guidelines. For example:
  - an antipseudomonal cephalosporin (e.g. ceftazidime 2 g tds IV) or antipseudomonal carbapenem (e.g. imipenem 0.5–1.0 g qds or meropenem 1 g tds IV) or a β-lactam/β-lactamase inhibitor (e.g. piperacillin-tazobactam 4.5 g qds IV);
  - ***plus*** an antipseudomonal fluoroquinolone (e.g. ciprofloxacin 400 mg tds IV or levofloxacin 750 mg od IV) or aminoglycoside (e.g. gentamicin 7 mg/kg od IV, adjusted to maintain monitored trough levels <1 μg/ml);
  - ***plus*** vancomycin 15 mg/kg bd (adjusted to maintain monitored trough levels 15–20 μg/ml) or linezolid 600 mg bd IV.
- Adjunctive therapy with inhaled aminoglycosides or polymyxin should be considered in patients not improving with systemic therapy.

If the clinical response is good, a seven-day course of therapy is adequate. However, aggressive or resistant pathogens (e.g. *P. aeruginosa*, *S. aureus*) may require treatment for 14–21 days. Therapy should be directed at causative organisms when culture data are available and unnecessary antibiotics withdrawn. Sterile cultures (in the absence of new antibiotics in the previous 72 hours) virtually rules out the presence of HAP. Although there is some evidence for a reduction in ICU-acquired HAP/VAP with prophylactic antibiotic administration, this strategy is not recommended.[4,5]

Conclusion

The most likely diagnosis in this case was HAP as the pneumonic process began >2 days after hospital admission. The differential diagnosis included peri-operative aspiration pneumonia or acute lung injury/ARDS secondary to a systemic inflammatory response syndrome (SIRS) associated with the initial peritonitis. HAP is associated with serious morbidity and a high mortality and getting 'the treatment regimen correct the first time' is important as effective initial therapy is associated with a better outcome. This patient had been in hospital <4 days and the risk of MDR organisms was low, so antibiotic monotherapy with a broad-spectrum agent (see above) would have been appropriate.

Further Reading

1 British Thoracic Society Standards of Care Committee. British Thoracic Society guidelines for the management of community acquired pneumonia in adults. *Thorax* 2001; **56** (Suppl 4): 1–68.

2 American Thoracic Society. Guidelines for the management of adults with community-acquired pneumonia. Diagnosis, assessment of severity, antimicrobial therapy, and prevention. *Am J Respir Crit Care Med* 2001; **163**: 1730–54.

3 British Thoracic Society. BTS guidelines for the management of community acquired pneumonia in adults – 2004 update. www.brit-thoracic.org.uk/Clinical-Information/Pneumonia/Pneumonia-Guidelines.aspx (accessed 01 06 11).

4 American Thoracic Society. Guidelines for the management of adults with hospital-acquired, ventilator-associated, and healthcare-associated pneumonia. *Am J Respir Crit Care Med* 2005; **171**: 388–416.

5 Tarsia P, Aliberti S, Cosentini R, Blasi F. Hospital-acquired pneumonia. *Breathe* 2005; **1**: 297–301.

PROBLEM

4 Lemierre's Disease

Boris Lams, Christopher Kosky

Case History

A 22-year-old Caucasian male presented to the emergency department complaining of neck and left-sided chest pain. He was well until five days previously when he developed a sore throat. This was followed by left-sided neck pain, fevers, left-sided pleuritic chest pain and shortness of breath. He had no significant past medical history and took no medication. He had not travelled abroad recently and had no risk factors for human immunodeficiency virus (HIV). Examination revealed a respiratory rate of 35 breaths/min. Whilst breathing 60% oxygen his oxygen saturation (SaO_2) was 95%. He had tenderness over the left lateral side of his neck and left-sided cervical adenopathy. His pulse rate was 135 beats/min with a blood pressure of 96/43 mmHg. He had reduced breath sounds in both lung bases. There were crackles at the left lung base. Heart sounds were normal and he had a soft, non-tender abdomen. Blood tests showed an elevated white cell count (17.7×10^9/l) and thrombocytopenia (45×10^9/l). A renal profile revealed an elevated urea (17.6 mmol/l) and creatinine (113 μmol/l). Liver function tests revealed an elevated bilirubin (45 μmol/l) and gamma glutamyl transferase (134 IU/l), normal alanine transaminase (50 IU/l) and low albumin (15 g/l). The C-reactive protein was elevated at 211 mg/l.

He was given 1000 ml of colloid intravenously and started on intravenous cefuroxime and clarithromycin. His chest radiograph showed bilateral pleural effusions with clear lung fields. A pleural ultrasound confirmed a moderate left-sided effusion. A guided diagnostic aspiration revealed a turbid yellow fluid with a pH of 6.89. *Fusobacterium necrophorum* was isolated from the pleural fluid. A chest drain was inserted. Despite some improvement in his oxygenation he remained toxic and unwell. He underwent a computed tomography (CT) scan of his chest (Figure 4.1).

What is the initial management of suspected pleural infection?

What does the chest CT scan show and what is the diagnosis?

What is Lemierre's disease?

How can internal jugular vein thrombosis be confirmed?

What is the treatment of Lemierre's disease?

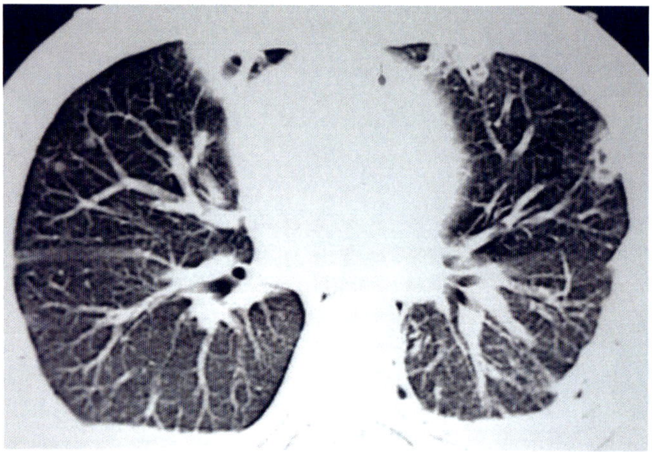

Figure 4.1 Chest CT scan.

Background

In a patient with suspected pleural infection, antibiotics should be started and a pleural ultrasound should be performed. If a pleural effusion is present, diagnostic aspiration should be performed under ultrasound guidance.[1] Sampling and analysis of pleural fluid from a parapneumonic effusion is important to determine whether the effusion will resolve without drainage. Clinical characteristics (e.g. peak temperature, white cell count, age) are not helpful in determining the future outcome of a parapneumonic effusion.

If the pleural aspiration reveals pus then an empyema is present and requires drainage with a chest tube. If serous fluid is present then this should be passed through a blood gas analyser to measure pH. Pleural fluid that has a pH less than 7.2 is defined as a complicated parapneumonic effusion and requires drainage. Large effusions (greater than half a hemithorax), loculated effusions or those associated with pleural thickening also usually require drainage. A CT scan of the chest should be performed for a small, loculated effusion, if the diagnostic aspirate fails or if the patient fails to improve.

Diagnosis

The chest CT scan shows a multiple bilateral lung abscess and bilateral pleural effusions. A previously fit man with pulmonary abscesses after an episode of sore throat and neck pain is consistent with a diagnosis of Lemierre's disease, also known as post-anginal sepsis or necrobacillosis.

Lemierre's disease

Lemierre's disease is due to septic thrombophlebitis of the internal jugular vein resulting in septicaemia and septic pulmonary emboli.[2] Lemierre's disease usually begins with pharyngitis, exudative tonsillitis, otitis media or odontogenic infection. Infection then spreads to the lateral pharyngeal space via the lymphatics. Infection of the internal jugular vein, which runs in the posterior aspect of the lateral pharyngeal space, results in thrombophlebitis. Internal jugular vein thrombophlebitis causes the characteristic neck pain and swelling along the sternomastoid muscle. The original pharyngitis may have resolved by the time the patient develops symptoms of internal vein thrombosis. Septic emboli from the infected internal jugular vein can result in pulmonary abscesses, pleural effusion and empyema. Septic emboli to the lungs occurs in 79% to 100% of cases.[3] Rarely, embolism results in septic arthritis or hepatic or cerebral abscesses. Other structures within the lateral pharyngeal space may also be involved. A Horner's syndrome may occur if there is involvement of the sympathetic trunk. Rupture of the carotid artery has been reported.[4–6]

The most common pathogens implicated in Lemierre's disease are *Fusobacterium necrophorum* and *Fusobacterium nucleatum*. Both bacteria are Gram-negative anaerobes that are normal oral bacteria. Other oral flora bacteria have also been implicated including *Streptococcus* and *Bacteroides* species. In some cases, the infection may be polymicrobial.

Internal jugular vein thrombosis

The presence and extent of the internal jugular vein thrombosis can be assessed by using ultrasonography, CT or magnetic resonance imaging.[7] Ultrasonography or CT may also be used to determine the spread of any metastatic infection to the lungs, brain or liver. Cultures of blood or pleural fluid may grow *Fusobacterium necrophorum* or *Fusobacterium nucleatum*. Underlying thrombophilia may contribute to jugular vein thrombosis.[8]

Treatment

If untreated, death from Lemierre's disease typically occurs within 7–15 days. Treatment is high-dose intravenous antibiotics aimed at β-lactamase-producing anaerobic organisms. Ticarcillin or imipenem can be used. Antibiotics should be modified once an organism is isolated and antibiotic sensitivities are known. The duration of therapy generally is for at least four weeks or until pulmonary abscesses have resolved. Anticoagulation should be considered if there is evidence of extension of thrombus or ongoing emboli. Surgical exploration, with ligation or excision of the internal jugular vein, has occasionally been employed.

In this patient the antibiotic regimen was changed to amoxicillin and clavulanic acid to which the cultured *Fusobacterium necrophorum* was sensitive. Despite a prolonged febrile course he slowly but fully recovered.

This previously rare infection appears to be becoming more common, perhaps related to a more parsimonious approach to the prescribing of antibiotics to those with pharyngitis.

Conclusion

Lemierre's disease should be suspected in patients who have had recent tonsillitis and present with a fever and neck pain. Neck pain arises from a thrombosed internal jugular vein and can lead to pulmonary and systemic septic emboli.

Further Reading

1 Davies HE, Davies RJO, Davies CWH. Management of pleural infection in adults. British Thoracic Society Pleural Disease Guideline 2010. *Thorax* 2010; **65**(Suppl 2): ii41–ii53.

2 Lemierre A. On certain septicaemias due to anaerobic organisms. *Lancet* 1936; **1**: 701–3.

3 Lu MD, Vasavada Z, Tanner C. Lemierre syndrome following oropharyngeal infection: a case series. *J Am Board Fam Med* 2009; **22**: 79–83.

4 Golpe R, Marin B, Alonso M. Lemierre's syndrome (necrobacillosis). *Postgrad Med J* 1999; **75**: 141–4.

5 Stokroos RJ, Manni JJ, de Kruijk JR, Soudijn ER. Lemierre syndrome and acute mastoiditis. *Arch Otolaryngol Head Neck Surg* 1999; **125**: 589–91.

6 Weesner CL, Cisek JE. Lemierre syndrome: the forgotten disease. *Ann Emerg Med* 1993; **22**: 256–8.

7 Auber AE, Mancuso PA. Lemierre syndrome: magnetic resonance imaging and computed tomographic appearance. *Mil Med* 2000; **165**: 638–40.

8 Riordan T. Human infection with *Fusobacterium necrophorum* (Necrobacillosis), with a focus on Lemierre's syndrome. *Clin Microbiol Rev* 2007; **20**: 622–59.

PROBLEM

5 Haemoptysis due to Bronchiectasis

Burhan Khan, Richard Leach

Case History

A 31-year-old woman was referred to the chest clinic from the emergency department after coughing up 100 ml of fresh red blood. She reports a 15-year history of intermittent haemoptysis in which she expectorates small quantities of blood mixed with bronchial secretions. Her previous chest radiographs (CXR) have been reported to be normal. Prior to this episode she had an upper respiratory tract infection with a cough productive of purulent sputum. Apart from whooping cough as a child there was no past medical history of chest disease or tuberculosis. She is a lifelong non-smoker. Chest and general examination were unremarkable. Routine blood tests, including an erythrocyte sedimentation rate (ESR) and C-reactive protein, and sputum microbiology including examination for tuberculosis (TB) were normal. Mantoux testing was consistent with immunity to TB. Her CXR is illustrated in Figure 5.1.

What are the principal causes of haemoptysis?

What factors determine where you would manage haemoptysis?

How is the cause of haemoptysis established in the outpatient setting?

How is massive haemoptysis managed?

Why does localized bronchiectasis occur and how is it best managed?

Background

Table 5.1 illustrates the principal causes of haemoptysis. Most episodes are mild or moderate and occur in the outpatient setting. Massive haemoptysis, defined as 500–1000 ml blood/day, accounts for ~15% of incidents and is a medical emergency. The majority of cases of haemoptysis are due to treatable causes including infection (e.g. tuberculosis) or bronchiectasis and <20% of episodes are due to malignancy or irreversible causes.[1–3] However, there is considerable geographic variation, with infective causes more common in the developing world. In a third of patients no cause is identifiable. In general, the high pressure bronchial, rather than the pulmonary, circulation is the source of bleeding.

Factors that determine management of haemoptysis

Small-volume haemoptysis is common and can be effectively investigated and managed in the outpatient setting. Most cases are due to minor upper or lower respiratory

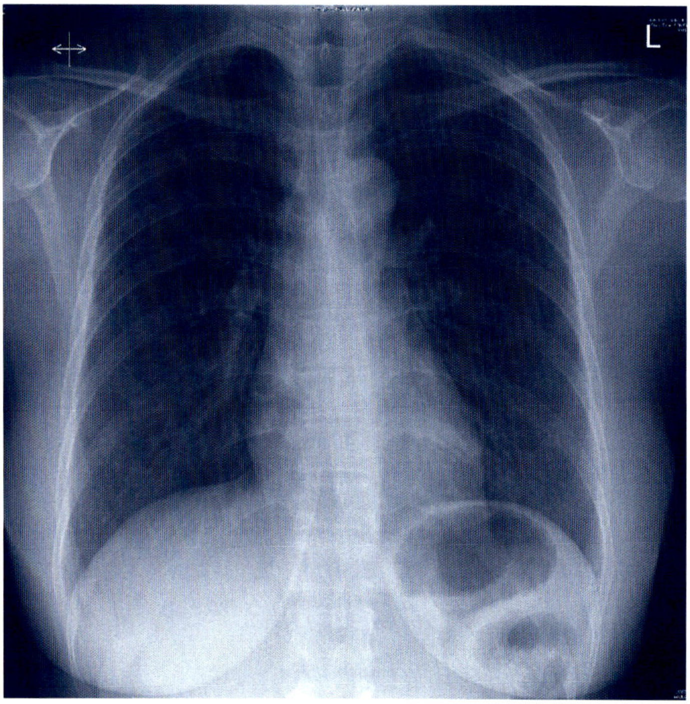

Figure 5.1 Chest radiograph.

Table 5.1 Common and rare causes of haemoptysis

Common causes	Less common causes
• Active tuberculosis • Pneumonia • Bronchiectasis • Fungal infections (*Aspergillus*) • Pulmonary embolism (PE) • Benign bronchial tumours (e.g. carcinoid) • Malignant bronchial tumours • Vasculitis (e.g. Wegener's granulomatosis, SLE) • Alveolar haemorrhage syndromes (e.g. Goodpasture's syndrome) • Anticoagulation (e.g. warfarin)	• Rare infections (viral/parasitic) • Lung abscesses • Mycetoma • Arteriovenous malformations • Pulmonary hypertension • Mitral stenosis • Congenital heart disease • Iatrogenic (lung biopsy) • Endometriosis • Coagulopathy (DIC) • Aortic aneurysm • Trauma including induced by diagnostic bronchoscopy

DIC, disseminated intravascular coagulation; SLE, systemic lupus erythematosus.

tract infections but in a third of cases the cause is not identified. These patients have a good prognosis and in most the haemoptysis resolves spontaneously without treatment. However, beware the sentinel bleed, which may herald a massive haemoptysis.

Overall, about 40% of cases presenting with haemoptysis are trivial (i.e. flecks of blood in sputum), 45% are moderate (i.e. <600 ml/day) and only about 15% are massive (i.e. >600 ml/day), though there is lack of consensus regarding cut-off volumes.[4,5]

Massive haemoptysis is usually encountered in the emergency department and should be regarded as a medical emergency requiring hospital admission. The mortality associated with massive haemoptysis is directly related to the underlying pathology and the rate and volume of blood loss. Patients expectorating >600 ml within 4 hours of onset have a mortality >70% compared to <5% in patients expectorating the same quantity over 16–48 hours. Death results from asphyxia, caused by alveolar flooding, and rarely from circulatory collapse.

Establishing the cause of haemoptysis in the outpatient setting

A good history and examination are essential; characteristic clinical features of diseases like TB, bronchiectasis and bronchogenic carcinoma may direct subsequent investigation and management. Chest examination can be helpful (i.e. localized crepitations) but may often be misleading (i.e. widespread crepitations due to extensive 'blood soiling' of the tracheobronchial tree). Examination of expectorated material provides clues. Food particles may suggest haematemesis but blood in nasogastric aspirates does not differentiate between haematemesis and haemoptysis, as coughed-up blood is often swallowed. Purulent sputum in the expectorated blood suggests bronchiectasis or lung abscesses. Associated haematuria raises the possibility of alveolar haemorrhage syndromes.

Routine blood tests should include ESR, C-reactive protein, d-dimers, *Aspergillus* precipitins and a vasculitis screen (e.g. anti-neutrophil cytoplasmic antibody [ANCA], anti-nuclear antibody [ANA], anti-glomerular basement membrane [anti-GBM]). Sputum must be sent for microbiology, acid-fast bacilli and cytology. A CXR is required in every patient and may identify consolidation, bronchiectasis, masses, cavities and abscesses. Contrast-enhanced or high-resolution computed tomography (CT) chest scans may be diagnostic (e.g. arteriovenous malformations, pulmonary emboli) and aid subsequent bronchoscopy or angiography by localizing the site of bleeding, tumours and other structural abnormalities. Bronchoscopy may independently identify a cause of haemoptysis not identified on CT scan (e.g. adenoma, inhaled foreign body) and facilitates sample collection and histological sampling (e.g. biopsy, bronchoalveolar lavage). Bronchoscopy following a CT scan has the highest diagnostic yield. Occasionally bronchial arteriography is required to detect the site of bleeding. If a cause is not found the prognosis is usually good and the haemoptysis resolves spontaneously.

In this case, the patient's age, recurrent haemoptysis and associated purulent sputum production suggested a potential clinical diagnosis of bronchiectasis. This was confirmed on the CT scan, which demonstrated two grossly dilated bronchi (>10 mm) adjacent to the left heart border, consistent with a diagnosis of localized bronchiectasis in the anteromedial segment of the left lower lobe (Figure 5.2).

Management of massive haemoptysis

Massive haemoptysis is a dramatic, life-threatening clinical emergency and can be distressing to patients, relatives and medical staff. Delayed and inappropriate treatment is common and consequently potentially treatable conditions are fatal.[1,2]

Figure 5.3 illustrates the management of massive haemoptysis, which requires a calm, systematic approach to reassure both the patient and attending staff. The key factors in the initial management are airway maintenance and high-flow oxygen therapy. Asphyxia, not blood loss, is the immediate, major risk to the patient. Protect the non-bleeding lung by placing the patient in the lateral decubitus (or Trendelenburg) position with the bleeding side down to prevent expectorated blood 'soiling' the unaffected lung.

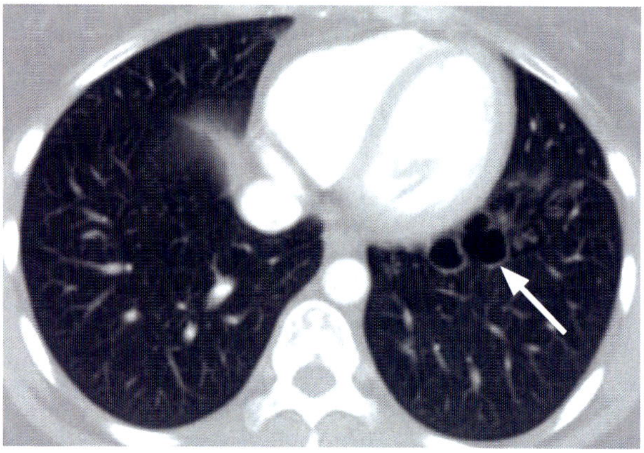

Figure 5.2 Chest CT scan demonstrating bronchiectasis with dilated bronchi adjacent to the heart (arrow).

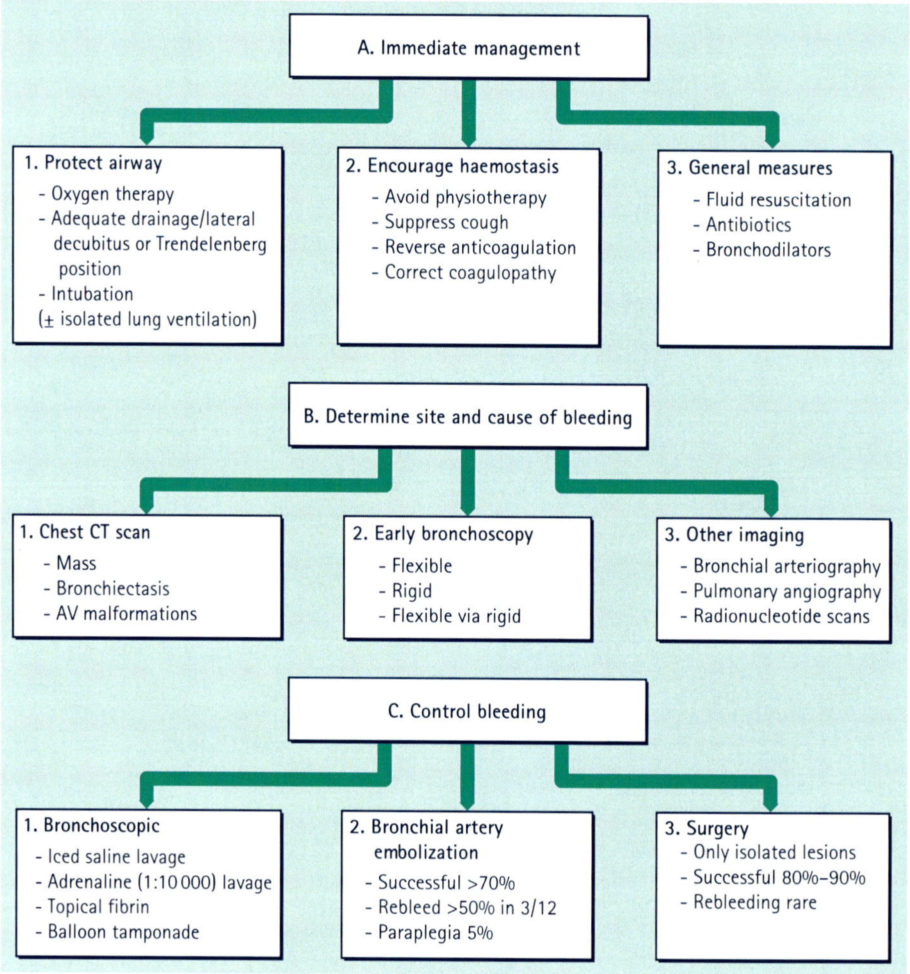

Figure 5.3 Management of massive haemoptysis. AV, arteriovenous.

Nebulized adrenaline (e.g. 5–10 ml of 1:10 000 adrenaline solution), oral tranexamic acid (i.e. 500 mg every 8 hours but not in renal failure) and cough suppression with codeine (i.e. 30–60 mg every 6 hours) may control haemoptysis by aiding clotting at the bleeding site. Circulatory support, correction of coagulopathy and reversal of anticoagulation should be addressed and appropriate antibiotics and bronchodilators considered. Avoid chest manipulation (e.g. physiotherapy) which can potentiate bleeding. Simple measures like nursing the patient on green linen can be reassuring.

If respiratory compromise necessitates urgent intubation, the unaffected lung may have to be ventilated independently until bleeding is controlled. In the emergency situation the endotracheal tube is advanced into the right main bronchus (which is in the same axis as the trachea) until breath sounds can no longer be heard in the left side of the chest. If bleeding is not on the right side, the endotracheal cuff is inflated and the right lung selectively ventilated. If bleeding is originating from the right lung, a Foley or Fogarty catheter should be positioned in the right main bronchus and inflated. The endotracheal tube is then withdrawn until the left lung is ventilated. Occasionally double-lumen tubes (e.g. Carlens, Robertshaw) may be used but require considerable technical expertise to position correctly and their small lumens limit adequate suctioning and prevent flexible bronchoscopy.

In these patients, obtaining a CT scan may be difficult due to haemodynamic instability, and urgent bronchoscopy may help establish the site and cause of bleeding.

- Rigid bronchoscopy (under general anaesthesia) is preferred when haemoptysis is severe as it allows rapid suctioning. However, visualization of the tracheobronchial tree is limited to the large airways.[6]
- Flexible bronchoscopy has the advantages of ready availability, introduction through an endotracheal tube (≥8.0 mm diameter) in the mechanically ventilated patient and it allows visualization of the subsegmental and upper lobe bronchi, which account for 80% of bleeding sites. The disadvantage is limited suctioning capability. Ideally, the flexible scope can be passed through the rigid bronchoscope to combine the benefits of both methods.

Temporary control of bleeding is achieved in over 90% of cases during bronchoscopy by directing boluses of iced saline, topical adrenaline (10 ml of 1:10 000 dilution), topical vasoconstrictors or fibrin at the bleeding site.[6,7] Balloon-tipped catheters can also be directed to tamponade bleeding airways. Laser photocoagulation, argon plasma coagulation, electrocautery cryotherapy and brachytherapy have all been used with varying success.[5]

Bronchial angiography and embolization (e.g. coils) is the established therapeutic technique for initial control of haemoptysis (Figure 5.4).[8,9] It is initially successful in >70% of cases, with the best results in patients with dilated bronchial arteries (e.g. bronchiectasis). Rebleeding is common and occurs in 20%–70% of cases over the following few weeks to months.[9] Infarction of the anterior spinal artery is the most serious complication of the procedure and occurs in 5% of cases.

Surgical therapy is mainly reserved for technical failure of arteriography.[5] Bleeding is permanently controlled in 82%–99% of surgically treated isolated lesions compared to 46%–68% of conservatively managed cases.[9,10] Primary medical management may be mandatory because bleeding is not localized (e.g. widespread *Aspergillus* infection) or amenable to surgical resection of a pulmonary segment. In some patients surgery is contraindicated because of end-stage lung disease (forced expiratory volume in 1 second [FEV_1] <40% predicted), poor cardiac reserve, unresectable cancer or severe bleeding diathesis.

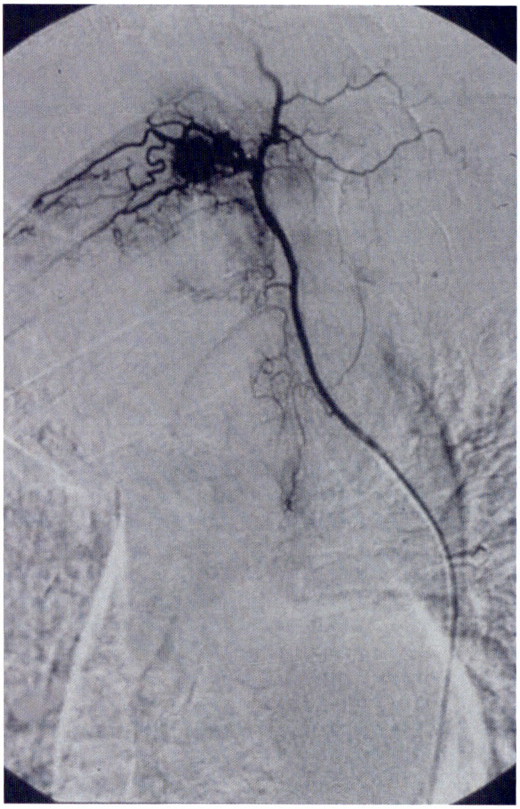

Figure 5.4 Bronchial angiogram showing blush at bleeding site.

Management of localized bronchiectasis

Bronchiectasis refers to irreversible, abnormal dilation of bronchi with associated chronic airways inflammation, sputum production, airflow obstruction and recurrent infection (± haemoptysis). An initial, usually infective, insult is required to damage the airway. Subsequent distorted anatomy results in sputum stagnation, recurrent infection, increasing airways damage and volume loss due to airways blockage by secretions. Bronchial neovascularization occurs within damaged airways causing hypertrophy and tortuosity of bronchial arteries. As these are at systemic pressure, vessel damage due to infection or mechanical factors leads to recurrent haemoptysis.

Bronchiectasis is usually generalized and is most commonly due to cystic fibrosis (i.e. a gene defect), immune deficiency (e.g. primary hypogammaglobulinaemia), infection (e.g. TB, pneumonia), toxic insults (e.g. aspiration, chemical inhalation) or systemic disease (e.g. rheumatoid arthritis, Crohn's disease). Table 5.2 lists causes of localized bronchiectasis.

Table 5.2 Causes of localized bronchiectasis

1. Luminal obstruction
Inhaled objects (e.g. teeth, peanut)
Slow-growing tumours (e.g. carcinoid, neurofibromas)
Post-tuberculous or pneumonic airways stenosis
2. Extraluminal compression
Enlarged nodes (e.g. mycobacteria, fungi, tumour)
Extramural tumour
3. Surgical distortion
Post-lobectomy
4. Generalized conditions with focal effects
Whooping cough (*Bordetella pertussis* infection)
Localized tuberculosis
Lobar pneumonia
Bronchopulmonary aspergillosis with mucous plugs

Management includes:

- Promotion of sputum clearance with postural drainage, 'huffing' (i.e. forced expiration at variable chest expansion), physiotherapy and cough augmentation. Oral N-acetylcysteine may reduce sputum viscosity.
- Antibiotic therapy decreases infection, inflammation and further airway damage. Antibiotics are usually given intermittently for exacerbations and at higher doses, for longer periods (i.e. two weeks), than in patients without bronchiectasis. They can be given orally, intravenously or as nebulizers depending on likely organisms and the results of sputum surveillance. The usual sequence of bacterial colonization is *Staphylococcus aureus*, *Haemophilus influenzae*, *Moraxella catarrhalis* and finally *Pseudomonas* species. Response to therapy is suggested by reduced sputum volumes, improved symptoms and spirometry, and a fall in C-reactive protein.
- Vaccination against influenza and pneumococcus.
- Bronchodilators and inhaled steroids to improve airflow obstruction.
- Nutrition and exercise to improve the patient's general condition.
- Lung resection surgery may be considered if disease is localized to a single lobe or segment. The incidence of localized disease due to severe childhood chest infections (e.g. whooping cough, tuberculosis) has fallen and the need for surgery is decreasing. Surgery is also indicated for life-threatening haemoptysis.

Conclusion

In this case, the history of childhood whooping cough suggests a previous infective cause for the localized bronchiectasis. As this patient was young and healthy, with normal spirometry (FEV_1 >70% predicted), and was experiencing increasingly frequent and severe episodes of haemoptysis, she was referred for, and underwent, successful surgical resection of her localized bronchiectasis.[11]

Further Reading

1 Thompson AB, Teschler H, Rennard SI. Pathogenesis, evaluation, and therapy for massive haemoptysis. *Clin Chest Med* 1992; **13**: 69–82.

2 Cahill BC, Ingbar DH. Massive hemoptysis. Assessment and management. *Clin Chest Med* 1994; **15**: 147–68.

3 Jones DK, Davies RJ. Massive haemoptysis. *BMJ* 1990; **300**: 889–90.

4 Hirshberg B, Biran I, Glazer M, Kramer MR. Hemoptysis: etiology, evaluation, and outcome in a tertiary referral hospital. *Chest* 1997; **112**: 440–4.

5 Sakr L, Dutau H. Massive hemoptysis: an update on the role of bronchoscopy in diagnosis and management. *Respiration* 2010; **80**: 38–58.

6 Conlan AA, Hurwitz SS. Management of massive haemoptysis with the rigid broncoscope and cold saline lavage. *Thorax* 1980; **35**: 901–4.

7 Tsukamoto T, Sasaki H, Nakamura H. Treatment of hemoptysis patients by thrombin and fibrinogen-thrombin infusion therapy using a fibreoptic bronchoscope. *Chest* 1989; **96**: 473–6.

8 Saumench J, Escarrabill J, Padró L *et al.* Value of fibreoptic bronchoscopy and angiography for diagnosis of the bleeding site in hemoptysis. *Ann Thorac Surg* 1989; **48**: 272–4.

9 Mal H, Rullon I, Mellot F *et al.* Immediate and long-term results of bronchial artery embolization for life-threatening hemoptysis. *Chest* 1999; **115**: 996–1001.

10 Bobrowitz ID, Ramakrishna S, Shim YS. Comparison of medical v surgical treatment of major hemoptysis. *Arch Intern Med* 1983; **143**: 1343–6.

11 Pasteur MC, Bilton, D, Hill AT. British Thoracic Society guideline for non-CF bronchiectasis. *Thorax* 2010; **65**(Suppl 1): i1–i58.

SECTION TWO **02**

Obstructive Lung Disease/Small Airways Disease

PROBLEM

6 Stable Chronic Obstructive Pulmonary Disease (COPD)

Burhan Khan, Richard Leach

Case History

A 64-year-old man with long-standing COPD and progressive breathlessness was referred for review of his clinical management. His exercise tolerance was limited to 50 metres on the flat or a flight of stairs. He was treated with full-dose inhaled ipratropium bromide and was using his salbutamol inhaler >10 times a day. Three COPD exacerbations in the last year had been treated with steroids and antibiotics. Burnt-out rheumatoid arthritis limited his hand function. He was a lifelong smoker of 20 cigarettes a day and had worked as a dock labourer.

On examination he was cachectic, barrel-chested and comfortable at rest but breathless on minimal exertion with a resting saturation (SaO_2) of 91%. He had minimal ankle oedema but the jugular venous pressure was fractionally elevated at 2 cm. Chest examination revealed poor air entry to both lungs and widespread soft expiratory wheeze. Spirometry recorded a forced expiratory volume in 1 second (FEV_1) of 0.9 l (35% predicted), forced vital capacity (FVC) of 2.6 l (74% predicted) and peak expiratory flow rate of 120 l/min. Recent oral steroid and bronchodilator trials had increased his FEV_1 by 4% and 3%, respectively. Blood gases on air were pH 7.37, partial pressure of arterial carbon dioxide ($PaCO_2$) 5.9 kPa and oxygen (PaO_2) 8.7 kPa, and bicarbonate (HCO_3) 33 mmol/l. A chest radiograph (CXR) revealed hyperinflation with small apical bullae and a cardiothoracic ratio at the upper limit of normal. Formal lung function tests demonstrated a residual volume (RV) of 198% predicted and a functional residual capacity (FRC) of 5.2 l or (184% predicted). Carbon monoxide gas transfer (TLCO) corrected for alveolar volume (KCO) was 42% of predicted. Desaturation occurred during exercise testing, and exercise tolerance and dyspnoea improved with ambulatory oxygen.

How is COPD defined and how severe is it in this patient?

What do you understand by the terms 'static' and 'dynamic' hyperinflation?

What non-pharmacological measures may help this patient?

What is the recommended hierarchy of pharmacological therapy in COPD?

Which bronchodilators are most effective and why?

Are inhaled corticosteroids effective in COPD?

What other pharmacological therapies may be helpful in COPD?

Background

Background and COPD definition

Chronic obstructive pulmonary disease is estimated to affect three million people in the UK but is often not diagnosed until the patient is >50 years old.[1] The principal cause is smoking. COPD is characterized by airflow obstruction that is not fully reversible and is usually progressive in the long term. Intermittent exacerbations cause rapid worsening of symptoms beyond normal day-to-day variation. COPD is defined as airflow obstruction with a reduction in the post-bronchodilator FEV_1/FVC ratio to less than 0.7. Surprisingly, disability in COPD is often poorly reflected by the FEV_1. If the FEV_1 is ≥80% a diagnosis of COPD should only be made in the presence of respiratory symptoms (e.g. breathlessness, cough, reduced exercise tolerance, exacerbations) and formal lung function testing.[1–4] As in this patient, airflow obstruction is irreversible following bronchodilator and steroid therapy (i.e. <15% increase in FEV_1), excluding a diagnosis of asthma. The severity of COPD is classified by (i) post-bronchodilator FEV_1 as a percentage of predicted[1–4] (e.g. National Institute for Health and Clinical Excellence [NICE] guidelines:[1] mild ≥80%; moderate 50%–79%; severe 30%–49%; and very severe <30% predicted) and (ii) by clinical picture (e.g. exercise capacity, breathlessness, PaO_2 and $PaCO_2$ in arterial blood gases, health status, body mass index [BMI], frequency of exacerbations, carbon monoxide transfer and severity of symptoms[5]).

There are two pathophysiological types of COPD:

- **Emphysema** occurs following alveolar septa and capillary destruction due to inadequate antiprotease defences against inhaled toxins. Tobacco smoke causes centrilobular emphysema with predominantly upper lobe involvement, whereas α_1-antitrypsin deficiency causes panacinar emphysema affecting the lower lobes. Lung function tests demonstrate impaired diffusion (DLCO, KCO) and increased lung volumes (total lung capacity, FRC, RV). Resting blood gases are often normal because alveolar septa and capillaries are destroyed in proportion to each other. Desaturation during exercise and increased minute ventilation are due to reduced diffusion capacity. CXR reveals hyperinflation (e.g. flat diaphragms), narrow mediastinum, bullae, hyperlucency and reduced peripheral vascular markings. Emphysematous patients tend to be relatively well oxygenated but breathless and cachectic with barrel chests due to hyperinflation. They are classically described as 'pink puffers'.
- **Chronic bronchitis** causes airways obstruction due to chronic mucosal inflammation (± airways damage), bronchospasm and mucous gland hypertrophy with hypersecretion, with the lung parenchyma less affected. Diffusion capacity and lung volumes are usually normal. The CXR shows less hyperinflation but increased vascular markings compared with CXR findings in emphysema. Ventilation-perfusion (V/Q) mismatch occurs due to poor alveolar ventilation as a result of early expiratory airways closure or alveolar collapse following airway obstruction. Breathlessness is unusual due to the development of brainstem insensitivity to $PaCO_2$. Consequently these patients are often hypoxaemic, hypercapnic and oedematous and are described as 'blue bloaters'. However, the concept of emphysematous 'pink puffers' and bronchitic 'blue bloaters' is outdated as most patients have coexistent elements of both disease processes and a mixed clinical picture (i.e. 'blue puffers').

'Static' and 'dynamic' hyperinflation

Emphysematous airways obstruction is caused by early distal airways collapse during expiration due to loss of the 'elastic' radial traction from the surrounding lung tissue that normally maintains airway patency (Figure 6.1).[6–8] The airway collapse prevents alveolar emptying causing air trapping and hyperinflation. Airway narrowing due to sputum, inflammation and bronchoconstriction can further increase air trapping. The hyperinflation enhances expiratory airflow, due to increased end-inspiratory alveolar pressure, but increases the elastic work of breathing because the inflated (i.e. horizontal) position of the ribs and the flattened diaphragm place the inspiratory muscles at a mechanical disadvantage. **'Static' hyperinflation** describes the alveolar air trapping that occurs at rest and is manifest as a barrel chest on clinical examination, increased RV and FRC on lung function tests and hyperinflation on chest radiographs. Emphysematous patients often breathe through 'pursed lips', which tends to hold open the collapsing airways for longer (i.e. by applying a small, distal airway pressure), allowing better emptying of the alveoli and reducing alveolar hyperinflation.

'Dynamic' hyperinflation describes air trapping that occurs (i.e. in addition to 'static' hyperinflation) during normal exercise or rapid ventilation (i.e. due to shorter breath cycle times), and is increased by airways obstruction (e.g. asthma, COPD exacerbations). For example, in a normal subject, an increase in respiratory rate during exercise reduces breath cycle time from 6 sec/breath at 10 breaths/min to 2 sec/breath at 30 breaths/min

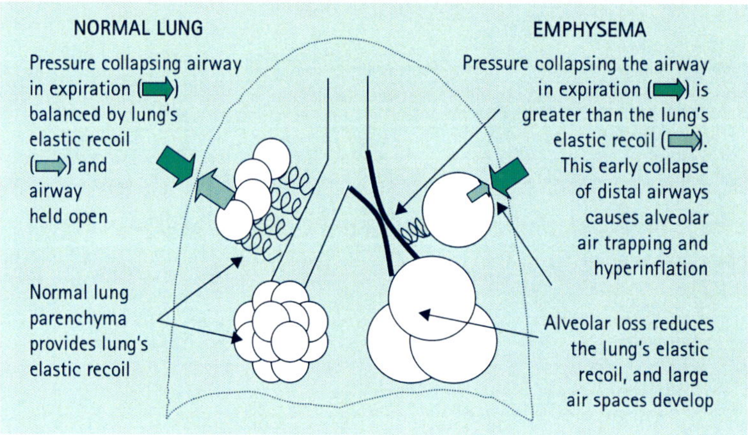

Figure 6.1 Pathophysiology of emphysema.

resulting in incomplete expiration (i.e. due to inadequate time), failure of alveolar emptying and, consequently, progressive hyperinflation. In COPD, inspiratory and expiratory times are prolonged due to airway narrowing, increasing normal exercise-induced hyperinflation and limiting exercise tolerance.

Non-pharmacological measures for COPD therapy

- **Smoking cessation** is the single most important intervention to prevent COPD and stop its progression. Even a three-minute period of counselling urging a smoker to 'quit' in a clear, strong and personalized manner can be effective and this should be done for every smoker at every visit. Further success is reported with support schemes (e.g. Action on Smoking and Health [ASH], National Health Service [NHS]) and anti-smoking pharmacotherapy (e.g. nicotine replacement therapy, bupropion, varenicline).
- **Vaccination** against influenza and pneumoccal infection is essential. In COPD patients, influenza vaccination reduces serious illness and death due to influenza by about 50%.
- **Nutrition**. BMI should be monitored and maintained in the range >20 kg/m^2 and <25 kg/m^2. When BMI is <20 kg/m^2, weight gain improves respiratory muscle strength and prognosis. Similarly, when BMI is >25 kg/m^2, reducing weight improves functional status and reduces dyspnoea.
- **Pulmonary rehabilitation** reduces symptoms, strengthens respiratory muscles, increases exercise tolerance, reduces hospitalizations, enhances quality of life and increases physical and emotional participation in everyday activities. These benefits are achieved by education (e.g. breathing techniques), addressing altered mood, reducing social isolation and by preventing weight loss, muscle wasting and exercise deconditioning.

The hierarchy of pharmacological therapy in COPD

Figure 6.2 illustrates the recently published NICE guidelines for COPD pharmacotherapy. Initially, short-acting bronchodilators – short-acting β_2 agonists (SABA; e.g.

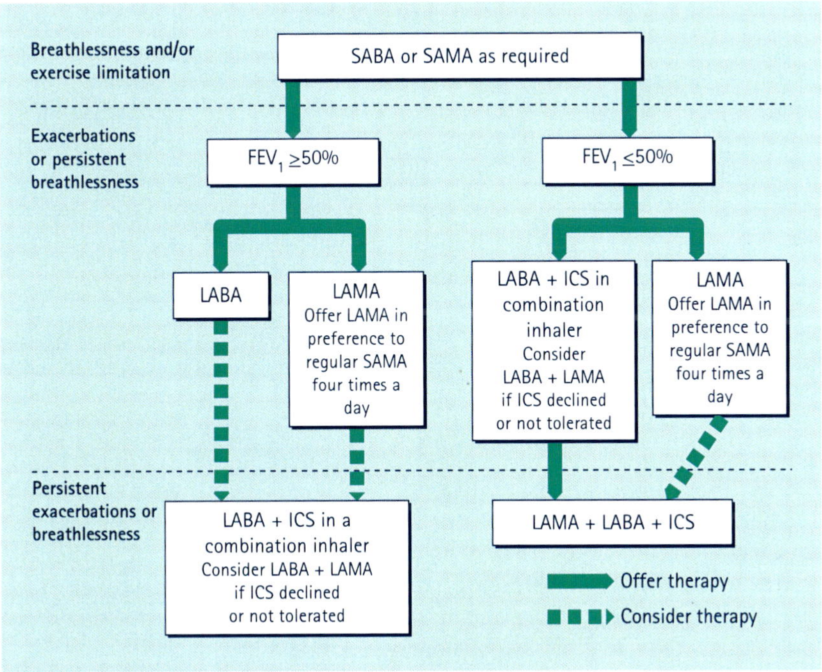

Figure 6.2 NICE guidelines (2010)[1] for inhaler therapy in stable COPD.

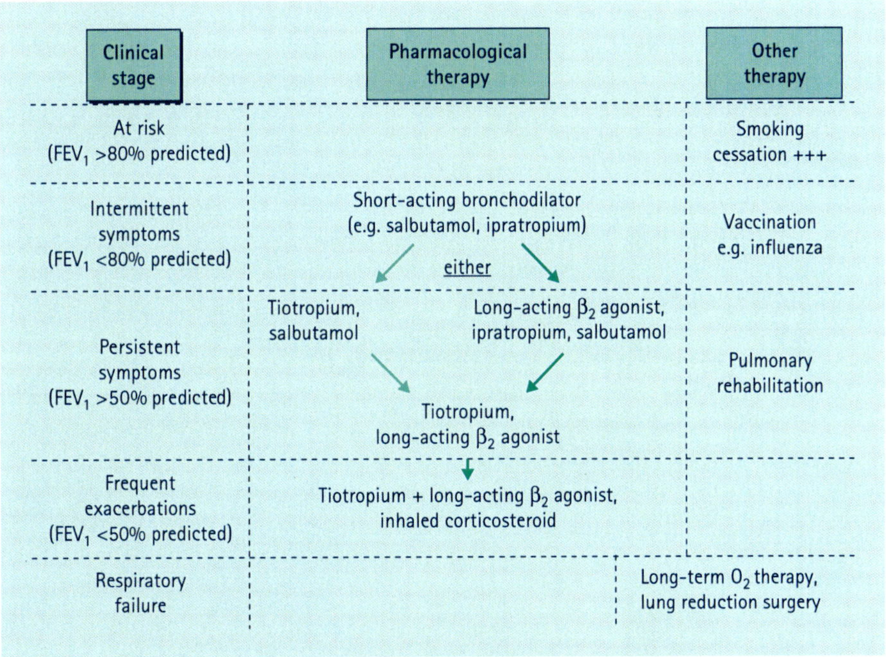

Figure 6.3 Algorithm for COPD management (modified from NICE 2010[1] and Cooper and Tashkin 2005[5]). The +++ indicates the importance of smoking cessation; the best way of treating COPD is to prevent it.

salbutamol) and anticholinergic agents (short-acting muscarinic antagonist [SAMA]; ipratropium bromide) – are prescribed on an as-required basis. In patients with exacerbations or persistent breathlessness and an FEV_1 ≥50% predicted, either a regular long-acting muscarinic antagonist (LAMA; e.g. tiotropium) or a long-acting β_2 agonist (LABA; e.g. formoterol, salmeterol) should be added to the treatment regime. SABA can be continued as required with the long-acting agents but SAMA (i.e. ipratropium bromide) should always be stopped when a LAMA (i.e. tiotropium) is started. As symptoms progress, LAMA and LABA can be combined. Current guidelines[1–4] only recommend regular inhaled corticosteroid (ICS) therapy in symptomatic COPD patients (i.e exacerbations and persistent breathlessness) with an FEV_1 ≤50% predicted or in patients who have had two or more exacerbations requiring oral steroid (± antibiotics) therapy over the preceding twelve months. Figure 6.3 shows a useful management algorithm for COPD.

Bronchodilators: mechanisms of action

Inhaled bronchodilators are central to the symptomatic management of COPD.[6–11] Although spirometric improvements are small, studies show reductions in FRC (i.e. hyperinflation) that correlate well with improved functional status, dyspnoea index and quality of life measures. Because β_2 agonists and anticholinergic agents have different mechanisms of action, acting on the sympathetic and parasympathetic systems, respectively, they act synergistically when used in combination. **β_2 agonists** have a rapid onset of action (<5 minutes) and are initially prescribed as short-acting agents (e.g. salbutamol). As COPD severity progresses, LABA (e.g. salmeterol, formoterol) are used and further improve health status.[5,6] **Anticholinergic agents** (i.e. muscarinic receptor antagonists) have a slower onset of action (maximum effect 30–40 minutes) but are equally effective (or better) than β_2 agonists. Both short-acting (e.g. ipratropium bromide) and long-acting (e.g. tiotropium bromide) anticholinergic agents improve health status and reduce hyperinflation.[6–9] However, once-daily tiotropium bromide is superior to ipratropium bromide as it acts specifically on the M_3 muscarinic receptor to produce bronchodilation, whereas ipratropium bromide acts on three receptors, where effects at M_1 and M_3 produce bronchodilation but action at M_2 causes bronchoconstriction. Consequently ipratropium could potentially neutralize the benefit of tiotropium and these two drugs should never be used in combination. Compared to ipratropium, tiotropium reduces COPD exacerbations by about 20% and hospital admissions by approximately 40%.[9]

Effectiveness of inhaled corticosteroids in COPD

In the ISOLDE Trial, ICS did not reduce the rate of decline in FEV_1 in COPD patients when compared with placebo.[10] However, ICS may reduce exacerbations and improve lung function, both alone and in combination with LABA, although this has not been found in all trials.[10–12] The TORCH study, a double-blind, prospective analysis of COPD survival in 6100 patients, demonstrated a reduction in exacerbations and hospital admissions and improved quality of life in patients treated with combination ICS/LABA therapy compared to ICS or LABA alone or placebo.[11] In the ISOLDE Trial, the reduction in exacerbations was greatest in patients with an FEV_1 <1.25 l. Subsequent *post hoc* analysis of the ISOLDE data and a number of retrospective database analyses of ICS and LABA combination therapy suggest a small survival benefit. In particular, a retrospective cohort study from the UK General Practice Research Database demonstrated that regular LABA (salmeterol) and/or ICS (fluticasone propionate) significantly improved three-year survival compared to controls (79% vs 63%; $P < 0.05$).[13]

Long-term ICS in mild/moderate COPD (i.e. FEV_1 >50% predicted) is only recommended if a previous trial of inhaled or oral steroids has shown a beneficial spirometric response. Long-term treatment with **oral corticosteroids** is not recommended in COPD; it benefits less than 25% of patients and steroid-induced myopathy and other systemic side effects may contribute to muscle weakness and early respiratory failure.

Other helpful pharmacological therapies in COPD

- **Methylxanthines** (e.g. theophylline, aminophylline) may be prescribed as slow-release oral preparations in stable COPD after trials of short- and long-acting bronchodilators. Plasma levels must be monitored at higher doses due to the narrow therapeutic index. Theophylline can improve exercise tolerance, respiratory drive, diaphragmatic strength, mucociliary clearance and blood gases but the effect on spirometry is negligible.
- **Mucolytics** therapy may be beneficial in patients with chronic cough productive of excessive sputum. If a short trial is not of symptomatic benefit, treatment should be stopped.
- **Conventional antidepressant pharmacotherapy** should be considered in severely depressed patients.
- **Benzodiazepines and narcotics** are respiratory depressants and may worsen hypercapnia. They are not recommended except as palliative measures in end-stage COPD when they may help relieve severe dyspnoea.
- **Diuretics (but not angiotensin converting enzyme inhibitors or calcium channel blockers)** should be considered in patients with peripheral oedema due to pulmonary hypertension (i.e. cor pulmonale).

Therapies that are not recommended in stable COPD include antitussive agents, as cough has a significant protective effect; α_1-antitrypsin replacement therapy in patients with α_1-antitrypsin deficiency; antioxidants; respiratory stimulants; regular antibiotics and immunoregulators.

The criteria for long-term oxygen therapy

Long-term oxygen therapy (LTOT) is only indicated in patients with a PaO_2 <7.3 kPa when stable or a PaO_2 >7.3 kPa and <8.0 kPa when stable with at least one of the following: secondary polycythaemia, nocturnal hypoxaemia (SaO_2 <90% for 30% of sleep time), peripheral oedema or pulmonary hypertension. Blood gases should be assessed on two occasions at least three weeks apart in stable patients receiving optimum therapy. However, ambulatory oxygen should be considered in patients with exercise desaturation (as in this case) and those with reduced breathlessness or improved exercise capacity with oxygen.

The use of spacer devices, dry powder inhalers and nebulizers in COPD

In most cases bronchodilator therapy is administered with hand-held inhaler devices.[1–4] In general, side effects are mild, predictable and dose dependent. However, inhaler technique is poor in >50% of patients. Regular instruction and reassessment are essential as technique deteriorates over time, especially in older subjects. Use of pressurized metered dose inhalers (pMDIs) in combination with large volume spacer devices improves drug delivery particularly in those with reduced dexterity or cognitive impairment. Spacers also reduce systemic absorption of ICS. Breath-activated devices (e.g. Easi-Breathe®) and dry powder inhalers demonstrated no significant differences in performance (e.g. FEV_1) when compared to MDIs, although ease-of-use and preference scores are better.

Nebulizer therapy (NT) should be considered when distressing or disabling breathlessness occurs despite maximal hand-held inhaler therapy.[1,14] Although FEV_1 is not improved with NT compared to hand-held inhalers (± spacer), NT may improve symptoms, exercise capacity and quality of life. However, NT should not be prescribed without confirming these benefits.

Conclusion

This patient has severe COPD (i.e. FEV_1 35% predicted), predominantly emphysema as indicated by the alveolar air trapping (i.e. raised RV and FRC), CXR hyperinflation, and reduced KCO due to loss of alveolar surface for gas transfer with associated exercise desaturation.

His management can clearly be improved and smoking cessation should be encouraged. He should be referred to a smoking cessation service for pharmacological and psychological support during attempts to stop smoking as 'quit rates' are improved. Pharmacological management should include the addition of tiotropium bromide and LABA inhalers. The LABA should be combined with an ICS as he has been treated with three courses of inhaled steroid in the last year. His poor hand function (due to the rheumatoid arthritis) suggests he would benefit from breath-activated inhaler devices. He may also benefit from pulmonary rehabilitation and encouragement to improve his nutritional status. Finally, portable oxygen may improve his exercise tolerance but ideally this should only be considered if the patient has stopped smoking due to the associated fire risks.

Further Reading

1 National Institute for Health and Clinical Excellence. Management of chronic obstructive pulmonary disease in adults in primary and secondary care. Clinical guideline 101. London: NICE, 2010. www.nice.org.uk (accessed 01 06 11).

2 Celli BR, MacNee W; ATS/ERS Task Force. Standards for the diagnosis and treatment of patients with COPD: a summary of the ATS/ERS position paper. *Eur Respir J* 2004; **23**: 932–46. www.ersnet.org (accessed 01 06 11).

3 Global Initiative for Chronic Obstructive Lung Disease (GOLD). Global strategy for diagnosis, management, and prevention of COPD. GOLD, 2009. www.goldcopd.org (accessed 01 06 11).

4 The COPD Guidelines Group of the Standards of Care Committee of the BTS. BTS guidelines for the management of chronic obstructive pulmonary disease. *Thorax* 1997; **52**(Suppl 5): S1–28. www.thorax.bmj.com (accessed 01 06 11).

5 Cooper CB, Tashkin DP. Recent developments in inhaled therapy in stable chronic obstructive pulmonary disease. *BMJ* 2005; **330**; 640–4.

6 Calverley PMA, Koulouris NG. Flow limitation and dynamic hyperinflation: key concepts in modern respiratory physiology. *Eur Respir J* 2005; **25**: 186–99.

7 O'Donnell DE, Flüge T, Gerken F *et al.* Effects of tiotropium on lung hyperinflation, dyspnoea, and exercise tolerance in COPD. *Eur Respir J* 2004; **23**: 832–40.

8 Celli B, ZuWallack R, Wang S, Kesten S. Improvement in resting inspiratory capacity and hyperinflation with tiotropium in COPD patients with increased static lung volumes. *Chest* 2003; **124**: 1743–8.

9 Barr RG, Bourbeau J, Camargo CA, Ram FSF. Tiotropium for stable chronic obstructive pulmonary disease: a meta-analysis. *Thorax* 2006; **61**: 854–62.

10 Burge PS, Calverley PMA, Jones PW, Spencer S, Anderson JA, Maslen TK. Randomised, double blind, placebo controlled study of fluticasone propionate in patients with moderate to severe chronic obstructive pulmonary disease: the ISOLDE trial. *BMJ* 2000; **320**: 1297–1303.

11 Vestbo J; TORCH Study Group. The TORCH (Towards a revolution in COPD health) survival study protocol. *Eur Respir J* 2004; **24**: 206–10.

12 Barnes PJ, Stockley RA. COPD: current therapeutic interventions and future approaches. *Eur Respir J* 2005; **25**: 1084–106.

13 Soriano JB, Vestbo J, Pride NB, Kiri V, Maden C, Maier WC. Survival in COPD patients after regular use of fluticasone propionate and salmeterol in general practice. *Eur Respir J* 2002; **20**: 819–25.

14 Boe J, Dennis JH, O'Driscoll BR *et al.* European Respiratory Society Guidelines on the use of nebulizers. European Respiratory Society Task Force on the use of nebulizers. *Eur Respir J* 2001; **18**: 228–42.

PROBLEM

7 Acute Ventilatory Failure in Chronic Obstructive Pulmonary Disease

Richard Leach, Craig Davidson

Case History

A 64-year-old man presented to the emergency room with an acute chronic obstructive pulmonary disease (COPD) exacerbation following a viral upper respiratory tract infection. His normal exercise tolerance was 50 metres on the flat and he had a long history of deteriorating breathlessness. He was on regular inhaled salmeterol and tiotropium bromide and he had been taking amoxicillin and prednisolone 30 mg daily for one day. Previous spirometry had recorded a forced expiratory volume in 1 second (FEV_1) of 0.7 litres (30% predicted), a forced vital capacity of 2.3 litres (74% predicted) and an oxygen saturation (SaO_2) of 89% on air. He had a 40 pack-year history of smoking.

At admission he was severely breathless at rest, exhausted and cyanosed (SaO_2 of 83% on 40% oxygen). His blood pressure was 110/60 mmHg. He had a soft systolic murmur over the left sternal edge, the central venous pressure was 4 cm and he had pitting peripheral oedema. Chest examination revealed very poor air entry with widespread soft expiratory wheeze. His peak expiratory flow was 60 l/min. Initial blood gases on air were partial pressure of oxygen (PaO_2) 5.7 kPa and carbon dioxide ($PaCO_2$) 7.8 kPa, and pH 7.25. Chest radiography demonstrated marked hyperinflation, cardiomegaly and alveolar infiltration in the left lower zone.

He was immediately started on non-invasive ventilation (NIV) but despite a good mask fit, reasonable compliance with ventilation and an initial improvement in blood gases, two hours later he was exhausted and his repeat blood gases were PaO_2 7.5 kPa, $PaCO_2$ 8.1 kPa and pH 7.23. Following intubation he was mechanically ventilated and transferred to the intensive care unit (ICU). Two hours later his PaO_2 was 8.5 kPa, $PaCO_2$ 12.4 kPa and pH 7.13, with the ventilator set to deliver a respiratory rate of 15 breaths/min, inspiratory to expiratory time ratio 1:3, no positive end-expiratory pressure (PEEP) and an inspired oxygen concentration (FiO_2) 0.6. The current tidal ventilation is 400 ml/breath with a minute ventilation of 6.0 l/min.

What are the causes of acute COPD exacerbations and why are they important?

What is the correct initial dose of oxygen in a COPD exacerbation?

Which patients benefit from non-invasive ventilation?

What non-ventilatory therapies improve outcome in COPD exacerbations?

What are the indications for mechanical ventilation (MV) and what proportion of patients survive?

How would you ventilate this patient and what do you understand by the term auto-PEEP?

How and when would you wean this patient from MV?

Background

Chronic obstructive pulmonary disease is a common, slowly progressive disease that causes a gradual, irreversible decline in lung function, chronic respiratory symptoms (e.g. cough, exertional dyspnoea), disability, intermittent exacerbations, respiratory failure and eventually death. It is usually due to cigarette smoke (>80% of cases) but other noxious gases or particles can cause COPD. Most smokers develop some degree of airway inflammation and, if they live long enough, up to 50% of smokers will develop the pathophysiological and clinical features of COPD. There is evidence of genetic susceptibility.[1–4]

An acute exacerbation of COPD (AECOPD) is defined as a sustained worsening of the patient's usual stable state that is acute in onset and includes worsening breathlessness, cough and an increase in discoloured sputum production. Exacerbations are common and when severe may require hospital admission. They are most commonly due to bacterial or viral infections. Environmental pollution is recognized to precipitate exacerbations. The differential diagnosis includes pneumothorax, ischaemic heart disease, heart failure and arrhythmias (e.g. atrial fibrillation due to medications, metabolic upset or atrial enlargement). Pulmonary embolism is difficult to exclude but recent studies suggest it is a rare event.

Frequent exacerbations probably accelerate the rate of decline in FEV_1 and have significant cost implications. In the UK the average length of hospital admission for an acute COPD exacerbation is 5–6 days and costs between £1500 and £3500. The readmission rate is >30% and mortality >10% within three months of the initial admission. Following ICU admission, twelve-month mortality is approximately 40%.

Controlled oxygen therapy in COPD exacerbations

Oxygen therapy (OT) is often vital in AECOPD. In most patients OT leads to a small increase in $PaCO_2$ which is of no consequence. Unfortunately, in about 10% of patients with severe COPD, OT causes a progressive increase in $PaCO_2$ due to impaired CO_2 elimination and reduced ventilatory drive, leading to hypercapnic respiratory failure (HCRF) and eventually hypercapnic coma. Nevertheless, these patients still benefit from low-dose 'controlled' OT (24%–28%) because even a small increase in PaO_2 on the steep part of the oxyhaemoglobin dissociation curve significantly increases arterial oxygen content without causing significant CO_2 retention. In 2008 the British Thoracic Society published guidelines for the acute use of OT[5] and recommended that the response to increased oxygen concentrations in AECOPD should be carefully monitored to achieve a PaO_2 >8 kPa on arterial blood gas (ABG) measurement without a substantial increase in $PaCO_2$.

Patients with a previous history of HCRF should be given an oxygen alert card (±24% Venturi mask) to present to health-care personnel in the event of a further AECOPD. In these patients the target oxygen saturation (SaO_2) should be 88%–92% pending ABG analysis to exclude a substantial rise in $PaCO_2$ (e.g. >1 kPa or pH <7.35). A higher SaO_2 has few advantages but may result in hypoventilation, hypercapnia and respiratory acidosis. In the absence of an oximeter, selecting the appropriate dose of pre-hospital OT can be difficult. During short periods (<20 minutes) of pre-hospital transport and emergency department assessment, 28%–35% OT should be started. If drowsiness develops or if HCRF has occurred previously (i.e. oxygen alert card), give 'controlled' OT using a fixed performance (24%–28%) Venturi mask. If initial ABG measurements confirm HCRF, OT should be titrated to the lowest concentration required to achieve an SaO_2 88%–92%. Continue to monitor ABG regularly.

If the $PaCO_2$ rises to >8 kPa or pH falls to <7.35, or if the patient becomes drowsy or fatigued, non-invasive positive pressure ventilation (NIPPV) should be initiated and is highly effective in many cases (see below). In those without correctable precipitants, progression to MV in the event of failure of NIPPV may not be appropriate, and in these cases limitation of treatment (i.e. to NIPPV) should be discussed with the responsible consultant. However, prolonged and satisfactory survival may follow a period of intubation and MV and historically many COPD patients have been denied access to the ICU.

If hypercapnia and respiratory acidosis progress despite NIPPV, and MV is considered inappropriate (i.e. end-stage disease), management should focus on increasing ventilatory drive. In these cases, FiO_2 is reduced to stimulate hypoxic respiratory drive and ventilation, thereby decreasing $PaCO_2$. Although SaO_2 will fall, aim to maintain PaO_2 at >6.5 kPa (SaO_2 <80%–85%).

In patients at risk of CO_2 retention, nebulized bronchodilators can be given using compressed air to drive the nebulizer, but in most cases using oxygen as the driving gas causes no problem as long as the nebulizer time is short and not given 'back to back'.

In COPD patients at low risk of developing HCRF, or if $PaCO_2$ is normal on the initial ABG measurement, OT should aim for the normal target SaO_2 range of 94%–98% if aged <70 years and 92%–98% if aged >70 years (i.e. a wider normal range in the elderly). Haemoglobin is almost fully saturated in these ranges and further increases in PaO_2 have no impact on oxygen delivery as little oxygen dissolves in plasma. Nasal prongs may be more comfortable than facemasks in these patients and allow normal communication, drinking and eating. ABG should be checked 30–60 minutes after a change in oxygen dose.

Criteria for non-invasive positive pressure ventilation

NIPPV is effective in hypercapnic AECOPD,[6] reducing hospital mortality from 20% to 10%. Careful case selection, an appropriate setting with experienced staff (e.g. high dependency unit) and early decisions regarding escalation of therapy (i.e. intubation/MV) are all important.

Criteria for NIPPV include severe dyspnoea, moderate acidosis (pH 7.25–7.35), hypercapnia ($PaCO_2$ 6–8 kPa) and respiratory rate >25 breaths/min. Exclusion criteria include severe acidosis (pH <7.15), profound hypotension, cardiovascular instability, impaired consciousness (Glasgow Coma Scale <11), severe anxiety, respiratory arrest, confusion or lack of co-operation, active vomiting or risk of aspiration, facial surgery or other factors preventing use of facemasks. Unfortunately, many patients are not started on NIPPV in the UK until they have severe acidosis (pH <7.25), which is associated with a greater failure rate (>30%). Earlier intervention (i.e. when the pH is 7.25–7.35) is associated with improved outcomes.[6]

NIPPV should be considered a trial of treatment with an agreed policy of either removal and provision of palliative care or escalation to intubation if it fails.

Non-ventilatory therapies that improve outcome in acute COPD exacerbations

Treatment with high-dose nebulized β_2 agonist (± anticholinergic) bronchodilators, oral steroids and antibiotics is essential. Oral steroids (e.g. prednisolone 30 mg orally for 7–10 days) improve lung function and reduce hospital stay when used in addition to conventional therapy. Routine sputum culture is not indicated as it is rarely of value. The acquisition of *Pseudomonas* or *Staphylococcus* organisms in sputum is an adverse sign and sputum examination is recommended if there is a failure to improve. Antibiotics reduce the duration of an exacerbation but are overused, particularly in the community. Data meta-analysis suggests a small morbidity and mortality benefit with antibiotic therapy. Initial empirical therapy with an aminopenicillin, macrolide or tetracycline is directed against likely organisms (e.g. *Haemophilus influenzae*, *Streptococcus pneumoniae, Moraxella catarrhalis*). Theophyllines have not been shown to be effective in AECOPD. Electrolyte imbalance (e.g. hypophosphataemia, hypokalaemia) should be corrected. Nebulized saline and ensuring adequate hydration and humidification of oxygen may assist secretion clearance. The role of nutrition (i.e. providing 2000 calories per day intake) is unclear but may be important in limiting further muscle wasting. Thromboembolic prophylaxis should be given. Respiratory stimulants are no longer appropriate.

Indications for mechanical ventilation

Indications for MV include severe hypoxaemia (PaO_2 <5.3 kPa), respiratory rate >35 breaths/min, increasing acidosis (pH <7.25), hypercapnia ($PaCO_2$ >8 kPa), respiratory arrest, NIPPV failure, confusion, poor cough and haemodynamic instability.

Mortality in ventilated COPD patients is about 20%, with higher mortality in those requiring >72 hours MV (~37%) and those who failed an extubation attempt (~36%). Mean duration of ventilation is 5–9 days. Contrary to general opinion, mortality in ventilated COPD patients with respiratory failure is less than in many non-COPD cases admitted to intensive care and long-term survival is better.

Nevertheless, MV should be avoided when possible because most COPD patients tolerate hypoxaemia and acidosis well, spontaneously breathing patients have an effective cough, COPD patients are at particularly high risk of developing ventilator-associated complications (e.g. pneumothorax, infection) and weaning can be difficult due to respiratory muscle weakness and the associated increase in work of breathing associated with hyperinflation.

In end-stage COPD (i.e. reduced exercise tolerance, resting breathlessness, loss of independence) it may be appropriate to limit ventilatory support to NIPPV. The decision to withhold MV of a patient should be based on health status and an estimate of survival time based on previous functional status, body mass index, long-term oxygen therapy requirement when well, comorbidities and previous ICU admissions. Neither age nor FEV_1 should be used in isolation when assessing suitability for MV. A clear statement of the patient's wishes in the form of an advance directive or 'living will' always makes these difficult decisions easier.

Mechanical ventilation in obstructive airways disease

In COPD (or asthma) MV can be associated with 'dynamic' hyperinflation of the lungs, which occurs when expiratory time is inadequate (i.e. rapid ventilatory rates) or tidal volumes are too high (see Chapter 6).[7,8] Auto-PEEP refers to the component of PEEP that is due to this 'dynamic' hyperinflation and represents the pressure of trapped alveolar gas. The pressure applied to the airway during MV to prevent alveolar collapse is called PEEP (or 'applied' PEEP or 'extrinsic' PEEP). The pressure measured when all airflow is stopped at end expiration is termed the 'total' PEEP. Auto-PEEP is the difference between 'total' PEEP and PEEP. Confusingly, the term 'intrinsic' PEEP often refers to both auto-PEEP and 'total' PEEP.

'Total' PEEP, and thus auto-PEEP, is usually measured by occluding the expiratory port of the ventilator at end expiration for approximately two seconds. As there is considerable regional variation in auto-PEEP, the measured end-expiratory pressure is the mean. Unfortunately 'total' PEEP measured at end expiration may be misleadingly low, as it reflects only pressures in alveoli that communicate with the airway (i.e. it excludes the pressures in airways obstructed at end expiration). As the end-inspiratory plateau pressure is usually uniform (i.e. there is little regional variation), it may be a better indicator of gas trapping (i.e. at different respiratory rates) when tidal volume and PEEP are fixed. A high plateau pressure, despite normal or low tidal volumes, indicates widespread gas trapping. A marked disparity between a high plateau pressure and a low auto-PEEP measured by end-expiratory occlusion suggests extensive airways obstruction due to inflammation or mucous plugging. The raised intrathoracic pressure associated with this hyperinflation can reduce venous return to the heart, decreasing cardiac output and leading to cardiovascular instability.

In cases of airways obstruction, patients require both long inspiratory and expiratory times (i.e. to achieve adequate alveolar inflation and deflation). This can be achieved by reducing the respiratory rate (RR). For example, if the RR is reduced from 15 to 8 breaths/min, the breath cycle time increases from 4 to 7.5 seconds. In this patient the longer respiratory cycle increased tidal volume (Tv) from 400 to 650 ml/breath. Although minute ventilation (Tv × RR) fell from 6 l/min (i.e. 400 ml × 15) to 5.2 l/min (i.e. 650 ml × 8), the alveolar ventilation ([Tv – Td] × RR; where Td is deadspace of 250 ml/breath) increased from 2.25 l/min (400–250 ml × 15) to 3.2 l/min (650–250 ml × 8) and hence reduced the $PaCO_2$ from ~12 kPa to ~8.5 kPa and increased pH from 7.13 to 7.27.

Auto-PEEP adds to the work of breathing and patient-ventilator dyssynchrony by presenting an increased threshold load to inspiration and by depressing the trigger sensitivity of the ventilator. In these cases addition of a low level of PEEP (e.g. ~5 cm H_2O) effectively replaces the auto-PEEP, improving comfort, reducing work of breathing and marginally improving distribution of ventilation without increasing hyperinflation.[7,8] Haemodynamic instability and barotrauma (e.g. pneumothorax) are obvious risks of serious hyperinflation.

Weaning from mechanical ventilation

Cautious weaning is undertaken as soon as possible but this can be difficult and hazardous in COPD patients. The best method is debated but abrupt reductions in the level of ventilatory support that induce respiratory muscle fatigue must be avoided. Whether pressure support or a T-piece trial is used, weaning is shortened when a clinical protocol is adopted. Several recent trials indicate that NIPPV, when compared with invasive pressure support ventilation, can facilitate and shorten the weaning process in COPD patients with acute or chronic respiratory failure, may reduce ICU length of stay, decrease nosocomial pneumonia and improve survival rates. [9]

Conclusion

In this case an understanding of the respiratory physiology associated with AECOPD facilitated optimal mechanical ventilation. Reducing the respiratory rate and adding ventilator PEEP to 'offset' auto-PEEP improved gas exchange and corrected the respiratory acidosis. The patient improved with nebulized bronchodilator and intravenous steroid therapy over the next four days and was subsequently extubated without difficulty onto NIPPV.

Further Reading

1 National Institute for Health and Clinical Excellence. Management of chronic obstructive pulmonary disease in adults in primary and secondary care. Clinical guideline 101. London: NICE, 2010. www.nice.org.uk (accessed 01 06 11).

2 Celli BR, MacNee W; ATS/ERS Task Force. Standards for the diagnosis and treatment of patients with COPD: a summary of the ATS/ERS position paper. *Eur Respir J* 2004; **23**: 932–46. www.ersnet.org (accessed 01 06 11).

3 Global Initiative for Chronic Obstructive Lung Disease (GOLD). Global strategy for diagnosis, management, and prevention of COPD; NHLBI/WHO workshop report (GOLD guidelines). NIH Publication No2701A, 2001. www.goldcopd.org (accessed 01 06 11).

4 American Thoracic Society. Standards for the diagnosis and care of patients with Chronic Obstructive Pulmonary Disease. American Thoracic Society, 1995. www.thoracic.org (accessed 01 06 11).

5 O'Driscoll BR, Howard LS, Davison AG. BTS guideline for emergency oxygen use in adult patients. *Thorax* 2008; **63**(Suppl 6): vi1–vi68.

6 Ram F, Picot J, Lightowler J, Wedzicha J. Non-invasive positive pressure ventilation for the treatment of respiratory failure due to exacerbations of chronic obstructive pulmonary disease. *Cochrane Database Syst Rev* 2004; CD004104.

7 Calverley PMA, Koulouris NG. Flow limitation and dynamic hyperinflation: key concepts in modern respiratory physiology. *Eur Respir J* 2005; **25**: 186–99.

8 Calfee CS, Matthay MA. Recent advances in mechanical ventilation. *Am J Med* 2005; **118**: 584–91.

9 Nava S, Ambrosino N, Clini E *et al.* Noninvasive mechanical ventilation in the weaning of patients with respiratory failure due to chronic obstructive pulmonary disease. A randomized controlled trial. *Ann Intern Med* 1998; **128**: 721–8.

PROBLEM

8 Difficult Asthma

Lynette Linkson, Richard Leach

Case History

A 48-year-old man was referred to the chest clinic with uncontrolled adult-onset asthma and severe persistent cough despite repeated courses of oral steroids. Previously his asthma had been well controlled with a combined inhaled corticosteroid (ICS) and long-acting β_2 agonist (LABA). He had no history of childhood asthma or occupational dust or pet exposure. He was an ex-smoker and his home had been adapted to reduce allergens. Recent blood tests had confirmed that he was atopic with a raised total immunoglobulin E (IgE) of 499 kIU/l (normal <100 kIU/l) and blood eosinophilia (0.96×10^9/l; 13.3% of the white cell count). Chest examination revealed poor air entry to both lung bases with widespread expiratory wheeze but no crepitations. Spirometry reported a forced expiratory volume in 1 second (FEV_1) 2.16 l (72% predicted), forced vital capacity (FVC) 2.77 l (77% predicted) and peak expiratory flow rate (PEFR) of 438 l/min (92% predicted). The flow volume spirometry suggested small airways obstruction consistent with asthma. A chest radiograph (CXR) was normal. During the previous three months he had been on regular oral steroids and weaning attempts had resulted in severe cough, wheeze, nocturnal waking and breathlessness. He had been treated according to the British Thoracic Society (BTS) Guidelines[1] (Table 8.1). The addition of leukotriene receptor antagonists and oral theophyllines was unhelpful in weaning the steroids.

How would you assess this patient?

How can compliance with and delivery of inhaled maintenance therapy be improved?

How is difficult asthma managed and how effective are the newer therapies?

Does steroid-resistant asthma exist?

Table 8.1 BTS guidelines: management of asthma[1]

Step 1. Mild, intermittent asthma • Short-acting β_2 agonist • Check inhaler technique and compliance • Eliminate potential triggers
Step 2. Regular preventer therapy • Start beclomethasone (BDP) 200 μg twice/day • Titrate BDP dose to lowest that controls symptoms • BDP ≤800 μg/day may cause oral *Candida*, dysphonia • BDP ≥800 μg/day may cause osteoporosis
Step 3. Add long-acting β_2 agonist (LABA) • If >400–800 μg/day BDP add LABA (e.g. salmeterol) • Consider combination inhaler (e.g. Symbicort®, Seretide®)
Step 4. Continuing poor control • Add leukotriene receptor antagonist (e.g. montelukast); 33% patients respond; stop after a month if no response. Useful in atopic and exercise-induced asthma • Add theophylline (but side effects, e.g. indigestion). Monitor serum theophylline levels • Add slow-release oral β_2 agonist
Step 5. Continuous or frequent oral steroids • Aim for lowest oral steroid dose • Side effects if >3 months treatment or 3–4 courses/year • Warn about side effects (diabetes, hypertension, etc.) • Consider osteoporosis prophylaxis (e.g. bisphosphonate)

Background

Patients with difficult asthma represent a small subgroup of asthma patients (<5%) but are typical referrals to chest physicians.[2] Some have labile asthma with unexpected severe exacerbations and associated frequent hospital admissions, whilst others have persistent chronic airflow obstruction despite aggressive therapy. In these patients oral steroids often fail to completely reverse airways obstruction, β_2 agonist responses are poor, and airflow obstruction, bronchial hyperresponsiveness and diurnal PEFR variation are more severe. The likely cause is ongoing airway inflammation, remodelling and fibrosis but steroid resistance, β_2 receptor downregulation and other disease processes should be considered.

Initial assessment of difficult asthma patients should include a review of the diagnosis of asthma (i.e. check history and previous notes), confirmation that the patient is compliant with therapy (i.e. check pharmacy records, plasma steroid levels, inhaler technique) and demonstration that the airflow limitation is reversible (i.e. steroid trial). The possibility of occupational asthma should be considered, particularly if patients improve at weekends or when on holiday, as specific workplace 'sensitizers' (e.g. isocyanates, metals, disinfectants, wood dusts, biological enzymes, animal antigens) account for approximately 10% of adult asthma.

Other diagnoses for cough, breathlessness and wheeze should be excluded including chronic obstructive pulmonary disease, bronchiectasis, vasculitis (e.g. Churg–Strauss syndrome, eosinophilic syndromes), allergic bronchopulmonary aspergillosis (ABPA), sinus and upper airways disease, cardiac dysfunction, gastro-oesophageal reflux disease (GORD), hyperventilation syndrome or psychiatric disease.

Compliance with and delivery of inhaled maintenance therapy

The 1997 FACET and 2000 OPTIMA studies confirmed the efficacy of regular maintenance therapy with combined inhaled corticosteroid (ICS) and LABA compared to higher dose ICS alone in asthma control.[3,4] However, compliance with inhaled maintenance therapy (e.g. ICS alone or combined LABA/ICS) is poor. The 2006 INSPIRE study reported that patients tend to overuse β_2 agonists during worsening asthma rather than increasing maintenance therapy.[5] Strategies reported to improve compliance and asthma control include patient-adjusted maintenance dosing (i.e. in which the patient is taught to adjust the level of medication in response to symptom severity) and once-daily maintenance dosing. Compared to metered dose inhalers (MDI), dry powder inhalers (DPI) – and in particular the turbohaler – have been shown to improve inhaler technique and lung drug deposition (i.e. lung deposition of ~8%–10% with MDI vs 18%–25% with DPI) although spacer devices increase deposition of MDI drug delivery to approximately 20%.[1]

The 'SMART' concept was recently introduced, in which Symbicort® (a combined formoterol [LABA]/budesonide [ICS] turbohaler) was used to provide a low-dose background maintenance therapy and 'reliever' therapy by using the combined inhaler when symptoms occur (i.e. no use of short-acting β_2 agonists like salbutamol). This regime attempts to tailor the intake of ICS to symptoms and improved asthma control despite a reduction in total ICS dose. Presumably this was achieved by ensuring ICS delivery during worsening asthma (i.e. at a time when the patient might normally resort to short-acting β_2 agonist use instead of increasing the dose of inhaled steroid), the simplified drug regime involving a single inhaler, and because the LABA, formoterol, can be used as a 'reliever' because of its rapid onset of action, which is comparable with that of salbutamol.[6]

Management of difficult asthma

Standard therapy with high-dose ICS, LABA, leukotriene antagonists and oral theophyllines is continued as recommended in the BTS guidelines.[1] Non-pharmacological factors including allergen avoidance (e.g. house dust mite control measures), smoking cessation, weight loss in obese asthmatics and breathing exercises may also aid asthma control. Initial management strategies for difficult asthma might include adjustable ICS maintenance dosing regimes and the 'SMART' concept of asthma management (as described above).

The oral steroid dose should be titrated to the lowest dose compatible with symptom control. If this remains >15 mg/day, with no obvious cause for increased steroid clearance (e.g. rifampicin therapy), steroid sparing agents and alternative therapies should be considered.

- **Steroid sparing agents** include methotrexate, ciclosporin, macrolide antibiotics and oral gold. All have potentially serious adverse effects and drug interactions which limit their use in clinical practice. Response is variable but steroid dose reductions of up to 50% over 3–6 months have been reported.[7,8] Unfortunately, there have been no confirmatory, randomized controlled trials. Haematological, renal and liver function monitoring is required.
- **New 'safer' steroids**. Research is ongoing into 'dissociated' steroid therapy in which the anti-inflammatory effects, mediated by transcription factor inhibition, are dissociated from the side effects mediated by glucocorticoid DNA binding.[2] Ciclesonide, a once-daily inhaled steroid, is activated by airway esterases and has fewer side effects due to high levels of protein binding.
- **Monoclonal antibody immunotherapy**
  1. **Anti-IgE**. Omalizumab is a humanized anti-IgE antibody that is effective in moderate to severe asthma associated with atopy and high serum IgE levels. Allergens bind to IgE and precipitate the release of proinflammatory mediators.[9] Targeting IgE blocks the allergic response rather than specific allergens or triggers, which are often unknown. IgE blockade has been shown to reduce eosinophilia in sputum, reduce bronchial hyperresponsiveness and improve symptom control.[10] Two randomized controlled trials of omalizumab reported reduced frequency of exacerbations by 28% and 58%, respectively, in addition to a reduction in inhaled steroid use. Although expensive to use, safety profiles were excellent.[2,9]
  2. **Anti–IL-5 (eosinophil inhibitors)**. Eosinophils are found in sputum, bronchoalveolar lavage (BAL) fluid and mucosal biopsies in asthma and influence bronchial hyperresponsiveness and airway remodelling. Interleukin-5 (IL-5) is essential to their formation. Inhalation of IL-5 by asthmatics induces bronchial hyperresponsiveness and sputum eosinophilia and high serum IL-5 levels are associated with decline in FEV_1. Intravenous infusion of monoclonal antibody against IL-5 produced long-term suppression of serum and sputum eosinophilia during allergen exposure but did not prevent bronchial hyperresponsiveness to allergens. In contrast, in previous studies in mice in which IL-5 genes were deleted, bronchial

hyperresponsiveness to allergens was prevented. Further work is required to determine whether IL-5 blockade has any role in asthma therapy.[11]

- **Cytokine modulation (anti-tumour necrosis factor alpha).** Atopic asthma is usually considered as an eosinophilic disorder involving helper T cell type 2 (Th2) cytokines (see anti-IgE and anti-IL-5 above) and is highly responsive to inhaled corticosteroids in mild disease. In difficult asthma the inflammatory pattern is more heterogeneous, with increased neutrophil and distal lung involvement and greater airways remodelling. This inflammatory response is more like a helper T cell type 1 (Th1) cytokine response, which is associated with increased tumour necrosis factor alpha (TNF-α) production.[12] In severe, steroid-dependent asthmatics, TNF-α is increased in BAL fluid and mast cells have raised TNF-α gene expression. Small, preliminary studies show upregulation of the TNF-α axis in refractory asthma, which can be decreased by TNF-α blockade using etanercept therapy. Improvements in asthma-related quality-of-life scores, lung function, bronchial hyperresponsiveness and symptoms were reported.[12]
- **Phosphodiesterase-4 inhibitors** (e.g. roflumilast) have broad anti-inflammatory actions with neutrophil inhibition. Clinical trial data are encouraging.[2]

Difficult asthma syndromes

Specific difficult asthma syndromes include:

- **Brittle asthma** is either type 1 with marked PEFR variability (>40% diurnal variation for 50% of the time) despite appropriate therapy; or type 2 with sudden severe attacks during good background control.
- **Steroid-resistant asthma** is rare and usually occurs in middle-aged, overweight women. Diagnoses other than asthma (e.g. psychogenic) are likely and treatment is usually supportive avoiding high-dose steroids.

Conclusion

In this patient a two-week course of high-dose oral steroid (i.e. prednisolone 30 mg daily) relieved the wheeze, breathlessness and cough. Almost complete reversibility was demonstrated on repeat spirometry with an FEV_1 3.34 l (112% predicted), FVC 3.93 l (109% predicted) and PEFR 501 l/min (106% predicted). The flow volume trace appeared normal and both F50 and F25 (indicators of small airways calibre) were within the normal ranges. Repeat blood tests confirmed a raised total IgE of 588 kIU/l (normal <100 kIU/l) and a significantly elevated eosinophil count of 1.16×10^9/l (15.2% of the white cell count) consistent with underlying atopy. The erythrocyte sedimentation rate was 22 mm/hr and anti-neutrophil cytoplasmic antibody (ANCA) was negative, excluding significant vasculitis and Wegener's granulomatosis. The *Aspergillus* serology was negative, ruling out ABPA. The normal CXR and subsequent computed tomography scan did not reveal an alternative cause for the patient's symptoms. A three-month trial of a proton pump inhibitor was initiated as the patient had some symptoms suggestive of GORD. This improved the cough fractionally but did not reduce the dependence on steroids for wheeze and breathlessness control. These results all supported the diagnosis of asthma and excluded steroid resistance.

Further Reading

1 British Thoracic Society. British guideline on the management of asthma. May 2011: www.brit-thoracic.org.uk

2 Chung KF, Godard P, Adelroth E *et al.* Difficult/therapy-resistant asthma: the need for an integrated approach to define clinical phenotypes, evaluate risk factors, understand pathophysiology and find novel therapies. ERS Task Force on Difficult/Therapy-Resistant Asthma. European Respiratory Society. *Eur Respir J* 1999; **13**: 1198–208.

3 Pauwels RA, Löfdahl CG, Rostma DS *et al.* Effect of inhaled formoterol and budesonide on exacerbations of asthma. Formoterol and Corticosteroids Establishing Therapy (FACET) International Study Group. *N Engl J Med* 1997; **337**: 1405–11.

4 O'Byrne PM, Barnes PJ, Rodriguez-Roisin R *et al.* Low dose inhaled budesonide and formoterol in mild persistent asthma: the OPTIMA randomized trial. *Am J Respir Crit Care Med* 2001; **164**: 1392–7.

5 Partridge MR, van der Molen T, Myrseth S-E, Busse WW. Attitudes and actions of asthma patients on regular maintenance therapy: the INSPIRE study. *BMC Pulm Med* 2006; **6**: 13.

6 Rabe KF, Atienza T, Magyar P, Larsson P, Jorup C, Lalloo UG. Effect of budesonide in combination with formoterol for reliever therapy in asthma exacerbations: a randomised controlled, double-blind study. *Lancet* 2006; **368**: 744–53.

7 Nizankowska E, Soja J, Pinis G *et al.* Treatment of steroid-dependent bronchial asthma with cyclosporin. *Eur Respir J* 1995; **8**: 1091–9.

8 Bernstein IL, Bernstein DI, Dubb JW, Faiferman I, Wallin B. A placebo-controlled multicenter study of auranofin in the treatment of patients with corticosteroid-dependent asthma. Auranofin Multicenter Drug Trial. *J Allergy Clin Immunol* 1996; **98**: 317–24.

9 Lanier BQ, Corren J, Lumry W, Liu J, Fowler-Taylor A, Gupta N. Omalizumab is effective in the long-term control of severe allergic asthma. *Ann Allergy Asthma Immunol* 2003; **91**: 154–9.

10 Solèr M, Matz J, Townley R *et al.* The anti-IgE antibody omalizumab reduces exacerbations and steroid requirement in allergic asthmatics. *Eur Respir J* 2001; **18**: 254–61.

11 Leckie MJ, ten Brinke A, Khan J *et al.* Effects of an interleukin-5 blocking monoclonal antibody on eosinophils, airway hyperresponsiveness, and the late asthmatic response. *Lancet* 2000; **356**: 2144–8.

12 Berry MA, Hargadon B, Shelley M *et al.* Evidence of a role of tumor necrosis factor alpha in refractory asthma. *N Engl J Med* 2006; **354**: 697–708.

PROBLEM

9 Asthma and Pregnancy

Lynette Linkson, Richard Leach

Case History

The obstetric team has asked you to review a 24-year-old woman who is 32 weeks pregnant with an acute exacerbation of her long-standing atopic asthma. She is currently on the obstetric ward for monitoring of her slightly raised blood pressure. Her asthma is normally well controlled on twice-daily inhaled beclomethasone (200 μg bd) with occasional use of a salbutamol inhaler. She has recently had a viral upper respiratory tract infection with cough and some wheeze but her peak expiratory flow rate (PEFR) has been stable at 400 l/min on the ward. She deteriorated rapidly overnight with increasing breathlessness and wheeze and her PEFR has fallen to 250 l/min despite increasing use of her metered dose inhaled salbutamol. Examination reveals widespread expiratory wheeze but her saturation is 92% on air.

Does pregnancy affect asthma and what are the associated risk factors?

Can asthma affect the fetus and the subsequent delivery?

How is asthma managed during pregnancy?

How should pregnant asthmatic women be managed during labour?

Is breast-feeding contraindicated in asthmatic mothers?

Background

Pregnancy can affect asthma and asthma can affect the outcome of pregnancy. One-third of pregnant, asthmatic women improve, one-third deteriorates and one-third stays the same. The course of asthma in successive pregnancies is usually similar. Severe asthma is more likely to deteriorate than mild asthma in pregnancy. Suggested mechanisms include changes related to maternal hormones, fetal sex, β_2 adrenoreceptor responsiveness and altered immune function.[1]

The main risk factor for development of an acute asthma exacerbation during pregnancy is severe asthma prior to pregnancy. Other factors include increased susceptibility to viral infection because of changes in cell-mediated immunity and inappropriate (i.e. patient initiated) discontinuation of inhaled corticosteroids. Exacerbations can occur at any time during pregnancy but usually occur predominantly late in the second trimester. Acute attacks are rare during labour due to endogenous steroid production.[2]

Effect of asthma on the fetus and the subsequent delivery

Meta-analysis of all studies demonstrated a twofold increase in risk of low-birth-weight babies in those suffering asthma exacerbations during pregnancy. This is the same as for maternal smoking during pregnancy.[2] Possible mechanisms include a maternal inflammatory response, steroid treatment, maternal hypoxia, altered placental function and fetal sex.[1] Pre-term delivery and pre-eclampsia are not significantly increased.[2]

Asthma management during pregnancy

Pregnant women should be advised to continue all their usual asthma medications. Both the maternal and fetal risks of poorly controlled asthma outweigh the small risks from standard acute treatment. There is a tendency for mothers to under-report symptoms and clinicians to undertreat acute exacerbations. Acute exacerbations should be treated as normal (i.e. as in non-pregnant women) with the addition of fetal monitoring. Thus steroids and nebulized bronchodilators should be used at normal dosages and oxygen saturations maintained above 95% during acute exacerbations.

Previous suggestions of an association between oral steroid use and pre-term labour and pre-eclampsia are probably unfounded.[1] Leukotriene antagonists should not be commenced during pregnancy due to limited safety data, although they should be continued in those who have failed to achieve adequate control with other agents in the past.

Management of pregnant asthmatic women during labour

Acute asthma is unusual during labour due to the associated high sympathetic drive and increased steroid production. Patients on more than 7.5 mg of oral steroid daily for longer than two weeks prior to delivery should be given intravenous hydrocortisone 100 mg 8-hourly during labour. Prostaglandin E_2 can be used to induce labour without risk but prostaglandin $F_2\alpha$ for post-partum haemorrhage may induce bronchospasm. Regional anaesthetic blockade (e.g. subdural anaesthesia) is preferable to general anaesthesia in asthmatic patients.

Breast-feeding in asthmatic mothers

Breast-feeding reduces the incidence of atopy in the children of asthmatic mothers and should be strongly encouraged. Even when the mother is taking high-dose prednisolone, which is secreted in breast milk, the child is only exposed to very small and clinically irrelevant doses of steroid.

Conclusion

In this patient the acute exacerbation was treated as normal with the usual doses of oral steroids and nebulized bronchodilators. A routine chest radiograph was performed and was normal. Oxygen saturations were maintained above 95% using high-flow oxygen. The patient made a rapid recovery and had a normal delivery a few weeks later.

Further Reading

1 Murphy VE, Gibson PG, Smith R, Clifton VL. Asthma during pregnancy: mechanisms and treatment implications. *Eur Respir J* 2005; **25**: 731–50.

2 Murphy VE, Clifton VL, Gibson PE. Asthma exacerbations during pregnancy: incidence and association with adverse pregnancy outcomes. *Thorax* 2006; **61**: 169–76.

PROBLEM

10 Allergic Bronchopulmonary Aspergillosis

Kate Brignall

Case History

A 50-year-old woman presented with non-pleuritic chest pain, cough and haemoptysis. She had been unwell for several weeks with intermittent fever and increasing breathlessness. She had been prescribed a salbutamol inhaler for suspected asthma and there was a history of recurrent chest infections. Despite a course of antibiotics a week earlier she had not improved. She had type 2 diabetes mellitus and a large goitre. Her regular medication included metformin and gliclazide. She was resident in the UK but was originally from India where she visited regularly. She had no history of tuberculosis (TB) or TB contacts. She was a lifelong non-smoker.

On examination she was unwell. She had a low-grade fever at 38.2°C and a slight tachycardia. Her respiratory rate was normal, oxygen saturation (SaO_2) was 95% and chest auscultation revealed coarse upper airway sounds. Examination was otherwise unremarkable. Investigations demonstrated a leukocytosis with a mild neutrophilia and a raised eosinophil count of 1.72×10^9/l; her renal function was normal. Spirometry showed an obstructive defect with a forced expiratory volume in 1 second/forced vital capacity (FEV_1/FVC) ratio of 55%. The chest radiograph (CXR) is illustrated in Figure 10.1. The initial computed tomography (CT) scan is shown in Figure 10.2.

What is the differential diagnosis?

How do *Aspergillus* species cause lung disease?

What is the pathophysiology of allergic bronchopulmonary aspergillosis (ABPA)?

What are the clinical features of ABPA?

How is ABPA diagnosed?

How is ABPA treated and monitored?

Background

Pulmonary eosinophilia encompasses a variety of conditions associated with transient pulmonary infiltrates and elevated blood eosinophil counts, although eosinophilic infiltration of the lung can occur without blood eosinophilia. In this case the history of asthma, recent respiratory symptoms, associated blood eosinophilia and a CXR demon-

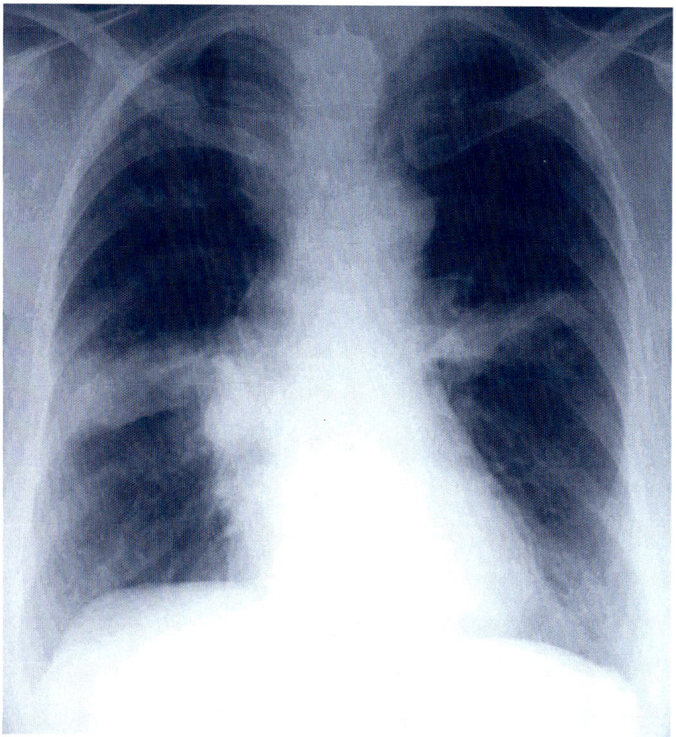

Figure 10.1 Chest radiograph.

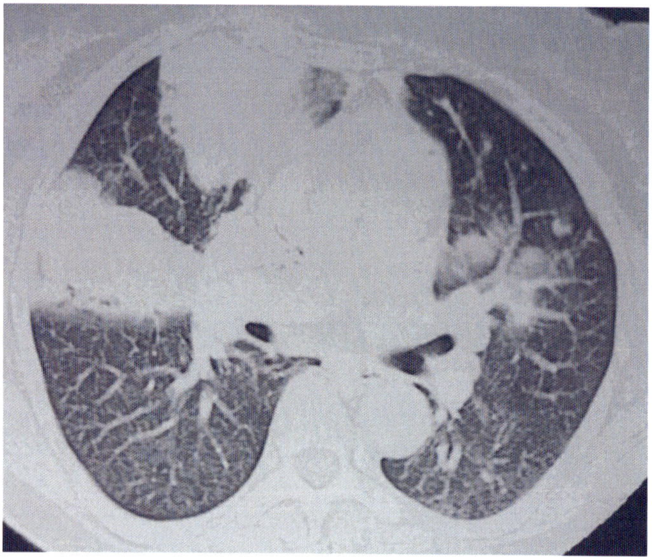

Figure 10.2 Chest CT scan.

strating air-space shadowing suggest a diagnosis of 'pulmonary eosinophilia'. Pulmonary eosinophilia is classified into idiopathic and secondary causes.[1–3]

Secondary causes include:

- **Fungal allergy**. Most commonly due to *Aspergillus fumigatus* (AF) causing the condition ABPA.
- **Helminth infections.** These occur throughout Southeast Asia, Africa and Central America. Simple pulmonary eosinophilia (Loffler's syndrome) is caused by parasitic infections (e.g. *Ascaris lumbricoides*, *Strongyloides*). Tropical pulmonary eosinophilia is caused by filarial worms (e.g. *Wucheria bancrofti*). Passage of larvae or filariae through the lungs may be associated with allergic reactions including fever and wheeze. Treatment requires anti-helminthic agents or filaricide, with steroids for severe pulmonary manifestations.
- **Drugs (e.g. penicillin, methotrexate), toxins and blood transfusions** may cause pulmonary eosinophilia which occurs within hours to days of the exposure and resolves within a week of removal of the cause.

Idiopathic causes include:

- **Chronic eosinophilic pneumonia**. This occurs in middle age, with a female to male ratio of 2:1. Onset is insidious over weeks to months with dyspnoea, cough, recent-onset asthma, occasional haemoptysis, weight loss, fever and night sweats. A CXR shows peripheral opacities and air-space infiltrates. Eosinophilia is present in sputum, bronchoalveolar lavage (BAL) fluid and blood. High-dose steroids result in rapid improvement but low-dose steroids should be continued for six months as relapses are common.
- **Acute eosinophilic pneumonia** presents at any age with a short history (<7 days) of fever, dyspnoea, cough and myalgia. Ventilatory support may be required in hypoxic respiratory failure. The CXR shows interstitial and alveolar infiltrates and although BAL detects eosinophils in over 25% of cases there is no blood eosinophilia. The response to high-dose steroids is prompt. Relapse is unusual if steroids are tapered over 2–4 months.
- **Churg–Strauss syndrome.** This is small/medium-sized vessel vasculitis associated with severe asthma, blood eosinophilia and pulmonary infiltrates. The anti-neutrophil cytoplasmic antibody (ANCA) is usually but not always positive. Treatment is with steroids and immunosuppressive agents.
- **Idiopathic hypereosinophilia syndrome** is a rare condition, more common in men aged 30–40 years, that presents with fever, weight loss, night sweats and pruritis. The blood eosinophilia ($>1.5 \times 10^9$/l; up to 70% of the white cell count) is persistent (>6 months) with associated eosinophilic tissue infiltration on histology and raised immunoglobulin E (IgE) levels. Heart (e.g. cardiomyopathy), skin (e.g. angio-oedema), central nervous system and gut manifestations can be life threatening. Treatment is with high-dose steroids and immunosuppressants.

Aspergillus lung disease

Aspergillus fumigatus and other *Aspergillus* moulds are ubiquitous and environmental load increases with humidity and building work. *Aspergillus* species cause a variety of clinical conditions[4–6] which depend largely on the host response and are classified as:

- **IgE-mediated allergic asthma**. This follows inhalation of *Aspergillus* spores with associated airways inflammation and bronchospasm. About 10% of asthmatics are skin-prick positive to *Aspergillus* species compared to 70% with house dust mite.
- **Extrinsic allergic alveolitis** (hypersensitivity pneumonitis). This occurs following inhalation of a large number of spores. For example, inhalation of *Aspergillus clavatus* from mouldy barley causes malt-worker's lung. Early removal from the source of exposure is curative but steroids may hasten recovery. Repeated exposure will eventually lead to lung fibrosis.
- **ABPA** describes the response to inhaled *Aspergillus* species in long-standing asthmatics who often present with deterioration.
- **Invasive *Aspergillus* pneumonia** occurs mainly during severe immunosuppression (e.g. chemotherapy). Macrophages normally destroy spores and neutrophils prevent tissue invasion. During severe neutropaenia, fungal digestive proteases allow hyphae to invade surrounding tissue. Invasion of blood vessels is associated with widespread dissemination (e.g. sinuses, eyes) and local haemorrhage (e.g. haemoptysis). Diagnosis is based on the detection of *Aspergillus* hyphae (e.g. sputum, BAL fluid, transbronchial biopsies) and characteristic features on a CT scan including honeycomb-like reticular changes with crescents of air at the edge of areas of consolidation ('halo' sign). AF immunoglobulin G (IgG) precipitins are usually negative. Galactomannan, an exoantigen of *Aspergillus*, may be detected but has a low sensitivity. Treatment requires aggressive, expensive and often toxic antifungal therapy (e.g. amphotericin, voriconazole).[6] A milder semi-invasive aspergillosis (previously known as chronic pulmonary aspergillosis or chronic necrotizing aspergillosis) occurs in middle-aged patients with chronic, pre-existing lung disease. Oral antifungals (e.g. itraconazole) may be effective but avoid oral steroids which cause further immunosuppression.
- **Aspergilloma**. This is a fungal ball which grows in a pre-existing lung cavity. Many are asymptomatic but there is often a local inflammatory response and 75% of cases present with haemoptysis due to damage to vessels on the inner surface of the cavity, with communication via a bronchus. Radical treatment with resection of the affected part of the lung may be necessary.

Pathophysiology of allergic bronchopulmonary aspergillosis

ABPA describes a hypersensitivity reaction to inhaled AF (although it can also occur in response to other fungi). Airway colonization by fungi causes recurrent symptoms but there is no relationship between the amount of exposure and the rate of sensitization. The condition occurs mainly in asthmatics, affecting 1%–2% of all asthmatics and 15% of patients with cystic fibrosis (CF). Although it occurs at any age, it is most common between the ages of 30 and 50 years old in the non-CF population. There is a wide spectrum of disease from mild asthma with occasional episodes of pulmonary eosinophilia to progressive lung damage and respiratory failure.

Humoral and cellular immune responses occur. The humoral response involves both IgE-mediated (type 1) and IgG-mediated (type 3) hypersensitivity reactions. The cellular response is through CD4 lymphocytes which produce interleukin-4 and interleukin-5, enhancing eosinophil-related inflammation.[3] Fungal enzymes and toxins, along with the host immune response, result in inflammation, impaired ciliary function, excessive mucous production and impaction of the airways with subsequent damage leading to proximal bronchiectasis.

The clinical features of allergic bronchopulmonary aspergillosis

Asthmatic patients with ABPA present acutely with wheeze and cough, sometimes productive of brown mucous plugs, and haemoptysis.[2,7–9] They often have atypical chest pains and systemic features of fever, anorexia and malaise. In its chronic form, acute episodes are superimposed on a chronic cough. Physical examination may be unremarkable or demonstrate local crepitations or wheeze.

Pulmonary function tests reveal air-flow limitation (reversible in <50%) with gas trapping, and a normal or reduced diffusing capacity. Later on in the disease, end-stage fibrosis and bronchiectasis will lead to a mixed obstructive and restrictive defect.

The CXR acutely shows hyperinflation, fleeting alveolar infiltrates due to eosinophilic pneumonia, and mucous plugging with segmental, lobar or even lung collapse. Characteristic radiographic findings include 'tram lines' due to thickened bronchial walls, 'toothpaste shadows' due to mucoid impaction and 'gloved finger shadows' due to bronchial exudates and bronchial wall thickening which extend from the hilum, which may all be migratory or fixed. Chronic radiographic changes are predominantly in the upper lobes with associated bronchiectasis (± fibrosis). High-resolution CT scanning may demonstrate proximal cylindrical bronchiectasis; however, this is neither a sensitive nor specific marker for ABPA

Diagnosis of allergic bronchopulmonary aspergillosis

ABPA is often under-diagnosed.[8,9] Early detection is important because treatment may slow or halt its progression. Current diagnostic criteria include clinical, radiographic and immunologic criteria classified into essential and minor features (Table 10.1).[3] Skin-prick testing is a good screening tool and a negative skin-prick test effectively excludes ABPA. Although total IgE levels and precipitins to AF are supportive they are neither sensitive nor specific. Specific IgG and IgE to AF are diagnostic. The CXR may be normal so if the skin-prick and serological tests are positive then a CT scan should be obtained to confirm the diagnosis.

Table 10.1 Current criteria for the diagnosis for ABPA

'Essential'
Asthma
Skin-prick test positivity for *Aspergillus fumigatus* (AF)
Elevated serum total IgE >1000 ng/ml
Elevated serum AF-specific IgE or IgG
Central bronchiectasis on CT scan
'Minor'
Positive precipitins to AF
Serum eosinophilia
History of pulmonary infiltrates on chest radiograph

Asthmatics frequently have features of ABPA but do not meet the full criteria for diagnosis:

- Positive skin-prick test (20%–30% of asthmatics);
- Positive serum precipitins to *Aspergillus* (10% of asthmatics);
- Recurrent mucoid impaction;

- Eosinophilia and high total IgE;
- Specific serology to AF should not be positive in asthmatics, nor should there be migratory areas of shadowing on CXR or evidence of bronchiectasis on CT.

Management of allergic bronchopulmonary aspergillosis

- **Corticosteroids** are the mainstay of treatment (based on observational studies).[7–9] The length of treatment and the dose have not been established. An acute flare warrants high-dose oral steroids for at least two weeks, then weaning over a period of weeks. Serial IgE concentrations correlate closely with clinical response and so can be used as a sensitive index of disease activity. Clinical and radiographic improvement has been associated with at least a 35% reduction in total IgE. Exacerbations are common and usually associated with a large rise in IgE levels. Steroid dependency may develop in advanced disease but steroids are of no value in end-stage fibrotic lung disease. Inhaled corticosteroids are of no benefit in ABPA but they are useful for the underlying asthma.
- **Antifungal agents**. Two randomized controlled trials of treatment with itraconazole (total daily dose of 400 mg) for 16 weeks demonstrated that it was well tolerated; reduced airway inflammation, markers of systemic inflammation and exacerbations; improved exercise tolerance; and decreased steroid requirements.[6,8] However, there was no significant change in lung function. The effect was temporarily sustained after stopping treatment, suggesting at least temporary eradication of the AF. Liver function should be monitored as itraconazole can cause liver dysfunction. It may also induce adrenal suppression in conjunction with the use of corticosteroids.

Some authors reserve the term ABPA only for those patients who develop inflammatory airways damage with bronchiectasis. Those IgG-positive patients without airways damage are classified as seropositive ABPA. An increase in inhaled steroids may be the only treatment required for seropositive ABPA. Oral steroids are highly effective in ABPA with and without airways damage, and appear to limit the host immune response without increasing tissue invasion by *Aspergillus*.

Conclusion

In this patient the differential diagnosis included asthma and associated fungal allergy, helminth infections (in view of her travel history) and tuberculosis. There was no obvious drug-related cause.[1] Extrinsic allergic alveolitis can cause a similar radiographic picture but the onset of symptoms is usually rapid following exposure to an antigen and is not often associated with eosinophilia.

In this case, further investigation revealed a raised total serum IgE of 9533 IU/ml, a positive skin-prick test to AF, positive precipitating IgG antibodies against AF, and specific IgE to AF. Sputum samples demonstrated a heavy growth of AF and *Pseudomonas*. Acid-fast bacilli and investigations for helminth infections were negative. Bronchoscopy revealed widespread mucous plugging suggesting bronchiectasis, which was confirmed on a repeat CT scan eight months later (Figure 10.3). These results confirmed the diagnosis of ABPA which responded to oral steroids and itraconazole.

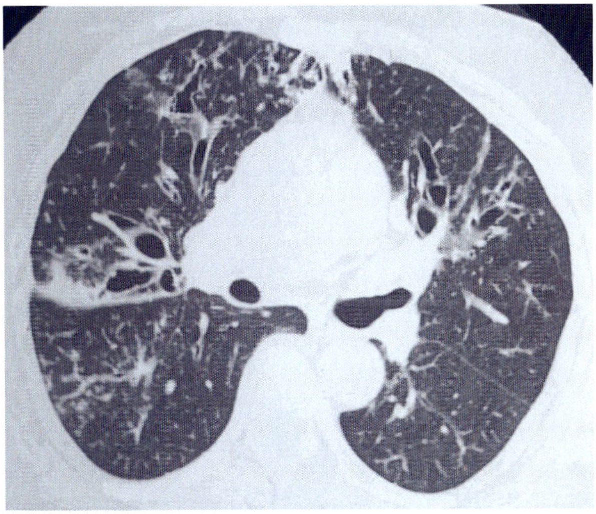

Figure 10.3 Proximal bronchiectasis in ABPA.

Further Reading

1 The Drug-Induced Lung Diseases. www.pneumotox.com (accessed 01 06 11).

2 Hinson KFW, Moon AF, Plummer NS. Broncho-pulmonary aspergillosis: a review and a report of eight new cases. *Thorax* 1952; **7**: 317–33.

3 Rosenburg M, Patterson, R, Mintzer R, Cooper BJ, Roberts M, Harris KE. Clinical and immunologic criteria for the diagnosis of allergic bronchopulmonary aspergillosis. *Ann Intern Med* 1977; **86**: 405–14.

4 Stevens DA, Moss RB, Kurup VP *et al.* Allergic bronchopulmonary aspergillosis in cystic fibrosis – state of the art: Cystic Fibrosis Foundation Consensus Conference. *Clin Infect Dis* 2003; **37**(Suppl 3): S225–64.

5 Patterson R, Greenberger PA, Radin RC, Roberts M. Allergic bronchopulmonary aspergillosis: staging as an aid to management. *Ann Intern Med* 1982; **96**: 286–91.

6 Wark PAB, Gibson PG, Wilson AJ. Azoles for allergic bronchopulmonary aspergillosis associated with asthma. *Cochrane Database Syst Rev* 2004; CD001108.

7 Wardlaw A, Geddes DM. Allergic bronchopulmonary aspergillosis: a review. *J R Soc Med* 1992; **85**: 747–51.

8 Vlahakis NE, Aksamit TR. Diagnosis and treatment of allergic bronchopulmonary aspergillosis. *Mayo Clin Proc* 2001; **76**: 930–8.

9 Akuthota P, Weller P. Allergic bronchopulmonary aspergillosis. UpToDate, 2010. www.uptodate.com (accessed 01 06 11).

PROBLEM

11 Chronic Cough

Jimstan Periselneris, Richard Leach

Case History

A 42-year-old man was referred to the chest clinic with a six-month history of recurrent paroxysmal cough and two episodes of cough syncope. He had minimal sputum production and no associated haemoptysis or breathlessness. The cough was most troublesome during the day and aggravated by cigarette smoke, strong perfumes, large meals and car fumes. It rarely disturbed sleep. He had no history of viral upper respiratory tract infection (URTI), atopy, asthma, sinusitis or childhood respiratory disease. There was no history of allergen, pet or bird contact, industrial dust contact or occupational asthma. Apart from occasional indigestion he had no past medical history of note. He was on no medication and he had never smoked. The cough interfered with his work as a salesman and he had avoided social engagements for many months.

Apart from being overweight (body mass index 28 kg/m^2), examination was normal. He had taken many proprietary cough medicines and his family general practitioner (GP) had treated him with antibiotics, antitussive agents, and oral and inhaled steroids. Routine blood tests, total immunoglobulin E and chest radiograph (CXR) were normal. Spirometry was normal with a forced expiratory volume in 1 second (FEV_1) >80% predicted.

How is cough classified and what are the commonest causes?

How is chronic cough assessed?

How is cough treated?

Are specialist cough clinics beneficial?

Background

Cough is a distressing symptom and occurs in many diseases (Table 11.1). Excessive cough can prevent sleep, cause social embarrassment and interrupt communication. The associated high pressures and rapid airflow may have haemodynamic effects (e.g. syncope), rupture blood vessels (e.g. eyes) and cause hernia, headache, pneumothorax, urinary incontinence and rib fractures. Respiratory disease reduces sputum clearance by 50% and the cough reflex acts as a reserve system increasing clearance by up to 20% (normally approximately 2.5%).[1]

Table 11.1 Causes of cough

Respiratory tract
Upper airways
Sinusitis*, post-nasal drip*, URTI*
Lower airways
LRTI (viral/bacterial)*, TB, pertussis
COPD*, chronic bronchitis*
Asthma*, cough variant asthma*
Eosinophilic bronchitis
Foreign body, airways irritants (e.g. smoke)
Bronchiectasis, ILD, lung cancer, OSA
Airway compression (e.g. lymph nodes)
Mediastinal masses
Gastrointestinal tract
GORD*
Oesophageal dysmotility or stricture with recurrent aspiration
Oesophago-bronchial fistula
Drugs
ACE inhibitors*, steroid inhalers*
Other
Left ventricular failure
Left atrial enlargement (e.g. mitral stenosis)
CNS disease with aspiration (e.g. MS, MND)
Psychogenic, idiopathic

* common; ACE, angiotensin converting enzyme; CNS, central nervous system; COPD, chronic obstructive pulmonary disease; GORD, gastro-oesophageal reflux disease; ILD, interstitial lung disease; MND, motor neurone disease; MS, multiple sclerosis; OSA, obstructive sleep apnoea; TB, tuberculosis; U/LRTI, upper/lower respiratory tract infection.

Cough is classified as:[1,2]

- **Acute cough**: defined arbitrarily as a cough lasting less than 3–8 weeks. Most are due to viral URTI and usually resolve within three weeks. Acute cough occurs in 40%–50% of patients with URTI, which equates to 48 million cases each year, half of whom self-medicate. Of the 12 million who consult their GP, twice as many are women due to their increased cough reflex sensitivity. Acute cough is usually benign and self-limiting but has a major economic impact due to absenteeism.[1] However, patients with haemoptysis, prominent systemic illness, a suspected inhaled foreign body or malignancy require further investigation.
- **Chronic cough**: defined as a cough lasting more than eight weeks. It usually refers to patients with a persistent dry cough and a normal CXR. Significant sputum production usually indicates primary lung pathology. All causes are reported in Table 11.1 but in practice over 90% are due to cough variant asthma (or eosinophilic bronchitis), gastro-oesophageal reflux disease (GORD) and post-nasal drip due to allergic rhinitis or chronic sinusitis. Post-viral coughs occasionally linger for 3–24 weeks. Epidemiologically, chronic cough will affect 10%–20% of adults and is more common in smokers, asthmatics, the obese and women.[1] Quality of life (QoL) is often impaired. The cause may be difficult to establish but specialist clinics, using management protocols, aid diagnosis and treatment in more than 80% of patients.

Assessment of chronic cough

Cost-effective management of chronic cough uses protocols combining selective diagnostic testing with empirical treatment trials determined by the clinical scenario (Figure 11.1). The cause of the cough and impact on QoL should be evaluated.

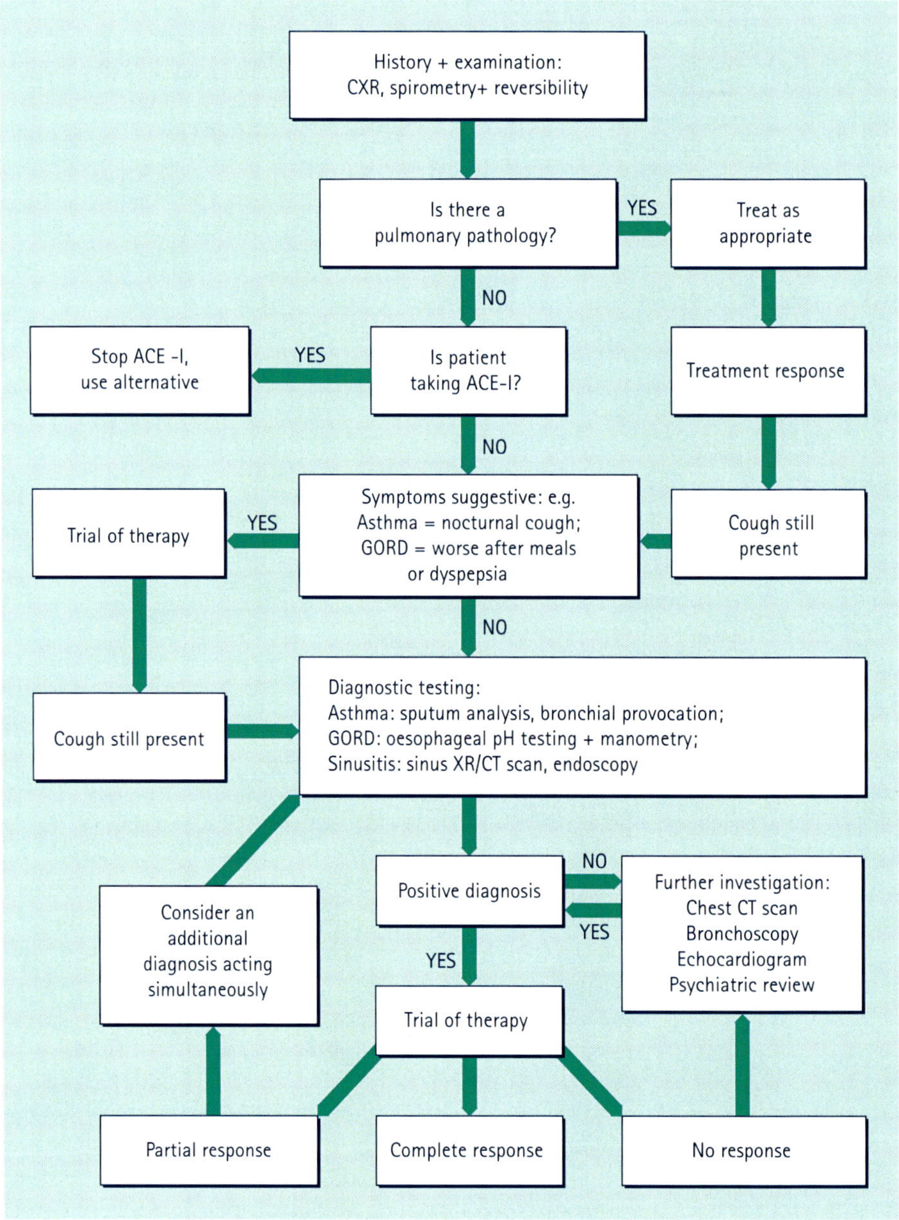

Figure 11.1 Management algorithm for chronic cough. ACE-I, angiotensin converting enzyme inhibitor; XR, radiology; CT, computed tomography.

A detailed history including onset, severity, timing and triggers for cough, with drug and occupational review, may suggest possible causes. For example, early morning or nocturnal cough or cough after exposure to dust, pollen or cold suggest asthma whereas cough after meals or with bending suggests GORD. However, characteristic symptoms are not always present.[1,2]

Examination should focus on sites most commonly associated with cough (e.g. larynx, nasal passages, chest). Evaluation of cough and impact on health status should be assessed with visual analogue scores and cough-specific QoL questionnaires. Routine investigation should include serial peak expiratory flow rate measurements, CXR and spirometry. If a potential cause is identified, a trial of treatment should be considered (see below).

If the aetiology is unclear (i.e. normal spirometry, no history of GORD) further investigations should include bronchial provocation (e.g. histamine, methacholine) tests, oesophageal pH and manometry, fibreoptic laryngoscopy and sinus radiology. Bronchoscopy has a low diagnostic yield (1%–6%) if included as part of an investigative algorithm but should be performed in all patients with suspected foreign body aspiration. If other tests are normal, a high-resolution computed tomography scan may provide diagnostic information in 24%–42% of patients with a normal CXR (e.g. bronchiectasis).[1,2] Treatment effects should be measured and recorded.

Treatment of cough

Acute cough may not require prescribed treatment. Home remedies (e.g. honey and lemon) often relieve distressing symptoms although many show little evidence of pharmacological effect. Proprietary, over-the-counter medications contain a number of potential antitussive agents:[3–5]

1. **Dextromethorphan** is a non-sedating, pharmacologically effective, long-acting cough suppressant (single meta-analysis[3]). Maximum cough-reflex suppression occurs at 60 mg. Most proprietary medications deliver subtherapeutic doses (i.e. approximately 15 mg) but caution is required when advising higher doses as many preparations contain other drugs (e.g. pseudoephedrine, paracetamol).
2. **Menthol** causes brief cough suppression by inhalation or capsules.
3. **Sedative antihistamines** suppress cough but also cause drowsiness.
4. **Codeine or pholcodine** are opiate antitussives with significant side effects (e.g. constipation, drowsiness, confusion in the elderly) but are no more effective than dextromethorphan and must be used with caution.

Chronic cough due to pulmonary disease (e.g. bronchiectasis) is debilitating but suppression may be contraindicated, especially when sputum clearance is important.[3,4] Specific chronic cough syndromes include:

1. **Cough variant asthma and eosinophilic bronchitis** account for approximately 30% of referrals to cough clinics. They represent one end of the asthma spectrum, with isolated cough but minimal airways inflammation or bronchoconstriction. Cough is typically nocturnal and worse in the mornings, after exercise and in cold air. Spirometry may be normal but bronchial challenge tests are usually positive in cough variant asthma. Eosinophilic bronchitis is steroid sensitive. It is associated with airway eosinophilia but no airway hyperresponsiveness and a negative bron-

chial challenge test does not exclude corticosteroid-sensitive cough. A trial of steroids (e.g. prednisolone 30 mg/day for two weeks) is required in all chronic cough patients. If there is no response the cough is unlikely to be due to asthma or its cough variants and an alternative diagnosis should be sought. If the cough responds to oral steroids, treatment with ongoing high-dose inhaled steroids, leukotriene receptor antagonists and antihistamines is required.[2–4] There is no evidence supporting long-acting β_2 agonist use.

2 **GORD** causes 5%–40% of chronic cough according to the British Thoracic Society guidelines[1] and up to 60% in the American College of Chest Physicians guidelines.[2] GORD-induced cough may be due to microaspiration of gastric contents or a vagally mediated oesophageal reflex stimulated by lower oesophageal sphincter (LOS) distal acid or non-acid volume reflux. Oesophageal dysmotility may contribute to both these mechanisms. GORD is usually long-standing and associated with daytime cough, worsening after meals and on sitting (due to increased intra-abdominal pressure), intermittent dysphonia and sore throat. Dyspepsia and reflux are common but not always present. Controlled trials of twice-daily proton pump inhibitors (e.g. omeprazole 20 mg twice daily) for eight weeks reduce GORD-induced cough in 40%–60% of cases. Prokinetic agents (e.g. metoclopramide 10 mg three times daily) are helpful in a proportion of patients. Medications that worsen reflux (e.g. nitrates, theophyllines) should be stopped. Baclofen increases LOS tone and decreases reflux and in a recent study reduced GORD-related cough resistant to other treatments. Antireflux surgery (i.e fundoplication) was effective in treating cough in carefully selected cases.

3 **Upper airways disease** causes cough associated with nasal congestion, sinusitis, 'recurrent throat clearing' and post-nasal drip syndrome. Treatment is with first-generation antihistamines, which have helpful anticholinergic properties, nasal ipratropium bromide and high-dose nasal steroids for three months, with an initial two-week course of antibiotic to cover *Haemophilus influenzae* (e.g. doxycycline) if sinusitis is suspected.

4 **Angiotensin converting enzyme (ACE) inhibitor cough** occurs in approximately 10% of people on ACE inhibitors following accumulation of lung bradykinin due to failure of its breakdown by ACE. It can occur within hours or more than a year after starting treatment. When the drug is stopped, the median time to cough resolution is 26 days but it can take up to 40 weeks. Most patients with ACE inhibitor-associated cough tolerate angiotensin II receptor blockers.

5 **Idiopathic or undiagnosed cough** is reported in 20% of referrals, despite extensive investigation, and typically occurs in middle-aged, overweight women, of whom about 30% have autoimmune disease (e.g. hypothyroidism). In psychogenic cough, cognitive behaviour therapy has proven benefit.

Specialist cough clinics

Poor diagnostic and treatment outcomes have been reported in hospital clinics without chronic cough management algorithms as extrathoracic causes of cough (e.g. GORD) are often overlooked. In contrast, specialist cough clinics report treatment success in 68%–100% of cases. Referral to a specialist clinic should be considered when there has been a failure of empirical treatment for asthma, GORD and rhinosinusitis or if serious cough complications occur (e.g. syncope, rib fractures).

Conclusion

In this case, the patient was treated for GORD-induced chronic cough with omeprazole 20 mg twice daily, on the basis of the daytime cough, indigestion and the previous failures of treatment with oral and inhaled steroid. The cough had resolved within eight weeks.

Further Reading

1 Morice AH, McGarvey L, Pavord I on behalf of the British Thoracic Society Cough Guideline Group. British Thoracic Society Guidelines: Recommendations for the management of cough in adults. *Thorax* 2006; **61**: i1–i24. www.thorax.bmj.com (accessed 01 06 11).

2 Irwin RS, Baumann MG, Bolser DC *et al.* Diagnosis and management of cough: ACCP evidence-based clinical practice guidelines. *Chest* 2006: **129**: 1s–292s.

3 Parvez L, Vaidya M, Sakhardande A, Subburaj S, Rajagopalan TG. Evaluation of antitussive agents in man. *Pulm Pharmacol* 1996; **9**: 299–308.

4 Chung KF. Currently available cough suppressants for chronic cough. *Lung* 2008; **186**(Suppl 1): S82–7.

5 Dicpinigaitis PV. Currently available antitussives. *Pulm Pharmacol Ther* 2009; **22**: 148–51.

PROBLEM

12 Aspiration Syndrome

Boris Lams, Richard Leach

Case History

A 45-year-old woman presented with a severe persistent cough that had not resolved with antibiotics or steroids. There was no sputum production, wheeze or haemoptysis. The patient was not aware of any potential precipitating events. She had no relevant past medical history or previous regular medication. She smoked ten cigarettes a day. Alcohol consumption was usually minimal but she did occasionally binge drink. She had been on a 'girls' night out' with her friend a few days before the onset of her symptoms.

On examination she appeared well but had a persistent cough. She was afebrile. There was a suggestion of mild left tracheal deviation but no cyanosis (saturation 94%), lymphadenopathy or clubbing. Cardiovascular examination was unremarkable and her blood pressure was 135/80 mmHg. Chest examination suggested some reduction in air entry at the left base but there was no wheeze or crepitations. The remainder of the examination was unremarkable.

Blood tests revealed a haemoglobin level of 12.3 g/dl and white cell count of 14.7×10^9/l (mainly neutrophils). C-reactive protein was raised at 38 mg/l. Biochemistry and renal and liver function tests were normal. All other investigations were normal. The chest radiograph suggested a degree of left lower lobe collapse with associated left mediastinal shift (Figure 12.1). A subsequent computed tomography (CT) scan demonstrated collapse of the posterior segment of the left lower lobe (Figure 12.2). The bronchoscopic appearance of the left lower lobe is illustrated in Figure 12.3.

What is the likely cause of these findings and how would you manage this patient?

How would you manage acute upper airways obstruction?

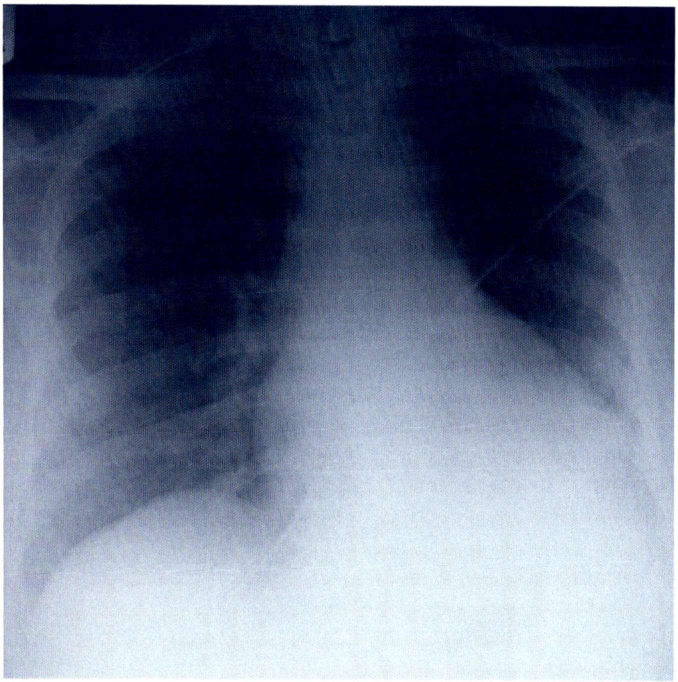

Figure 12.1 Chest radiograph.

Background

Partially masticated food is the most commonly aspirated solid particulate matter (the 'café coronary' syndrome) but coins, teeth or confectionary may also be inhaled. Upper airways may also be obstructed by vomit, sputum plugs, blood clots, laryngospasm or airway stenosis.[1,2] Inflammatory oedema due to inhaled toxic gases, burns, trauma, anaphy-

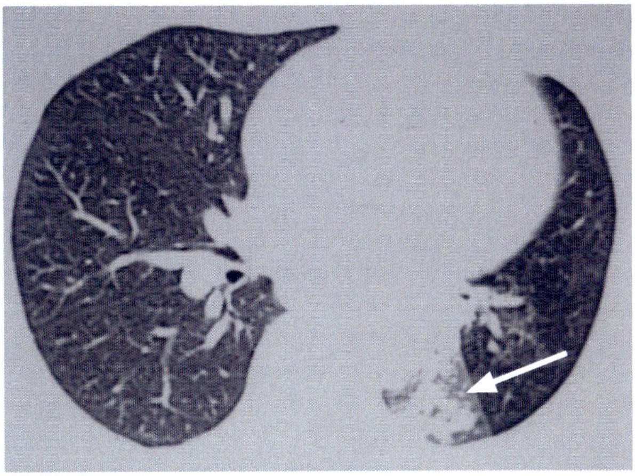

Figure 12.2 Chest CT scan. Collapse of the posterior segment of the left lower lobe is indicated by the arrow.

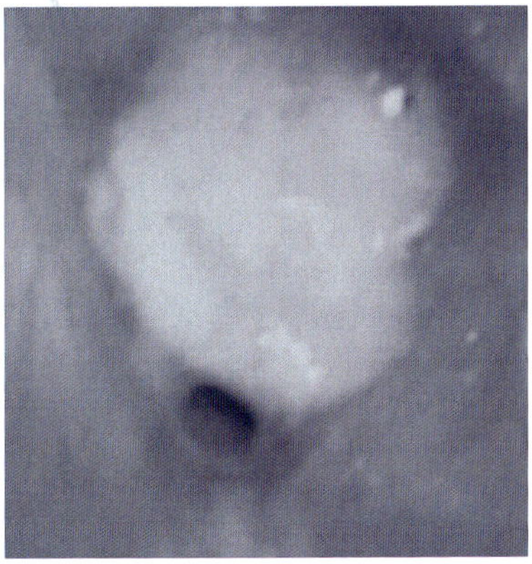

Figure 12.3 Bronchoscopic appearance of the left lower lobe bronchus *(see also inside front cover).*

laxis or laryngeal angio-oedema also occludes airways. Occasionally childhood infections including epiglottitis or diphtheria can cause acute laryngeal obstruction. Pharyngeal occlusion by the tongue should be excluded and is usually due to loss of pharyngeal muscle tone caused by drugs, alcohol, unconsciousness or neurological events.[3,4]

Management of acute upper airways obstruction

Upper airways obstruction is either:

- **Complete upper airways obstruction** with inability to speak, rapid-onset cyanosis and respiratory distress with paradoxical abdominal and chest-wall movement (classically described as see-saw breathing). If not rapidly corrected it causes collapse, coma, cardiovascular instability and finally cardiac arrest.[3,4]
- **Partial upper airways obstruction** causes noisy breathing with stridor, snoring, wheeze and cough.

If the episode of 'choking' is witnessed, consider sharp blows to the back of the chest to dislodge the obstructing particle. If this fails, attempt abdominal thrusts (i.e. the Heimlich manoeuvre). Stand behind the patient with your arms around the patient's costal margin and the hands clenched below the xiphoid process. Pull the hands backwards sharply, compressing the upper abdomen. The resulting increase in thoracic pressure may dislodge the obstructing particle, which is then exhaled by the patient.[3,4]

If these manoeuvres fail and the patient loses consciousness, call for help and then:

- **Inspect the oral cavity** for obstructions and remove with a finger sweep. Suction out secretions. Leave well-fitting dentures in place.
- **Open the airway** with backwards head tilt, chin lift and jaw thrust. In trauma only use jaw thrust to avoid further injury to the cervical spine.
- **Maintain oxygenation** with supplemental oxygen (10–15 l/min) if available. If there is no spontaneous respiratory effort, attempt mask ventilation with a self-inflating bag. If this fails, consider a laryngeal mask or endotracheal intubation. Insert an oropharyngeal (or nasopharyngeal) airway if the patient is breathing.
- **Consider emergency cricothyroidotomy** if the patient is not breathing and cannot be ventilated. It is only successful if the obstruction is at the level of the larynx. A large-bore needle, knife or hollow tube (e.g. ballpoint pen) is inserted through the cricothyroid membrane palpable just below the thyroid cartilage.
- **Urgent bronchoscopy or thoracic surgery** may be required to remove obstructing lesions. A history of recurrent cough or pneumonia with radiological changes following an episode of aspiration suggests the need for exploration to recover an obstructing foreign body (e.g. peanut, chicken bone).
- **Heliox**, a mixture of helium and oxygen, is a temporary measure to improve ventilation past an airways obstruction, as helium has a lower density than nitrogen.
- **Nebulized epinephrine/adrenaline** temporarily reduces airways obstruction due to laryngeal or airways oedema (e.g angio-oedema) whilst awaiting the effects of definitive treatment.

Irritation of the upper airways by blood, pharyngeal secretions, toxic inhaled gases, burns, aspirated food or vomit, and extubation can cause laryngeal spasm, oedema, stridor and respiratory distress. Immediate intubation may be required but in less critical situations, nebulized adrenaline (2–3 ml 1:1000 adrenaline), salbutamol and intravenous steroids may alleviate laryngeal oedema and airways spasm.

In some patients, life-threatening anaphylactic reactions with angio-oedema can occur within minutes of exposure to a specific antigen. Immediately treat cardiorespiratory emergencies with intravenous epinephrine (0.5–1.0 mg), hydrocortisone (200 mg) and chlorpheniramine (10 mg). Start fluid resuscitation in hypotensive shock and treat bronchospasm with nebulized salbutamol (± intravenous aminophylline). Consider early endotracheal intubation in cases with severe upper airways obstruction.

Conclusion

In this case, the history, clinical findings and further history from the patient's friends determined that the patient was rather inebriated on the 'girls' night out' that preceded the onset of her symptoms.

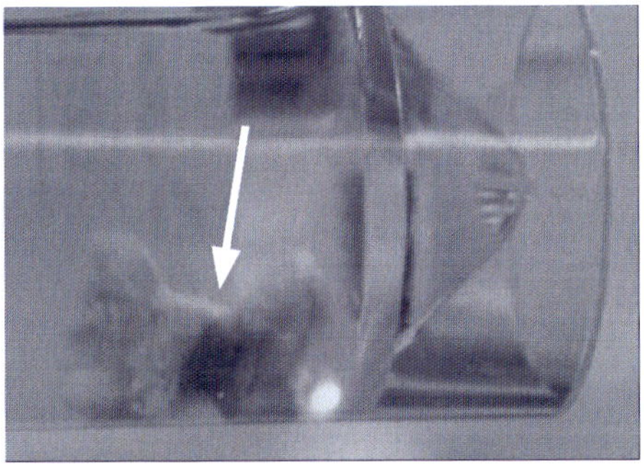

Figure 12.4 Chicken bone (arrow) retrieved from the left lower lobe bronchus *(see also inside front cover).*

On their way home they had been to a fast food chicken diner and whilst there the patient had an episode of paroxysmal coughing after aspirating her food. The patient did not remember the episode! The inhaled chicken bone that was completely obstructing the posterior segment of the left lower lobe was dislodged at bronchoscopy and lifted out using a wire bronchial retrieval cage (Figure 12.4).

Further Reading

1 Lomotan JR, George SS, Brandstetter RD. Aspiration pneumonia. Strategies for early recognition and prevention. *Postgrad Med* 1997; **102**: 229–31.

2 Reza Shariatzadeh M, Huang JQ, Marrie TJ. Differences in the features of aspiration pneumonia according to site of acquisition: community or continuing care facility. *J Am Geriatr Soc* 2006; **54**: 296–302.

3 Resuscitation Council (UK). 2010 Resuscitation Guidelines. www.resus.org.uk/pages/GL2010.pdf (accessed 01 07 11).

4 American Heart Association. American Heart Association Guidelines for Cardiopulmonary Resuscitation and Emergency Cardiovascular Care. *Circulation* 2010; **122**(18 Suppl 3): S640–861.

Interstitial Lung Disease/Sarcoid

PROBLEM

13 Classification of the Idiopathic Interstitial Pneumonias

Richard Leach, John Rees

Case History

A 35-year-old man presented with a three-year history of slowly progressive cough and exercise-induced dyspnoea. He was breathless on mild inclines and could only climb one flight of stairs. Apart from a recent chest infection, he had no previous medical or family history of note. In particular there had been no childhood respiratory disease and no evidence of tuberculosis, vasculitis or connective tissue disease (CTD). He was on no medication. He smoked 20–30 cigarettes per day (approximately 15 pack years). There was no previous drug, industrial dust or allergen exposure including pets or bird contact. On examination he appeared well and oxygen saturation (SaO_2) was 94%. He had marked finger clubbing. Chest examination revealed poor air entry to both bases with soft inspiratory ('Velcro') crepitations in both lungs.

Initial blood tests including serum angiotensin converting enzyme, anti-nuclear antibody, rheumatoid factor and autoantibody screens were normal. Lung function revealed a forced expiratory volume in 1 second (FEV_1) of 1.49 l (40% predicted), a forced vital capacity (FVC) of 1.74 l (39% predicted) and a peak expiratory flow rate (PEFR) of 6.6 l/sec (74% predicted). Total lung capacity was 3.07 l (48% predicted), residual volume 0.95 l (54% predicted), carbon monoxide gas transfer (TLCO) 31% predicted and transfer coefficient (KCO) 99% predicted (i.e. corrected for alveolar volume).

Chest radiography detected bi-basal and left upper lobe reticular shadowing, and high-resolution computed tomography (HRCT) scan (Figure 13.1) demonstrated bilateral, patchy, peripheral ground glass opacification (GGO) affecting mainly the left upper lobe and both bases with minimal fibrotic change (minor cystic change and septal thickening) and no adenopathy. At bronchoscopy the bronchial tree was normal; bronchoalveolar lavage (BAL) detected increased numbers of pigment-laden macrophages, neutrophils and eosinophils. Lower lobe transbronchial biopsies did not detect granulomas but insufficient tissue was obtained for precise histological classification.

What is the most likely diagnosis?

How are the idiopathic interstitial pneumonias (IIPs) classified?

Does this patient require further histological confirmation of the diagnosis?

How would you manage this case?

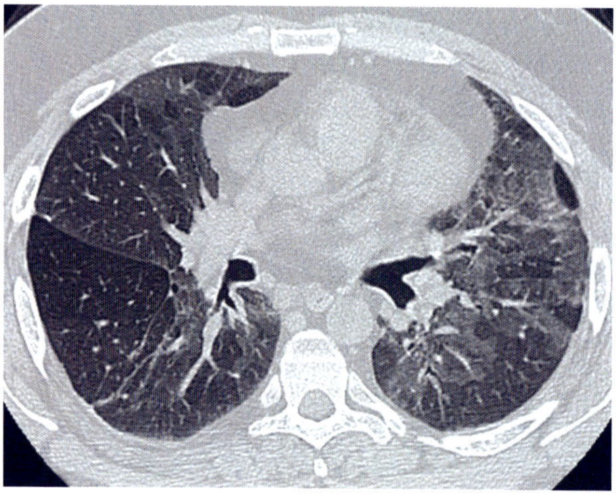

Figure 13.1 HRCT scan.

Background

The term diffuse parenchymal (interstitial) lung disease (DPLD/ILD) describes a group of disorders characterized by inflammation and/or fibrosis primarily involving the pulmonary interstitium (i.e. the tissue between the alveolar epithelium and the capil-

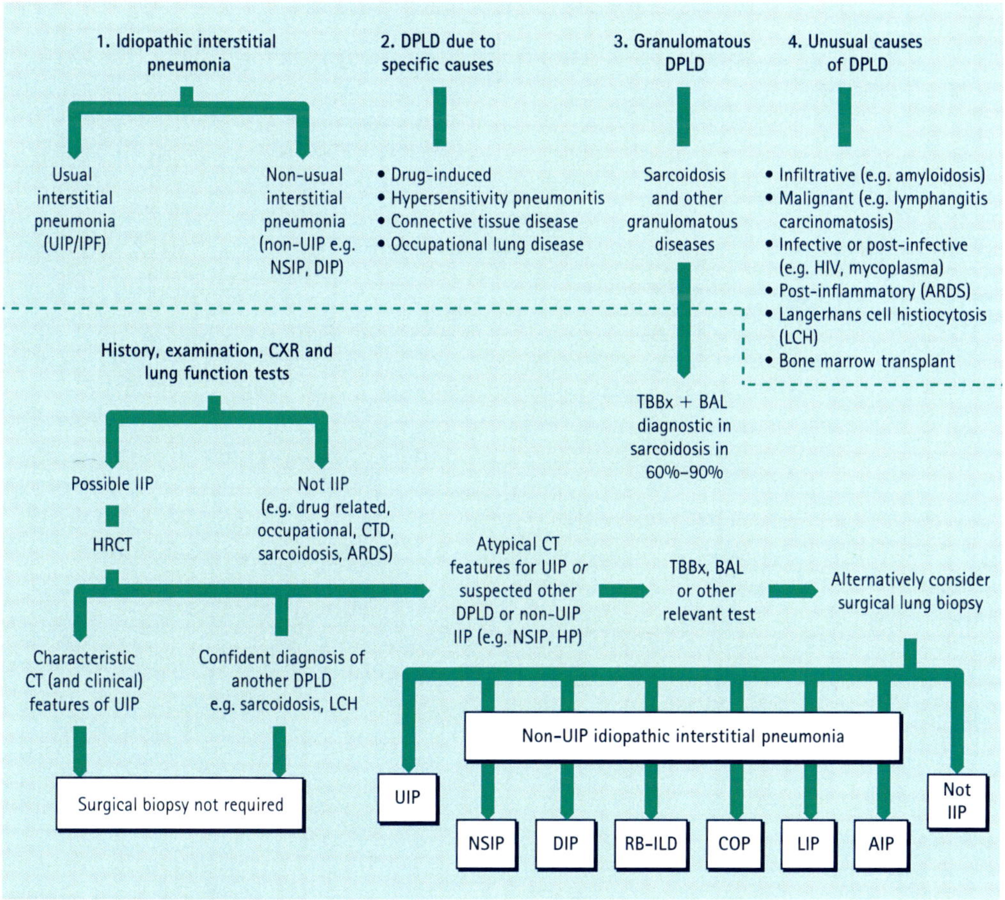

Figure 13.2 Classification (above dotted line) and suggested diagnostic process (below dotted line) in DPLD. AIP, acute interstitial pneumonia; ARDS, acute respiratory distress syndrome; BAL, bronchoalveolar lavage; COP, cryptogenic organizing pneumonia; CT, computed tomography; CTD, connective tissue disease; CXR, chest radiograph; DIP, desquamative interstitial pneumonia; DPLD, diffuse parenchymal lung disease; HP, hypersensitivity pneumonitis; IIP, idiopathic interstitial pneumonia; IPF, idiopathic pulmonary fibrosis; HIV, human immunodeficiency virus; LIP, lymphocytic interstitial pneumonia; NSIP, non-specific interstitial pneumonia; RB-ILD, respiratory bronchiolitis-associated interstitial lung disease; TBBx, transbronchial biopsy; UIP, usual interstitial pneumonia.

lary endothelium) and/or the bronchovascular and septal tissues comprising the lung's fibrous framework.[1–4] The alveolar air spaces, distal airways and vasculature are also frequently involved.

Figure 13.2 illustrates a diagnostic approach to DPLD/ILD. The main objective is to identify the most likely diagnosis in the fewest steps. DPLD due to drugs, CTD, occupational exposure and hypersensitivity pneumonitis can be identified from a comprehensive history including recreational and work experience, thorough examination for features suggestive of a CTD, appropriate blood tests (e.g. anti-nuclear antibodies, rheumatoid factor), serology (e.g. avian precipitins), lung function testing and radiological imaging. Similarly the clinical, radiological and histological features of sarcoidosis are diagnostic.

Classification of the idiopathic interstitial pneumonias

Differences in clinical course, histopathological pattern and prognostic outcome suggest that individual IIPs are separate clinicopathological entities. Diagnosis of IIP is initially one of exclusion having failed to detect an alternative cause. However, subsequent classification is difficult on clinical grounds alone. Guideline consensus panels emphasize an integrated clinical, radiological and pathological approach to final diagnosis and classification.[1–3] There are two principal subgroups of IIP distinguished by the presence or absence of the features of usual interstitial pneumonia (UIP):

- Idiopathic pulmonary fibrosis (IPF) accounts for about 70% of IIPs. It is a chronic, progressive, fibrosing interstitial pneumonia of unknown cause associated with the histopathologic and/or radiologic pattern of UIP (see below).[1–6] IPF/UIP is not steroid sensitive and has a relatively poor prognosis.
- IIP not associated with the radiological/histological features of UIP (non-UIP diseases) accounts for approximately 30% of IIP (e.g. non-specific interstitial pneumonia [NSIP], desquamative interstitial pneumonia [DIP], acute interstitial pneumonia [AIP]). About half of these IIPs are steroid sensitive with a good prognosis (median survival >10 years), although a few like AIP have a worse prognosis than IPF/UIP (see below).

Consequently, distinguishing IPF/UIP from the other IIP subgroups has important therapeutic and prognostic implications. The pathogenesis of IIP is usually thought to involve widespread interstitial inflammation, progressive parenchymal fibrosis and a gradual decline in pulmonary function.[7,8] This 'inflammatory' model is probably correct in most 'non-UIP' steroid-sensitive IIP (e.g. NSIP, DIP) but not for patients with UIP. Recent research suggests that UIP is associated with minimal inflammation and is due to abnormal, parenchymal wound healing, characterized by chronic fibroproliferation, following alveolar epithelial damage.[7,8]

The clinical nomenclature, associated histological pattern and radiographic features associated with individual IIPs are presented in Table 13.1.

1. Idiopathic pulmonary fibrosis is synonymous with usual interstitial pneumonia (IPF/UIP). The clinical course is variable and unpredictable with progressive deterioration over several years, often with periods of stability but also with episodes of acute decline ('acute exacerbations'). Median survival times are 2–3 years with a five-year survival of 30%–50%.[3] A minority of patients with mild to moderate IPF/UIP may remain stable for relatively long periods, whereas others experience accelerated phases, with rapid decline and subsequent death.[3] Patients are usually >50 years old, often male, with a gradual onset of symptoms (>6 months), clubbing (in approximately 25%–50%) and Velcro-type fine, end-inspiratory, basal crepitations. Characteristic radiological features of UIP include a bilateral, predominantly basal and subpleural pattern of septal reticulation with 'tractional' airway changes and subpleural honeycombing. Ground glass opacities are common but less extensive than the reticulation. BAL fluid contains increased neutrophils and eosinophils. Lymphocytosis is not a feature and lymphocytes comprising >15% of the white cell count suggests another diagnosis (e.g. NSIP, cryptogenic organizing pneumonia [COP], sarcoidosis). Likewise if eosinophils are >20% of the white cell count, consider eosinophilic lung diseases. The key histological features in UIP are architectural destruction, fibrosis with honeycombing, scattered fibroblastic foci, patchy dis-

Table 13.1 Clinical nomenclature, histologic pattern and radiographic features of idiopathic interstitial pneumonias

Clinical nomenclatures	Histologic pattern	Typical CT findings	CT distribution
UIP/IPF	UIP	Reticular abnormality + volume loss, honeycombing, traction bronchiectasis, focal ground glass	Peripheral, basal + subpleural
NSIP	NSIP	Ground glass attenuation, consolidation, reticular opacities	Peripheral, subpleural, basal, symmetrical
DIP	DIP	Ground glass attenuation, reticular lines	Lower zone, mainly peripheral
RB-ILD	RB	Bronchial wall thickening, patchy ground glass opacity, centrilobular nodules	Diffuse
AIP	DAD	Consolidation, ground glass opacity (often lobular sparing), late traction bronchiectasis	Diffuse
COP	OP	Patchy consolidation and/or nodules	Subpleural, peribronchial
LIP	LIP	Centrilobular nodules, ground glass attenuation, bronchovascular + septal thickening	Diffuse

AIP, acute interstitial pneumonia; COP, cryptogenic organizing pneumonia; DAD, diffuse alveolar damage; DIP, desquamative interstitial pneumonia; IPF, idiopathic pulmonary fibrosis; LIP, lymphocytic interstitial pneumonia; NSIP, non-specific interstitial pneumonia; OP, organizing pneumonia; RB, respiratory bronchiolitis; RB-ILD, respiratory bronchiolitis-associated interstitial lung disease; UIP, usual interstitial pneumonia.

tribution and involvement of the peripheral lung. At low magnification the appearance is heterogeneous with alternating areas of normal lung, interstitial fibroblastic change, fibrosis and honeycomb change. These histological changes can be similar to those seen in CTD, drug-induced diseases, hypersensitivity pneumonitis and asbestosis. During acute exacerbations, areas of diffuse alveolar damage (DAD) and organizing pneumonia may be detected.

2. Non-specific interstitial pneumonia recognizes that some patients with IIP do not fit into a well-defined histological pattern. It identifies a group of IIPs with a more favourable prognosis that need to be distinguished from UIP but that also differ from DIP, COP and AIP. NSIP represents a heterogeneous group of disorders and subsets of patients with different clinical courses. It may precede the onset of collagen vascular disorders by months to years, or be associated with occupational exposure and hypersensitivity pneumonitis. Before 1994, NSIP was classified as 'cellular UIP' or 'mixed cellular and fibrotic UIP'. NSIP is characterized by varying degrees of inflammation and fibrosis with some forms being predominantly cellular (cellular NSIP) and others primarily fibrotic (fibrotic NSIP). Most investigators believe that cellular NSIP is the early form of fibrotic NSIP. Fibrosis can be extensive but it is usually uniform (i.e. rather than 'patchy' as in UIP). Fibroblastic foci and honeycombing are rare but nevertheless NSIP can be difficult to distinguish from UIP and both patterns may coexist in the same patient. NSIP presents a problem for clinicians because there is no distinctive clinical phenotype for patients with this histological pattern. Age of onset is earlier than for UIP, at about 40–50 years old, with no sexual predominance or association with smoking. Onset is usually gradual with symptoms for 6–30 months before diagnosis, although it can be subacute. Clinical features are otherwise similar to UIP. BAL fluid lymphocytosis occurs in approximately

50% of cases. On HRCT scans bilateral, symmetrical GGO occurs mainly in subpleural parenchyma. Prognosis is better than for UIP, especially in those with a predominantly cellular pathology. Complete recovery can occur with steroid therapy but most patients improve or stabilize.

3. Respiratory bronchiolitis-associated interstitial lung disease (RB-ILD). Respiratory bronchiolitis occurs mainly in smokers. The histopathology is characterized by pigmented intraluminal macrophages in first- and second-order bronchioles. Although often asymptomatic, it can present with pulmonary symptoms, abnormal lung function and imaging abnormalities and is then described as RB-ILD. The invariable relationship with smoking means that it is often associated with emphysema. Most patients are male (male:female ratio 2:1), current smokers (>30 pack years) who present in the fourth and fifth decades with mild to moderate dyspnoea, cough and occasional hypoxaemia. Heavy smokers may present earlier. The HRCT findings include centrilobular nodules, patchy ground glass attenuation and thickening of the walls of central or peripheral bronchi. Many patients improve after cessation of smoking but steroid therapy may be required.

4. Desquamative interstitial pneumonia was initially thought to be a precursor stage of UIP with desquamation of epithelial cells. However, it is now recognized as severe RB-ILD with characteristic accumulation of pigment-laden alveolar macrophages which diffusely fill alveolar spaces. It is almost invariably associated with cigarette smoking although rare cases due to environmental exposures or passive smoke inhalation are described. It affects mainly men in their forties and fifties. Onset is insidious with dyspnoea and cough progressing to respiratory failure over weeks or months. Clubbing occurs in 50% of cases. Lung physiology usually shows normal or mildly restrictive lung volumes with a moderately decreased diffusing capacity (DLCO). BAL fluid contains many macrophages with intracellular granules of yellow, golden or brown smoker's pigment. Neutrophils, eosinophils and lymphocytes may also be increased. HRCT scans invariably show GGO with a lower zone predilection (>70%) and peripheral distribution (>50%). Mild, uniform reticular fibrosis occurs in many cases but honeycombing affects <30% and is limited in extent. Prognosis is good following smoking cessation and/or corticosteroid therapy, with resolution of GGO and a 70% ten-year survival rate. Progression to fibrosis occurs in <20% of cases.

5. Cryptogenic organizing pneumonia is now preferred to the previous term bronchiolitis obliterans organizing pneumonia. It describes the histopathological pattern of organizing pneumonia within the alveolar ducts and alveoli with or without organization within the bronchioles ('polypoid bronchiolitis obliterans'). 'Organizing pneumonia' is often idiopathic but it also occurs with many infective (e.g. viral) and non-infectious conditions (e.g. rheumatoid arthritis, drugs). At onset, patients are usually about 55 years old. Non-smokers outnumber smokers by 2:1. Typically, presentation is a short history of cough, dyspnoea, intermittent fever, weight loss and myalgia, following several courses of antibiotic therapy for suspected lower respiratory tract infections. Localized crepitations and hypoxaemia are common but clubbing is absent. Inflammatory markers (e.g. C-reactive protein, erythrocyte sedimentation rate) are usually raised and lung function tests confirm a mild to moderate restrictive pattern with reduced gas transfer. Radiological imaging shows bilateral, patchy consolidation (90%), nodular opacities along the bronchovascular bundles (15%–50%) and GGO (~60%) mainly in the subpleural lower zones. Most patients recover completely with oral steroids but some require prolonged (>6 months) therapy.

6. Acute interstitial pneumonia, previously known as Hamman–Rich syndrome, is a rapidly progressive, histologically distinct form of IIP. The histopathological picture is described as an organizing form of DAD indistinguishable from acute respiratory distress syndrome. It affects all age groups (mean 50 years old) with no sex predominance or smoking association. Patients often present shortly (<3 weeks) after a suspected viral upper respiratory tract infection, with severe dyspnoea, widespread consolidation and diffuse crepitations. Radiological imaging reveals bilateral opacities, GGO and architectural distortion. There is no effective therapy and mortality is high (>50%). Most deaths occur within 4–8 weeks of onset. Recurrence or progressive pulmonary fibrosis may occur in survivors.

7. Lymphocytic interstitial pneumonia (LIP) is associated with diffuse lymphocytic and plasma cell alveolar infiltration. Previously LIP was considered pre-neoplastic and a precursor of pulmonary lymphoma. However, only a few cases undergo malignant transformation and many cases previously labelled as 'LIP' were probably non-Hodgkin's low-grade B-cell (mucosal-associated lymphoid tissue [MALT]) lymphomas. Differentiation is now possible with immunohistochemical stains. Idiopathic LIP is rare and many previous cases are now classified as NSIP. LIP is often associated with an underlying systemic condition (e.g. systemic lupus erythematosus, rheumatoid arthritis, autoimmune thyroid disease, primary biliary cirrhosis, acquired immune deficiency syndrome, myasthenia gravis, etc.) which must be excluded. BAL reveals many lymphocytes without clonality. Most patients respond to steroid therapy but about a third progress to diffuse fibrosis.

Indications for histological confirmation in idiopathic interstitial pneumonitis

In the absence of contraindications, surgical biopsy is advised in suspected IIP when the clinical course and radiological HRCT scan features are not typical of UIP. HRCT scanning is an integral part of IIP evaluation. Its primary role is to separate patients with the characteristic radiological features of UIP from those with radiological features of other IIPs (e.g. NSIP, DIP). The presence of characteristic UIP features is sufficient to allow a confident diagnosis of IPF and to eliminate the need for surgical biopsy. HRCT scan diagnosis is based on finding a bilateral, mainly basal and subpleural reticular pattern associated with honeycombing and/or traction bronchiectasis.[9] Consolidation, GGO and nodules are absent.

The development of video-assisted thoracoscopic lung biopsy has made it more acceptable to recommend surgical biopsy in DPLD. Yield is high (92%) and morbidity (2.5%) and mortality (0.3%) low. Biopsies should be taken from at least three sites, including the transition from normal to abnormal lung tissue, guided by HRCT findings. The surgeon should try to avoid deflation of the specimen as this complicates the histological appearance.

Conclusion

In this case, the progressive dyspnoea, cough, finger clubbing, inspiratory crepitations, restrictive lung function with reduced gas transfer and radiographic features were all consistent with a diagnosis of DPLD. The medical history and screening tests excluded DPLD due to drug therapy, occupational exposure or CTD. Sarcoidosis was unlikely in view of the absence of granulomas on transbronchial biopsies or lymphadenopathy on computed tomography scan. Consequently the most likely diagnosis was IIP. The patient's age, clinical picture and HRCT scan (i.e. ground glass shadowing with minimal reticular shadowing) indicated the need for a surgical biopsy. A histological diagnosis of DIP was subsequently established.

In DIP, approximately 70% of cases improve with smoking cessation and/or steroid therapy. This patient stopped smoking but failed to improve. Subsequent treatment with high-dose steroid (prednisolone 40–60 mg daily) for six months did not alter lung physiology nor HRCT scan appearances. Significant steroid side effects occurred including hyperglycaemia. He was subsequently treated with a steroid sparing regime using prednisolone 10 mg daily, azathioprine 150 mg daily and the antioxidant and mucolytic carbocisteine 650 mg three times daily. His respiratory function and HRCT scan findings are unchanged three years after diagnosis. These findings suggest that he is one of the 20% of DIP cases that fail to improve and eventually progress to pulmonary fibrosis.

Further Reading

1 Joint statement of the American Thoracic Society (ATS) and the European Respiratory Society (ERS). Idiopathic pulmonary fibrosis: diagnosis and treatment. International Consensus Statement 1999. *Am J Respir Crit Care Med* 2000; **161**: 646–64.

2 Wells AU, Hirani N. Interstitial lung disease guideline. British Thoracic Society in collaboration with Thoracic Society of Australia and New Zealand and the Irish Thoracic Society. *Thorax* 2008; **63**(Suppl 5): v1–v58.

3 An official ATS/ERS/JRS/ALAT Statement. Idiopathic pulmonary fibrosis: evidence-based guidelines for diagnosis and management. *Am J Respir Crit Care Med* 2011; **183**: 788–824.

4 King TE. Clinical advances in the diagnosis and therapy of the interstitial lung diseases. *Am J Respir Crit Care Med* 2005; **172**: 268–79.

5 MacDonald S, Rubens M, Hansell DM *et al.* Nonspecific interstitial pneumonia and usual interstitial pneumonia: comparative appearances and diagnostic accuracy of thin-section CT. *Radiology* 2001; **221**: 600–5.

6 Swiggris JJ, Kuschner WG, Kelsey JL, Gould MK. Idiopathic pulmonary fibrosis: challenges and opportunities for the clinician and investigator. *Chest* 2005; **127**: 275–83.

7 Selman M, King TE Jr. Pardo A. Idiopathic pulmonary fibrosis: prevailing and evolving hypotheses about its pathogenesis and implications for therapy. *Ann Intern Med* 2001; **134**: 136–51.

8 Adamson I, Young L, Bowden D. Relationship of alveolar epithelial injury and repair to the induction of pulmonary fibrosis. *Am J Pathol* 1988; **130**: 377–83.

9 Wells AU, Desai SR, Rubens MB *et al.* Idiopathic pulmonary fibrosis: a composite physiologic index derived from disease extent observed by computed tomography. *Am J Respir Crit Care Med* 2003; **167**: 962–9.

PROBLEM

14 Treatment of Idiopathic Pulmonary Fibrosis/Usual Interstitial Pneumonias

Lucy Schomberg, Richard Leach

Case History

Following a twelve-month history of dry cough and increasing exercise-induced dyspnoea, a 65-year-old man presented with deterioration in his symptoms after an upper respiratory tract infection. Despite three recent courses of antibiotics, regular inhaled bronchodilators and a course of oral steroid therapy he remained breathless on minimal exercise (<50 metres on the flat). There was no past medical or family history of note. He was on no other regular medication. A review of systems was unremarkable and there were no features of vasculitis or connective tissue disease. He smoked ten cigarettes a day (approximately 20 pack years) and had no previous occupational exposure or drug, avian or allergen contact.

On examination he was comfortable at rest. There was no cyanosis (oxygen saturation [SaO_2] 92%) or lymphadenopathy. He had early finger clubbing. Chest examination revealed bilateral, soft inspiratory crepitations at both lung bases. Blood tests including serum angiotensin converting enzyme, anti-nuclear antibody, rheumatoid factor and autoantibody screens were normal. Lung function tests revealed a forced expiratory volume in 1 second (FEV_1) 1.72 l (55% predicted), forced vital capacity (FVC) 1.95 l (58% predicted), total lung capacity 3.78 l (59% predicted)) and reduced gas transfer (KCO 60% predicted). Chest radiography demonstrated bi-basal reticular shadowing with volume loss. Bronchoscopy was normal and bronchoalveolar lavage (BAL) detected mainly neutrophils and occasional eosinophils. Transbronchial biopsies excluded granulomatous change but were otherwise unhelpful for histological classification. High-resolution computed tomography (HRCT) scan showed early bilateral, patchy, peripheral interstitial shadowing with some traction bronchiectasis and volume loss (Figure 14.1). These changes were more marked at the lung bases. Honeycomb changes were present in the subpleural areas (arrows in Figure 14.1). There was no lymphadenopathy, consolidation or ground glass shadowing.

What is the likely diagnosis and is histological confirmation required?

What are the histological features and would BAL be helpful?

Is this an inflammatory condition?

What treatment would you recommend?

What is the prognosis for this patient?

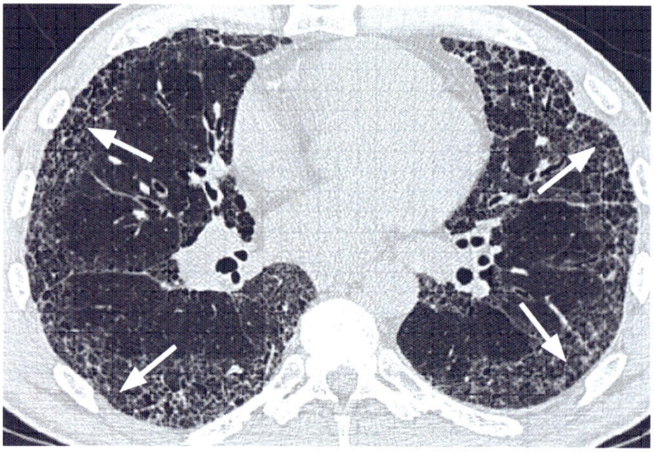

Figure 14.1 Chest HRCT scan. Honeycomb changes in the subpleural areas are indicated by the arrows.

Background

Idiopathic pulmonary fibrosis (IPF) is the commonest idiopathic interstitial pneumonia (IIP). It is a chronic, progressive, fibrosing interstitial pneumonia of unknown cause, occurring primarily in older adults, limited to the lungs, and associated with the histopathologic and/or radiologic pattern of usual interstitial pneumonia (UIP; see below).[1–3] The definition of IPF requires the exclusion of other forms of interstitial lung disease (ILD; Chapter 13) including other idiopathic interstitial pneumonias and those associated with environmental exposure, medication or systemic disease.[1–3] IPF has an estimated incidence of approximately 4.6–16.3 per 10^5 population.[3] Patients are usually >50 (median 70) years old, male, with dyspnoea of longer than six months, digital clubbing (in approximately 25%–40%) and fine 'Velcro-like' inspiratory crepitations. Smoking, some environmental exposures (e.g. metal dust, farming, masonry) and gastro-oesophageal reflux disease (GORD) are associated with a worse outcome. Familial forms of IPF are rare (<5%), and are mainly autosomal dominant with variable penetrance.

The HRCT scan is an integral part of the evaluation of patients with ILD. Its principal role is to distinguish IPF from other IIP (e.g. non-specific interstitial pneumonia [NSIP], desquamative interstitial pneumonia [DIP]) by establishing the presence of UIP. Characteristic radiological features of UIP include a bilateral, predominantly basal and subpleural pattern of septal reticulation with 'tractional' airway changes and honeycombing. Ground glass opacification (GGO) is common but less extensive than the reticulation. Specific criteria for HRCT diagnosis of UIP have been reported (Table 14.1). Consolidation, other pleural abnormalities (e.g. plaques), non-honeycomb cysts, extensive GGO or nodules suggest an alternative diagnosis.

When based on these criteria, the accuracy of UIP diagnosis on HRCT scan has a reported sensitivity of 43%–78% and specificity of ≥90%. When expert radiologists interpret HRCT scans, sensitivity is 77%, specificity 72% and positive predictive value (PPV) 85% for biopsy-proven UIP. However, when the same radiologists were confident in the diagnosis of UIP, which occurred in 50% of cases, the sensitivity was 87%, specificity

95% and PPV 96%.[4] On this basis, the presence of classical HRCT features of UIP, in the right clinical context, is considered diagnostic of IPF and obviates the need for surgical biopsy in >50% of cases. When the HRCT criteria for UIP are not fulfilled, surgical lung biopsy may be required (Figure 14.2).[3]

Table 14.1 High-resolution computed tomography criteria for UIP pattern

UIP pattern (all 4 features)	Possible UIP pattern (all 3 features)	Inconsistent with UIP (any)
• Subpleural, basal predominance • Reticular abnormality • Honeycombing with or without traction bronchiectasis • Absence of features listed as inconsistent with UIP pattern	• Subpleural, basal predominance • Reticular abnormality • Absence of features listed as inconsistent with UIP pattern	• Upper or mid-lung predominance • Peribronchovascular predominance • Extensive ground glass abnormality (i.e. > reticular abnormality) • Profuse micronodules (bilateral, predominantly upper lobes) • Discrete cysts (multiple, bilateral, away from areas of honeycombing) • Diffuse mosaic attenuation/air trapping (bilateral in 3 or more lobes) • Consolidation in bronchopulmonary segments/lobe

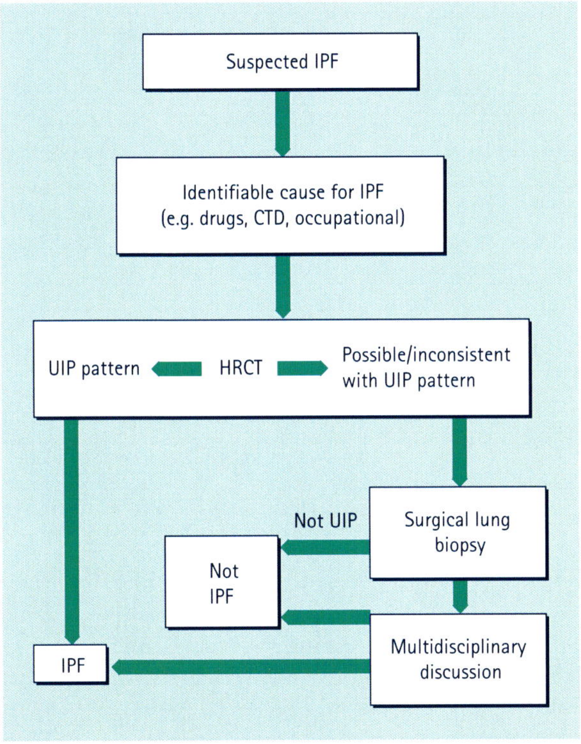

Figure 14.2 Diagnostic algorithm for idiopathic pulmonary fibrosis. CTD, connective tissue disease.

Histological features of IPF/UIP

Histological features in UIP include prominent fibroblastic foci and a distribution of fibrosis that is spatially heterogeneous (i.e. adjacent fibrotic and normal lung) but also temporally variable (i.e. areas of fibrosis of varying ages). Micro- and macrocystic honeycombing are expected. In suspected IPF the most important application of BAL is exclusion of other diagnoses. It is not necessary in the majority of cases. In IPF, BAL usually reveals an excess of neutrophils and eosinophils. Lymphocytosis is uncommon and a lymphocytosis of >40% should prompt exclusion of chronic hypersensitivity pneumonitis. Eosinophilia of >20% should prompt consideration of an eosinophilic lung disease.[3]

Pathophysiological mechanism of fibrosis in UIP

For many years the prevailing pathological theory was that IPF/UIP represented a generalized inflammatory condition leading to widespread parenchymal fibrosis and progressive decline in pulmonary function. In the corticosteroid-sensitive idiopathic interstitial pneumonias including DIP and NSIP (Chapter 13) this model appears to hold true.

However, recent pathologic and clinical data suggest that inflammation does not play a prominent role in the pathogenesis of UIP[1,3,5] and suggest that it is a distinct pathophysiological entity, best termed 'epithelial-fibroblastic disease', which is characterized by minimal inflammation and chronic fibroproliferation due to abnormal wound healing.

As previous pharmacological treatment strategies have aimed to eliminate or suppress inflammation, the poor responses to previous therapy may simply reflect the underlying fibrotic rather than inflammatory pathophysiology of UIP.

Treatment of IPF/UIP

The evidence supporting the use of any pharmacological, anti-inflammatory or immunosuppressive therapy in IPF/UIP is poor.[1–3] No individual regime has been proven to alter the course of or improve survival in IPF/UIP although clinical trials of some agents have suggested a possible benefit. To date most studies have been confounded by the heterogeneity of patient groups (e.g. combined UIP/NSIP) and varying study designs.

Treatment failure is most likely in older men (>50 years), with an extensive smoking history, severe dyspnoea, poor lung function, reduced gas transfer and honeycomb changes on HRCT scan. Current therapy does not reverse established fibrosis and as potential benefit diminishes in later disease, the associated and frequent therapeutic side effects become less acceptable. The physician should be prepared to discuss potential treatment options with the patient and help them make a decision consistent with their own values.

The 2008 British Thoracic Society guidelines recommend initial treatment of IPF/UIP with:

- **Combination 'triple therapy'** using low-dose prednisolone (initially 0.5 mg/kg/daily tapering to 10 mg daily over three months), azathioprine (50 mg daily increasing by 25–50 mg at 1–2-weekly intervals to 2 mg/kg or a maximum dose of 150 mg) and N-acetylcysteine (NAC; 600 mg three times daily), especially in patients with a potentially favourable outcome (i.e. young patients [<50 years old] with no contraindications to therapy, early disease with mild lung impairment and increased GGO and less fibrosis on HRCT scan). In a small trial (27 patients), low-dose prednisolone and azathioprine were compared with prednisolone alone. Lung function was reported to have stabilized in the azathioprine group after one year and there was a non-statistically significant reduction in mortality (43% vs 77%) after nine years.[1,6,7] Although usually well tolerated, azathioprine use must be monitored for hepatotoxicity, renal dysfunction and bone marrow suppression with regular blood tests at two-weekly then six-weekly intervals.

The 2011 ATS/ERS/JRS/ALAT guidelines[3] for diagnosis and management of IPF are less supportive of the use of 'triple therapy' as described above and recommend that the majority of patients with IPF should not be treated but that it may be a reasonable choice in a minority of patients. A similar recommendation is given for:

- **N-acetylcysteine monotherapy**. NAC is a precursor of the antioxidant glutathione and may restore depleted lung glutathione. In a one-year study, addition of NAC to regular therapy with prednisolone and azathioprine reduced decline in vital capacity and gas transfer but did not affect mortality compared with placebo (9% vs 11%)[7] Small trials of oral or nebulized monotherapy also suggest reduced lung function decline.[3]
- **Pirfenidone**. This is a pyridone molecule that inhibits transforming growth factor β-stimulated collagen synthesis and blocks fibroblast proliferation. A small trial in 54 patients with UIP who had failed other therapeutic measures suggested some stabilization of lung function over two years[3,7] A subsequent randomized controlled trial (RCT) in 109 Japanese patients demonstrated some improvement in lung function and was controversially aborted in favour of pirfenidone because there were fewer (0% vs 14%) acute exacerbations.[8] Reduction in lung function decline has been reported in a further RCT.[3]
- **Anticoagulation**. A small survival benefit was reported in the anticoagulation arm of a Japanese unblinded RCT comparing corticosteroid and anticoagulant therapy with corticosteroid therapy alone. However, the evidence is very limited.

The 2011 ATS/ERS/JRS/ALAT guidelines do not recommend the use of:

- **Steroid monotherapy**. Neither survival nor disease course are improved and side effects are universal.[1–3] There are no prospective controlled trials of steroid monotherapy, as most previous studies were invalidated by the incorrect classification of NSIP with UIP. The reported response rates of 10%–30% in these studies may simply reflect the effect in steroid-sensitive NSIP rather than UIP.[1,2] Trials of pulsed steroid therapy had no additional benefit. When there is genuine doubt about the diagnosis, a steroid trial with monitoring of benefit (i.e. vital capacity, diffusing capacity [DLCO]) and side effects may be warranted. Pre-treatment tuberculin testing and osteoporosis prophylaxis are recommended.
- **Colchicine**. This inhibits fibroblast proliferation and collagen synthesis.[2] Several retrospective and randomized and non-randomized prospective studies have failed to show a significant reduction in lung function decline when corticosteroids were compared with colchicine therapy.[2,6]
- **Ciclosporin**. There are limited data with minimal evidence of benefit.[2,3]
- **Combination corticosteroid and immunomodulator therapy** (e.g. cyclophosphamide or azathioprine). There are no convincing data to suggest benefit and treatment toxicity is a major factor in many patients.[3,7]

- **Interferon gamma-1b (Iγ-1b)**. This is a glycoprotein that inhibits the proliferation of fibroblasts and reduces collagen synthesis in pulmonary fibrosis.[7,9] A double-blind trial in 330 patients with severe, steroid-unresponsive UIP showed no benefit with Iγ-1b over twelve months compared to placebo and it did not affect disease progression or quality of life.[7] Likewise, a large trial examining the role of Iγ-1b in 800 patients with less advanced UIP showed no difference in overall mortality.
- **Etanercept** is a soluble human tumour necrosis factor (TNF) receptor that binds to TNF and neutralizes its activity. TNF has been implicated in the pathogenesis of IPF but a RCT failed to show a difference in FVC over 48 weeks, although non-significant benefits were reported in gas transfer and walking distance.
- **Bosentan** is an endothelin receptor A and B antagonist. Endothelin-1 is a powerful vasoconstrictor and growth factor involved in the pathogenesis of pulmonary hypertension and potentially IPF. However, a RCT failed to demonstrate benefit using change in walking distance as the primary end-point but there were trends favouring bosentan use in secondary end-points of disease progression, dyspnoea and quality of life.[3]

Non-pharmacological treatments

Good nutrition, pulmonary rehabilitation, long-term oxygen therapy in patients with resting hypoxaemia, treatment of comorbidities and GORD, and early referral for lung transplantation may improve outcome.[3]

- **Lung transplantation** reduces risk of death in IPF/UIP by 75% following single lung transplantation compared with patients on the transplant waiting list.[2,3,10] A retrospective review of 821 lung transplants reported improved survival in single rather than bilateral lung transplants.[10] Early referral for lung transplantation, even before the outcome of medical therapy is established, is warranted.[2]

Clinical course and prognosis in IPF/UIP

IPF is a fatal lung disease but the clinical history is variable and unpredictable. The clinical course is one of progressive deterioration over several years, often with periods of stability but also with episodes of acute decline. Recent clinical series, in well-defined UIP cases, suggest median survival times of 2–3 years with a five-year survival range of 30%–50%.[1–3] A minority of patients with mild to moderate UIP may remain stable for relatively long periods, whereas others experience accelerated phases, with rapid decline and subsequent death. These accelerated phases ('acute exacerbations') characterize the course of UIP and portend a poor prognosis.[11] They are associated with a histological pattern of acute lung injury (i.e. diffuse alveolar damage) on a background of UIP.

Factors that predict worse survival at the time of diagnosis include age, male sex, smoking history (proportional to number of pack years), severity of breathlessness, lung function, gas exchange and hypoxaemia, degree of radiographic abnormality and HRCT honeycomb fibrosis, BAL-associated neutrophilia, eosinophilia and extent/severity of the fibroblastic foci on histology. Combinations of these factors may be used to predict survival.[1,2]

Conclusion

In this case the HRCT features were consistent with a diagnosis of UIP. In the context of the characteristic clinical presentation and HRCT scan, the guidelines suggest that a confident diagnosis can be made without a formal histological diagnosis.[1–3]

Further Reading

1. Joint statement of the American Thoracic Society (ATS) and the European Respiratory Society (ERS). Idiopathic pulmonary fibrosis: diagnosis and treatment. International consensus statement. *Am J Respir Crit Care Med* 2000; **161**: 646–64.
2. Wells AU, Hirani N. Interstitial lung disease guideline. British Thoracic Society in collaboration with Thoracic Society of Australia and New Zealand and the Irish Thoracic Society. *Thorax* 2008; **63**(Suppl 5): v1–v58.
3. Raghu G, Collard HR, Egan JJ *et al*. An official ATS/ERS/JRS/ALAT statement: idiopathic pulmonary fibrosis: evidence-based guidelines for diagnosis and management. *Am J Respir Crit Care Med* 2011; **183**: 788–824.
4. King TE Jr. Clinical advances in the diagnosis and therapy of the interstitial lung diseases. *Am J Respir Crit Care Med* 2005; **172**: 268–79.
5. Selman M, King TE Jr, Pardo A. Idiopathic pulmonary fibrosis: prevailing and evolving hypotheses about its pathogenesis and implications for therapy. *Ann Intern Med* 2001; **134**: 136–51.
6. Richeldi L, Davies HR, Ferrara G, Franco F. Corticosteroids for idiopathic pulmonary fibrosis. *Cochrane Database Syst Rev* 2003; CD002880.
7. Davies HR, Richeldi L, Walters EH. Immunomodulatory agents for idiopathic pulmonary fibrosis. *Cochrane Database Syst Rev* 2003; CD003134.
8. Azuma A, Nukiwa T, Tsuboi E *et al*. Double-blind, placebo-controlled trial of pirfenidone in patients with idiopathic pulmonary fibrosis. *Am J Respir Crit Care Med* 2005; **171**: 1040–7.
9. Raghu G, Brown KK, Bradford WZ *et al*. A placebo-controlled trial of interferon gamma-1b in patients with idiopathic pulmonary fibrosis. *N Engl J Med* 2004; **350**: 125–33.
10. Meyer DM, Edwards LB, Torres F, Jessen ME, Novick RJ. Impact of recipient age and procedure type on survival after lung transplantation for pulmonary fibrosis. *Ann Thorac Surg* 2005; **79**: 950–7.
11. Sung A, Swigris J, Saleh A, Raoof S. High-resolution chest tomography in idiopathic pulmonary fibrosis and nonspecific interstitial pneumonia: utility and challenges. *Curr Opin Pulm Med* 2007; **13**: 451–7.

PROBLEM

15 Acute Eosinophilic Pneumonia

Boris Lams, Christopher Kosky

Case History

A 50-year-old Afro-Caribbean woman reported a 48-hour history of breathlessness and dry cough. She was well until ten days earlier, when she developed fevers and anorexia. She had a history of hypothyroidism and was receiving levothyroxine. She said she did not use alcohol, tobacco or illicit drugs. There was no history of dust inhalation or animal exposure. She was born in Jamaica and at the age of fifteen had immigrated to the United Kingdom. There was no other history of travel.

On examination her temperature was 40.3°C. Respiratory rate was 38 breaths/min. Her jugular venous pressure was not elevated, heart sounds were normal and there was no peripheral oedema. She had crackles in the mid and lower zones of both lungs. Oxygen saturations were 77% on air. The white blood cell count was 14.6 (normal range 4.0–11.0 × 10^9/l) with an eosinophil count of 6.9 (normal range 0–0.4 × 10^9/l). Arterial blood gas analysis on air showed partial pressures of oxygen (PaO_2) 7.4 kPa and carbon dioxide ($PaCO_2$) 4.1 kPa, and base excess of –4. A chest X-ray showed diffuse alveolar shadowing (Figure 15.1). She was intubated and ventilated. A portable echocardiogram showed the left ventricle was hyperdynamic but functioning normally. A chest computed tomography (CT) scan showed patchy bilateral consolidation, air bronchograms and tiny pleural effusions (Figure 15.2).

What is the differential diagnosis?

Which tests would be useful?

How would you manage acute eosinophilic pneumonia?

What is the prognosis of acute eosinophilic pneumonia?

Background

In this case, the most likely diagnosis was an acute eosinophilic pneumonia (AEP). Acute eosinophilic pneumonia is an idiopathic condition characterized by pulmonary infiltration of eosinophils. Reported secondary causes of AEP include venlafaxine, H1N1 virus,[1] inhalation of concrete dust[2] and daptomycin.[3] It typically presents with the rapid onset, usually over a period of less than three weeks, of cough, dyspnoea, fever, night sweats,

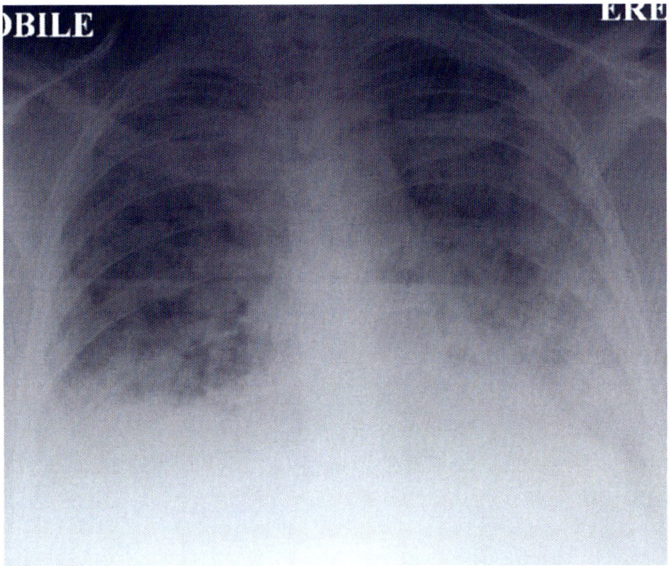

Figure 15.1 Chest radiograph at presentation.

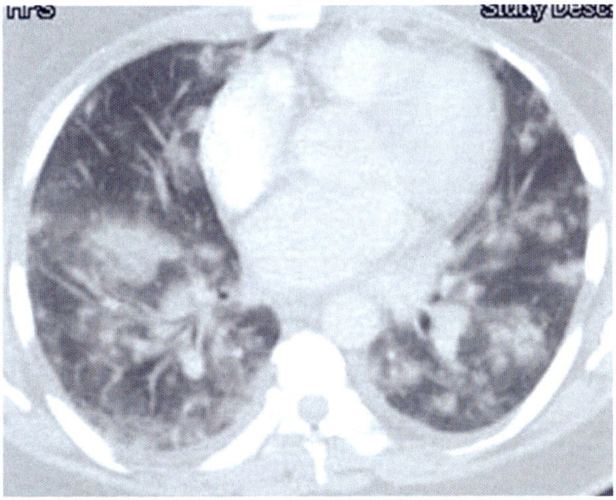

Figure 15.2 Chest CT scan at presentation.

pleuritic chest pain, myalgias and malaise. Examination reveals fever and bi-basal crackles. Blood eosinophilia may be preceded by a neutrophil leukocytosis in some patients.[4] High immunoglobulin E levels have been reported in those in whom it has been measured.[5]

In AEP the chest radiograph usually shows diffuse alveolar or reticular shadowing. Bilateral random areas of ground glass opacity and consolidation with septal lines are commonly seen on the CT scan.[6] Small pleural effusions are common, often bilateral and are eosinophil rich.

Differential diagnosis

In this case, the patient has a rapidly progressive pulmonary eosinophilia. Pulmonary eosinophilia can be defined as the combination of pulmonary infiltrates and a peripheral eosinophilia, or the presence of eosinophils in bronchoalveolar lavage (BAL) fluid or lung tissue at biopsy. Pulmonary eosinophilia may occur without a peripheral eosinophilia and in early stages the pulmonary infiltration may not be visible on a standard chest radiograph. A number of different processes may cause pulmonary eosinophilia (Table 15.1).

Table 15.1 Causes of pulmonary eosinophilia

Drugs/toxins	NSAIDs Nitrofurantoin Phenytoin Crack cocaine Heroin 1,1,1-trichloroethane (Scotchgard®)
Helminth and fungal infection	Transpulmonary *Ascaris lumbricoides* Hookworm *Strongyloides stercoralis* Direct invasion *Paragonimus* *Echinococcus* Cysticercosis Haematogenous seeding Schistosomiasis Trichinellosis
Filaria	*Wuchereria bancrofti* *Brugia malayi*
Vasculitis	Churg–Strauss syndrome
Allergic	Allergic bronchopulmonary aspergillosis
Idiopathic	Acute eosinophilic pneumonia Chronic eosinophilic pneumonia
Other	Hypereosinophilic syndrome

NSAIDs, non-steroidal anti-inflammatory drugs.

Helminthic infections are a cause of pulmonary eosinophilia. Löffler's syndrome is characterized by cough, retrosternal discomfort, pulmonary infiltrates and a peripheral eosinophilia.[7] Löffler's syndrome is caused by the transpulmonary passage of bloodstream larvae of *Ascaris lumbricoides* during their normal life cycle. Less commonly, Löffler's syndrome is due to hookworm or *Strongyloides stercoralis*. The diagnosis can be confirmed by identifying larvae in respiratory secretions.

Direct invasion of the pulmonary parenchyma by *Paragonimus* lung flukes, cysticerci or *Echinococcus* can cause haemoptysis, pleural effusions and a peripheral eosinophilia. Rarely, haematogenous spread of schistosomiasis and trichinellosis can elicit pulmonary eosinophilia. Tropical filarial pulmonary eosinophilia is caused by an immune response to circulating microfilariae. It occurs in 0.5% of patients with lymphatic filariasis due to *Wuchereria bancrofti* or *Brugia malayi*.[8]

In this case, the absence of history of recent travel made parasitic infection unlikely. Furthermore, parasitic infection usually gives rise to self-limited pulmonary symptoms. Rapid progression to ventilatory failure is not seen.

Pulmonary eosinophilia may be related to medication, especially non-steroidal anti-inflammatory drugs and antibiotics, but no causative drug could be identified in this case.

Chronic eosinophilic pneumonia is an idiopathic condition that usually presents subacutely with progressive dyspnoea, night sweats, weight loss and occasionally wheeze. The chest radiograph shows a characteristic peripheral pattern of consolidation termed 'photographic negative of pulmonary oedema'. In this case, the short duration of symptoms and chest radiograph are not in keeping with a chronic eosinophilic pneumonia.

Allergic bronchopulmonary aspergillosis usually presents with worsening asthma, expectoration of mucous plugs, fleeting eosinophilic pulmonary infiltrates on chest X-ray and proximal bronchiectasis. Churg–Strauss syndrome is an eosinophilic vasculitis occurring in a patient with asthma. Features may include pulmonary infiltrates, sinusitis, mononeuritis multiplex, and cardiac and skin involvement. An anti-neutrophil cytoplasmic antibody (ANCA) test is often positive. In this case there was no history of asthma.

Hypereosinophilic syndrome usually presents insidiously, often with an incidentally raised eosinophil count. Gradual progression with eosinophilic infiltration of the skin, heart, lungs, nervous system and gastrointestinal system occurs. It is important to remember that tuberculosis and neoplasms may also give rise to a peripheral eosinophilia.

Investigations

Bronchoalveolar lavage was performed and specimens showed fluid containing high numbers of eosinophils, typical of AEP. There were no visible parasites or organisms in BAL specimens. Serology for *Strongyloides stercoralis* was weakly positive. Stool samples were negative for parasites and ova. Serology for human immunodeficiency virus was negative. ANCA was negative.

Management

The acute presentation with rapid onset of respiratory failure is characteristic of AEP. In one series, 14 of 22 patients (64%) developed respiratory failure and required mechanical ventilation.[7]

In AEP, there is usually a dramatic improvement with oral or intravenous corticosteroids.[9] However, if pulmonary eosinophilia is due to *Strongyloides*, corticosteroid therapy may precipitate hyperinfection. *Strongyloides* hyperinfection is characterized by overwhelming parasitic infection and organ invasion. Active *Strongyloides* infection was thought unlikely in this case, given the absence of larvae in the BAL specimen and weakly reactive serology. Stool examination for parasites is usually not positive during the transpulmonary passage of *Strongyloides* larvae.

In this case the weakly positive serology to *Strongyloides stercoralis* may have been due to childhood exposure in Jamaica. The patient was commenced on intravenous methylprednisolone (250 mg once a day for three days) followed by 60 mg of prednisolone once a day. Ivermectin 2 mg was given to treat possible coexisting *Strongyloides* infection.

There was a strikingly rapid resolution in her symptoms, peripheral eosinophilia, radiology and oxygenation. She was extubated after three days. There was a complete resolution in symptoms and chest X-ray at two weeks. Corticosteroids were reduced and stopped at six weeks.

Prognosis

The prognosis of AEP is excellent, without relapse after withdrawal of corticosteroids.

Conclusion

Acute eosinophilic pneumonia presents with acute respiratory failure, bilateral lung infiltrates and blood eosinophilia. Treatment with corticosteroids usually results in an excellent prognosis.

Further Reading

1 Jeon EJ, Kim KH, Min KH. Acute eosinophilic pneumonia associated with 2009 influenza A (H1N1). *Thorax* 2010; **65**: 268–70.

2 Hines SE, Schwartz DA, Groshong SD, Rose CS. Eosinophilic pneumonia recurrence following inhalation exposure to concrete dust. *Am J Resp Crit Care Med* 2010; **181**; A4075.

3 Miller B, Gray A, LeBlanc TW, Sexton DJ, Martin AR, Slama TG. Acute eosinophilic pneumonia secondary to daptomycin: a report of three cases. *Clin Infect Dis* 2010; **50**: e63–8.

4 Philit F, Etienne-Mastroïanni B, Parrot A, Guérin C, Robert D, Cordier JF. Idiopathic acute eosinophilic pneumonia: a study of 22 patients. *Am J Respir Crit Care Med* 2002; **166**: 1235–9.

5 Umeki S. Reevaluation of eosinophilic pneumonia and its diagnostic criteria. *Arch Intern Med* 1992; **152**: 1913–9.

6 Daimon T, Johkoh T, Sumikawa H *et al.* Acute eosinophilic pneumonia: thin-section CT findings in 29 patients. *Eur J Radiol* 2008; **65**: 462–7.

7 Löffler W. Transient lung infiltrations with blood eosinophilia. *Int Arch Allergy Appl Immunol* 1956; **8**: 54–9.

8 Ottesen EA, Nutman TB. Tropical pulmonary eosinophilia. *Annu Rev Med* 1992; **43**: 417–24.

9 Jantz MA, Sahn SA. Corticosteroids in acute respiratory failure. *Am J Respir Crit Care Med* 1999; **160**: 1079–100.

PROBLEM

16 Cryptogenic Organizing Pneumonia

Boris Lams, Christopher Kosky

Case History

A 27-year-old Caucasian nurse presents to hospital with a two-month history of gradually increasing dyspnoea, dry cough and a 2 kg weight loss. She was previously well. She says that one month ago she had night sweats but that these settled. She was given a course of amoxicillin by her general practitioner two weeks ago. She is currently taking ciprofloxacin but this has also had no effect on her symptoms. She has no other past medical history. She keeps no pets. She travelled to Lake Malawi a year ago on a diving trip and was well during and after this trip. She takes no medications. She does not smoke.

On examination she looks well. Her temperature is 36.9°C, pulse is 94 beats/min, blood pressure 130/80 mm Hg, oxygen saturation (SaO_2) 93% on air. Her jugular venous pressure is not elevated and heart sounds are normal. She has widespread fine crackles throughout both lung fields.

Investigations reveal a raised white cell count (12.2×10^9/l), raised neutrophil count (9.3×10^9/l), normal eosinophil count (0.2×10^9/l), normal haemoglobin (12.2 g/dl) and raised platelet count (472×10^9/l). Renal profile is normal. Liver profile is normal except for a low albumin (37 g/l), raised alkaline phosphatase (136 IU/L) and raised gamma glutamyl transferase (135 IU/l). C-reactive protein is elevated (125 mg/l). A chest radiograph (CXR) is performed (Figure 16.1).

What does the CXR show and what is the differential diagnosis?

What investigations help in the diagnosis of cryptogenic organizing pneumonia (COP)?

What causes COP?

What is the treatment of COP?

Background

Cryptogenic organizing pneumonia is usually idiopathic. An organizing pneumonia can be secondary to connective tissue disorders such as systemic lupus erythematosus and rheumatoid arthritis. Drugs such as amiodarone, bleomycin and nitrofurantoin can also cause an organizing pneumonia. Organizing pneumonia can coexist adjacent to pulmo-

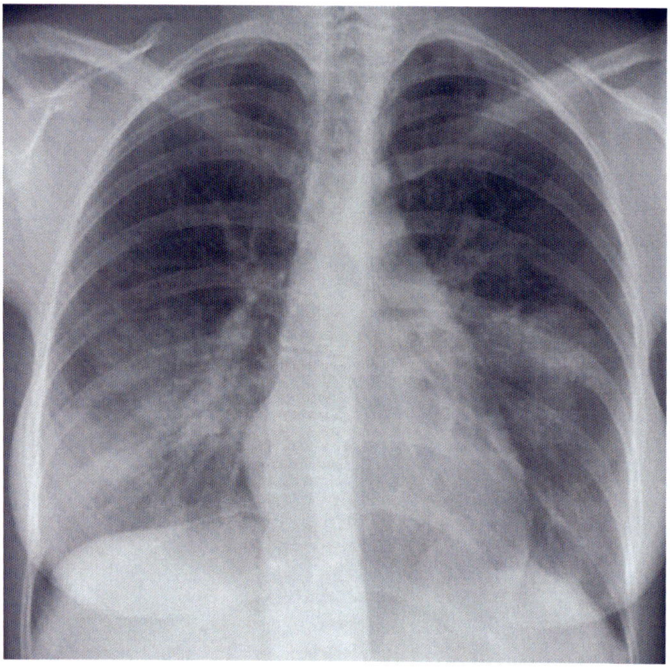

Figure 16.1 Chest radiograph at presentation.

nary malignancy or be secondary to malignancy elsewhere in the body, for example cutaneous lymphoma.[1]

In this case, secondary causes of COP are unlikely in the absence of arthralgias, rash and other symptoms or causative drugs.

Differential diagnosis

The CXR shows bilateral shadowing, more marked in the lower than the upper zones. She has a mass-like lesion in the left mid zone. The differential diagnosis includes:

- **Community-acquired pneumonia**. Her symptoms of cough and breathlessness together with the mild elevation in neutrophils may represent a community-acquired pneumonia. It would be odd for these symptoms not to have improved with her previous amoxicillin and her current course of ciprofloxacin. Although she may have been exposed to tuberculosis (TB) in her work as a nurse, TB typically affects the upper zones of the lung.
- ***Pneumocystis jirovecii*** infection is possible, although the CXR appearances are not typical and she has no obvious risk factors for human immunodeficiency virus infection. Diving in Lake Malawi may have exposed her to schistosomiasis. However, acute pulmonary eosinophilia from haematogenous seeding of schistosomiasis usually presents within eight weeks of exposure and is normally associated with blood eosinophilia.
- **Malignancy**. The combination of weight loss and lower zone pulmonary infiltrates raises the possibility of metastatic cancer. Diffuse alveolar shadowing is also seen in bronchoalveolar cell carcinoma and in primary pulmonary lymphoma.

- **Non-specific interstitial pneumonia.** The presence of progressive dyspnoea and cough could be explained by non-specific interstitial pneumonia although the time course is a little short for this and the CXR appearances are uncharacteristic. She has no known antigen exposure to account for a hypersensitivity pneumonitis, which predominantly affects the upper lobes of the lung. The absence of a blood eosinophilia makes chronic eosinophilic pneumonia unlikely.
- **Cryptogenic organizing pneumonitis.** Her clinical picture and radiograph are most consistent with COP. Clinical presentation of COP is similar to that of community-acquired pneumonia, with cough, dyspnoea and weight loss often preceded by a viral-like prodrome. COP is unaffected by antibiotics. Presentation is usually subacute and within three months of onset of symptoms. Radiographic findings in COP are those of bilateral alveolar shadowing which is usually more marked basally. Occasionally peripheral changes predominate when distinction from a chronic eosinophilic pneumonia is not possible radiologically. Other patterns have been described including unilateral disease (10% of cases) and presentations with mass lesions.[2]

Investigations

A high-resolution computed tomography (CT) chest scan should be performed in patients with suspected COP.[3] In this case, the patient's CT chest scan (Figure 16.2) shows areas of consolidation with air bronchograms in the lower zones. Multiple ground glass ring shadows are also seen throughout the lung fields. These have been described as the CT reverse halo sign or atoll sign, and are characteristic of COP.[4] The CT reverse halo sign has also been described in Wegener's granulomatosis and in pulmonary paracoccidioidomycosis.

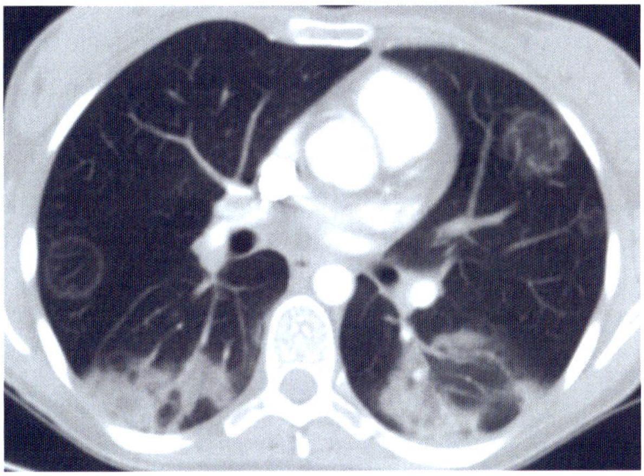

Figure 16.2 Chest CT scan.

In this patient, anti-neutrophil cytoplasmic antibody was not detected, making the diagnosis of Wegener's granulomatosis unlikely. Connective tissue disease causing an organizing pneumonia was also unlikely as anti-nuclear antibodies, extractable nuclear antibodies and rheumatoid factor were not detected.

Transbronchial lung biopsy showed features typical of COP. Histological specimens showed excessive proliferation of granulation tissue within small airways (proliferative bronchiolitis) and alveolar ducts, associated with chronic inflammation in the surrounding alveoli.

COP and idiopathic bronchiolitis obliterans organizing pneumonia (BOOP) are the same disease. The preferred term is COP. The term BOOP has raised confusion as it suggests that the disease is characterized by a clinical bronchiolitis, whereas in fact COP has the features of a parenchymal pneumonic process rather than an airways-based disease. BOOP is also confused with obstructive bronchiolitis, a completely different condition.

Transbronchial lung biopsy is recommended to confirm the diagnosis of COP.[3] Bronchoscopic alveolar lavage can also be performed during the bronchoscopy to exclude infection. In COP, lavage specimens typically reveal an increased mixed cellularity with occasional foamy macrophages. When transbronchial lung biopsy is non-diagnostic, or in a case of atypical COP, a biopsy should be obtained by video-assisted thoracic surgery or open lung biopsy may be required.

The clinical, radiological and histological features do not usually allow one to distinguish between COP and a secondary organizing pneumonia. The histological diagnosis of an organizing pneumonia should prompt a search for other causes of an organizing pneumonia such as post-infection, aspiration, drug reactions, collagen vascular disease (particularly rheumatoid arthritis and myositis), hypersensitivity pneumonitis and as a reaction to an underlying malignant disorder (particularly haematological malignancy).

Treatment

Typical COP has a good prognosis and treatment with corticosteroids is usually successful. However, relapse requiring reintroduction of steroid therapy occurs in over half of patients with COP and cannot be predicted. Relapses are uncommon with prednisolone doses >20 mg daily and are rarely associated with a poor prognosis.[5] The length of initial treatment with corticosteroids is usually 6–12 months. Immunosuppressive therapy for relapsing disease may be required. A small group of patients have a fibrosing COP that is associated with a worse outcome.

In this case the patient was started on prednisolone 60 mg a day. Her symptoms improved within 48 hours of treatment. A CXR one month after commencing prednisolone was normal. The prednisolone dose was tapered and stopped after six months without a relapse in symptoms.

Conclusion

Idiopathic cryptogenic organizing pneumonia should be suspected in patients with pulmonary consolidation that does not improve with antibiotics.

Further Reading

1 Cordier JF. Cryptogenic organising pneumonia. *Eur Respir J* 2006; **28**: 422–46.

2 Epler GR, Colby TV, McLoud TC, Carrington CB, Gaensler EA. Bronchiolitis obliterans organizing pneumonia. *N Engl J Med* 1985; **312**: 152–8.

3 Wells AU, Hirani N. Interstitial lung disease guideline. British Thoracic Society in collaboration with the Thoracic Society of Australian and New Zealand and the Irish Thoracic Society. *Thorax* 2008; **63**(Suppl 5): v1–58.

4 Kim SJ, Lee KS, Ryu YH *et al.* Reversed halo sign on high-resolution CT of cryptogenic organizing pneumonia: diagnostic implications. *AJR Am J Roentgenol* 2003; **180**: 1251–4.

5 Lazor R, Vandevenne A, Pelletier A, Leclerc P, Court-Fortune I, Cordier JF. Cryptogenic organizing pneumonia. Characteristics of relapses in a series of 48 patients. The Groupe d'Etudes et de Recherche sur les Maladles "Orphelines" Pulmonaires. *Am J Respir Crit Care Med* 2000; **162**; 571–7.

PROBLEM

17 Sarcoidosis (Radiographic Stage I)

Anne Collett, Richard Leach

Case History

A 35-year-old male Caucasian barrister presented with a four-week history of dry cough, breathlessness and fatigue. There was no past medical history. He was a non-smoker with no industrial dust contact, travel abroad, antigenic exposure or family history of chest disease. An occupational radiograph five years earlier was normal. On examination he was afebrile. There was no palpable lymphadenopathy. He was not clubbed and saturation (SaO_2) was 96%. The cardiovascular system was unremarkable. Chest examination was normal with good air entry to both bases and no crackles or wheeze. Fundoscopy and urinalysis detected no abnormalities. Routine blood tests including lymphocyte count, liver function tests, calcium and lactate dehydrogenase were normal. The erythrocyte sedimentation rate was 8 mm/hr and serum angiotensin converting enzyme (ACE) was fractionally raised at 95 IU/l (normal 0–82 IU/l). Pulmonary function tests (PFT) were forced expiratory volume in 1 second (FEV_1) 2.64 l (68% predicted), forced vital capacity (FVC) 4.66 l (99% predicted) and peak expiratory flow rate (PEFR) 390 l/min (76% predicted). The functional residual capacity was 87% predicted and gas transfer (DLCO) 85% predicted. The chest radiograph (CXR) is illustrated in Figure 17.1.

What is the most likely diagnosis in this case and is histological confirmation required?

What is the aetiology of this condition and is it likely to affect the patient's children?

What is the natural clinical course of this disease and are there any prognostic indicators in this case?

How are the radiological changes classified and do they have prognostic significance?

Is a computed tomography (CT) scan required and how would you establish a histological diagnosis?

How would you explain the obstructive pattern of PFT in this case?

Will steroid therapy benefit this patient?

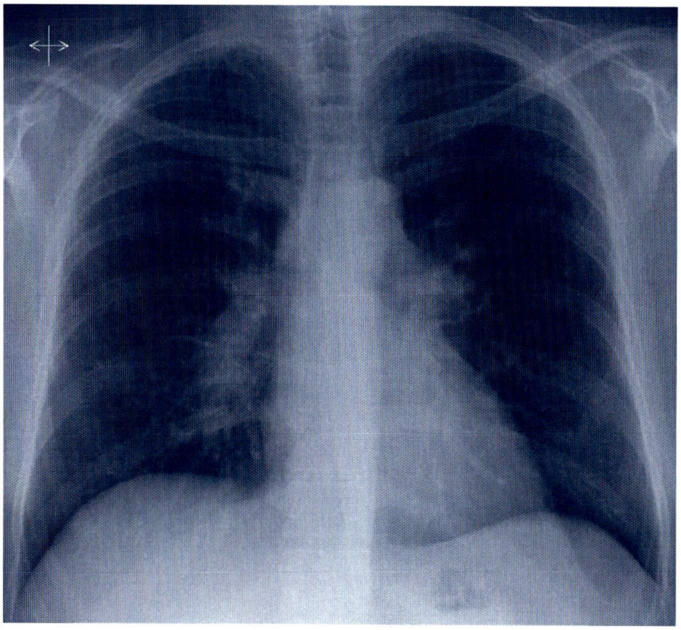

Figure 17.1 Chest radiograph.

Background

Sarcoidosis is a benign, multisystem inflammatory disorder of unknown cause that affects most organs but most commonly the respiratory system.[1–3] It typically occurs in 20–40 year olds and is unusual in children. African-Americans, Scandinavians and the Irish are most commonly affected, as are those with first- or second-degree relatives with sarcoidosis. Spontaneous resolution occurs in over 50% of cases over 1–5 years but it may lead to chronic progressive disease. Black people may develop an aggressive, systemic form of the disease. Geographically, incidence varies from 5 to 100 per 10^5 population and is approximately 10 per 10^5 population in the UK.

Establishing a diagnosis of sarcoidosis depends on demonstrating (i) a compatible clinical picture; (ii) histological confirmation of non-caseating granulomas and (iii) exclusion of other diseases that produce a similar clinical or histological picture.[1–3] If clinical presentation of sarcoidosis is unusual, histological confirmation of the diagnosis must be obtained. However, detection of granulomas in a single organ does not confirm a diagnosis of sarcoidosis, as granulomas are seen in other disease processes. It is the combination of the clinical picture and histological findings that is important. The recommended initial evaluation is shown in Table 17.1.[1–3] Diagnostic work-up aims to confirm the disease histologically, assess the extent of organ involvement, establish if the disease is progressive and determine if therapy will be beneficial.

Table 17.1 Recommended initial evaluation of patients with sarcoidosis

1	History (including occupational/environmental exposure)
2	Examination including fundoscopy
3	Full blood count including lymphocyte count
4	Biochemistry, calcium, LFT, LDH, serum ACE
5	ECG, CXR, urine analysis (± calcium excretion)
6	PFT; spirometry and DLCO
7	Mantoux test (to exclude TB)

ECG, electrocardiogram; LDH, lactate dehydrogenase; LFT, liver function tests; TB, tuberculosis.

The CXR in this patient shows bilateral hilar lymphadenopathy (BHL). The differential diagnosis includes sarcoidosis, tuberculosis, lymphoma, viral infection (e.g. Epstein–Barr, human immunodeficiency virus), fungal infection (e.g. histoplasmosis), toxoplasmosis, brucellosis and less common 'sarcoid-like' reactions due to carcinomas. In a study of 100 consecutive patients with BHL, sarcoidosis was confirmed in 95% of asymptomatic patients with a normal clinical examination. However, malignancy was the cause in 11 of the 100 BHL patients, all of whom were symptomatic.[4] Consequently, histological confirmation may not be needed in asymptomatic patients with symmetrical BHL or in those with a typical acute presentation (see below). However, histological confirmation is strongly recommended in symptomatic patients with asymmetrical or massive BHL or large paratracheal lymph nodes.

Aetiology

The cause of sarcoidosis is unknown despite considerable research. Current evidence suggests that sarcoidosis results from exposure of a genetically susceptible subject to an appropriate antigenic trigger.[2,5] It is also possible that the antigenic trigger differs between patients depending on individual genetic susceptibility. Recognition that certain races and ethnic backgrounds (e.g. black people, northern Europeans) are more susceptible and that familial clustering occurs, suggests a genetic predisposition to sarcoidosis. First- or second-degree relatives of a primary case have an increased risk of developing sarcoidosis in studies from the UK and USA.[2,5] Genetic studies identifying areas of the genome associated with sarcoidosis suggest a link with chromosomes 3 and 5 and the short arm of chromosome 6. There also appears to be an association with class II major histocompatibility complex (MHC) alleles, which determine presentation of antigens to T cells at the onset of the response that results in granuloma formation and sarcoidosis. Several alleles appear to confer susceptibility to the disease (e.g. class I human leukocyte antigen [HLA] B8 and class II HLA DRB1, HLA-DQ) and others confer protection (e.g. HLA DR 1).

Many potential environmental antigenic triggers have been proposed as the cause of sarcoidosis.[2,3,5] This is based on epidemiological data showing geographical (e.g. pine pollen exposure), occupational (e.g. health-care workers, firefighters, beryllium exposure), chemical exposure (e.g. insecticides, inorganic particles, moulds) and seasonal (e.g. winter, spring) clustering. Two potential infective triggers have been described, mycobacteria and propionibacteria. The role of mycobacteria has been examined in more than 20 studies and the degree of association varies from 0% to 89%. However, recent studies, using sensitive polymerase chain reaction methodology, detected no *Mycobacterium tuberculosis* DNA in tissue samples from sarcoid patients. However, higher levels of *Propionibacterium acnes* and *P. granulosum* DNA, an infection which occurs in early adult life, were detected in thoracic lymph nodes from sarcoid patients as compared to controls. Many other agents have been implicated as triggers including viruses (e.g. Epstein–Barr), *Borrelia burgdorferi*, aluminium, talc, clay and beryllium. Although the host may be a potential source of triggering antigens, the possibility that sarcoidosis is an autoimmune disease is now considered less likely.

Clinical course of pulmonary sarcoidosis

The clinical features most commonly associated with pulmonary sarcoidosis, either endobronchial or parenchymal, are non-productive cough, dyspnoea and chest discomfort which occur in 30%–50% of cases.[2,3,5] In contrast to idiopathic pulmonary fibrosis, physical findings are unusual. Crepitations occur in <20% of patients (even if radiographic infiltrates are extensive) and clubbing is infrequent. Constitutional symptoms including fever, weight loss and malaise occur in 30% and fatigue in 70% of cases. Fatigue correlated inversely with carbon monoxide diffusing capacity (DLCO) in one study. Although sarcoidosis can affect any organ system, pulmonary manifestations usually predominate. Onset may be acute as in Löfgren's syndrome (i.e. BHL, erythema nodusum, arthritis, constitutional symptoms) which usually resolves spontaneously; or insidious and progressive with pulmonary infiltration and organ-related symptoms requiring treatment.

Many patients with sarcoidosis are asymptomatic and detected on routine medical or occupational CXR. Radiographic abnormalities occur in 85%–95% of sarcoid patients,[1,2,5] but 30%–60% of these patients are asymptomatic with incidental CXR findings. Sarcoidosis resolves spontaneously without treatment in 65%–70%, a chronic course ensues in 10%–30% and death occurs in 2%–5% of cases. Chronic pulmonary sarcoidosis usually results in pulmonary fibrosis and respiratory failure. In the USA, 87% of sarcoid-related deaths are due to pulmonary complications whereas in Japan cardiac complications account for 77% of deaths.[1]

Acute inflammatory manifestations including erythema nodosum, polyarthritis and fever indicate a good prognosis with spontaneous remission rates of >85%. Factors associated with a poor prognosis and a chronic relapsing course include age >40 years old at onset, hypercalcaemia, ethnic origin (e.g. black race), extrathoracic disease, splenomegaly, lupus pernio, chronic uveitis, and bone, central nervous system and cardiac involvement. Lower family income is also associated with a worse outcome. At the onset, PFT have little prognostic value but serial measurements of FVC and DLCO detect progressive pulmonary fibrosis which has a poor outcome. Many cell markers and laboratory tests have been examined as potential markers of disease activity and apart from serum ACE, which may reflect granuloma burden, and the soluble interleukin-2 receptor, which may reflect T-cell activity, none has been recommended for routine assessment.[1–3,5] Even these are of limited value. Routine CXR and spirometry (± DLCO) are the most effective means of monitoring pulmonary disease.

Diagnosis

The CXR is abnormal in >85% of patients with sarcoid. BHL (± right paratracheal lymph nodes) occurs in 50%–85% of cases whereas unilateral hilar lymphadenopathy is rare occurring in <10%. Pulmonary parenchymal infiltrates, usually central or in the upper lobes, with or without BHL, occur in 25%–50% of cases. The radiographic staging system for pulmonary sarcoidosis was introduced 40 years ago and is illustrated in Table 17.2.[2,5,6] Prognosis is best with stage I and poorest in stage IV. Spontaneous remission occurs in 60%–90% of stage I, 40%–60% of stage II and 10%–20% of stage III. Spontaneous remission usually occurs within 2–3 years and failure to remit during this time predicts chronic or persistent disease. Spontaneous remission is associated with a low relapse rate. However, within different ethnic groups and geographical regions there is considerable variability. This patient has BHL with no evidence of parenchymal involvement and spontaneous remission is a strong possibility.

Table 17.2 Radiographic staging in sarcoidosis

Stage	Finding
0	Normal chest radiograph
I	Bilateral hilar lymphadenopathy (BHL)
II	BHL plus pulmonary infiltrates
III	Pulmonary infiltrates (without BHL)
IV	Pulmonary fibrosis (± bullae)

The CT scan is superior to CXR in delineating mediastinal, parenchymal and hilar structures but is not necessary for routine evaluation of pulmonary sarcoidosis.[1–3,5] It is helpful in about 30% of cases:

- When the CXR is normal but sarcoidosis is suspected;
- To discriminate between active inflammation and fibrosis in stage II or III disease;
- To detect specific complications (e.g. bronchiectasis, aspergilloma);
- To detect superimposed infection or malignancy.

Characteristic CT features of pulmonary sarcoid include mediastinal and hilar adenopathy, micronodules and nodular opacities along bronchovascular bundles, pleural and subpleural nodules, septal and non-septal lines and ground glass opacities. In later disease, traction bronchiectasis, fibrous bands, cystic/bullous changes and hilar retraction develop.

Flexible fibreoptic bronchoscopy with transbronchial lung biopsy establishes a histological diagnosis in 60%–90% of cases, including stage I disease (i.e. no CXR parenchymal involvement), provided four to five biopsy samples are obtained during the procedure.[1–3,7] Bronchial mucosal biopsies should also be taken as non-caseating granulomas are detected in 40%–60%, even if the mucosa appears normal. If mucosal nodularity, oedema or hypervascularity are present the diagnostic yield is as high as 90%. Transbronchial needle aspiration of mediastinal or hilar nodes has a diagnostic yield of >60%.[1]

Bronchoalveolar lavage (BAL) detects an increase in lymphocytes (>30%) in 90% of patients at presentation but this may occur in many other disorders. However, a BAL CD4+/CD8+ ratio of >3.5 is specific for sarcoidosis, with a sensitivity of 52%–59% and a specificity of 94%–96%.[8,9] Three independent studies have confirmed that a clinical/radiological picture typical of sarcoidosis and a CD4+/CD8+ ratio >3.5 provides reliable confirmation of the diagnosis of sarcoidosis and obviates the need for histological diagnosis.[2,8]

If bronchoscopic biopsies or BAL fail to establish a diagnosis and no other easily accessible lymph node or biopsy site is identified, cervical mediastinoscopy or a parasternal mini-thoracotomy (to biopsy para-aortic or aortopulmonary window nodes) or surgical lung biopsy may be indicated. Currently, video-assisted thoracoscopic surgical biopsy is preferred to traditional thoracotomy lung biopsy. Endoscopic bronchial ultrasound-guided needle biopsy of mediastinal nodes is increasingly performed. Liver biopsy is not specific and is not recommended as a routine procedure.

Pulmonary function tests

Abnormal PFT are seen in 20% of patients with radiographic stage I sarcoidosis, and 40%–70% of patients with parenchymal infiltrates (stages II, III, IV).[1–3] Although correlation with CXR is only moderate, PFT provide a baseline for monitoring disease progression or resolution and should be performed at presentation in every patient. The DLCO and the vital capacity are the most sensitive measures of disease progression.[1,3] A normal CXR is associated with a reduced FVC and DLCO in 15%–25% and 25%–50% of cases, respectively.

Although the typical finding is a restrictive pattern, obstructive defects (i.e. reduced FEV_1, FEV_1/FVC ratio) occur in approximately 30%–50% of patients, particularly those with parenchymal involvement.[1,3] In a study of 107 patients with newly diagnosed sarcoidosis, 61 (57%) patients had a reduced FEV_1/FVC ratio, 29 (27%) had reductions in DLCO and only 7 (6%) had a restrictive defect.[10,11] In advanced pulmonary sarcoidosis severe obstructive patterns can occur and this is associated with a higher mortality risk.

About 50% of stage I and II sarcoid patients have bronchial hyperreactivity on methacholine challenge, exhibited clinically as a 'hacking' cough.[1,2] Similarly, bronchial narrowing due to granulomatous lesions, compression by enlarged lymph nodes, airways distortion and peribronchial fibrosis may cause obstructive defects.

Treatment

Most patients with pulmonary sarcoidosis do not require treatment. Asymptomatic BHL or pulmonary infiltration on CXR (stage II, III) is usually monitored. The American Thoracic Society/European Respiratory Society recommendations for steroid therapy in sarcoidosis include progressive, systematic pulmonary or extrapulmonary disease, asymptomatic progressive loss of lung function, cardiac and neurological disease, eye disease not responding to topical therapy, and symptomatic hypercalcaemia. The use of steroid therapy varies between centres, with some treating only a third of cases and others up to two-thirds.[12]

Conclusion

In this case the CXR shows BHL. The acute onset, raised serum ACE and BHL without parenchymal involvement on CXR suggest that the most likely diagnosis is sarcoidosis and that spontaneous resolution is likely. However, the finding of considerable compression of the right main bronchus at bronchoscopy prompted a CT scan which demonstrated large mediastinal and paratracheal lymph nodes. One of these nodes measuring 4.5 cm was compressing the right main bronchus. In view of this extensive adenopathy, a limited thoracotomy with surgical node biopsy was performed. Following histological confirmation of the diagnosis as sarcoidosis, the patient was treated with high-dose steroid therapy with rapid resolution of the lymphadenopathy and relief of the obstructive defect on spirometry. Following steroid weaning over twelve months this patient remains well without relapse after three years.

Further Reading

1 Joint Statement of the American Thoracic Society (ATS), the European Respiratory Society (ERS) and the World Association of Sarcoidosis and Other Granulomatous Disorders (WASOG) adopted by the ATS Board of Directors and by the ERS Executive Committee, February 1999. Statement on sarcoidosis. *Am J Respir Crit Care Med* 1999; **160**: 736–55.

2 Iannuzzi MC, Rybicki BA, Teirstein AS. Sarcoidosis. *N Engl J Med* 2007; **357**: 2153–65.

3 Drent M, Costabel U (eds). Sarcoidosis. European Respiratory Society Monograph 2005; Volume 32.

4 Winterbauer RH, Belic N, Moores KD. Clinical interpretation of bilateral hilar lymphadenopathy. *Ann Intern Med* 1973; **79**: 65–71.

5 Baughman RP, Lower EE, du Bois RM. Sarcoidosis. *Lancet* 2003; **361**: 1111–8.

6 Scadding J. Prognosis of intrathoracic sarcoidosis in England. A review of 136 cases after five years' observation. *Br Med J* 1961; **2**: 1165–72.

7 Gilman MJ, Wang KP. Transbronchial lung biopsy in sarcoidosis. An approach to determine the optimal number of biopsies. *Am Rev Respir Dis* 1980; **122**: 721–8.

8 Costabel U, Zaiss AW, Guzman J. Sensitivity and specificity of BAL findings in sarcoidosis. *Sarcoidosis* 1992; **9**: 211–4.

9 Prasse A, Pechkovsky DV, Toews GB *et al.* A vicious cycle of alveolar macrophages and fibroblasts perpetuates pulmonary fibrosis via CCL18. *Am J Respir Crit Care Med* 2006; **173**: 781–92.

10 Harrison BD, Shaylor JM, Stokes TC, Wilkes AR. Airflow limitation in sarcoidosis – a study of pulmonary function in 107 patients with newly diagnosed disease. *Respir Med* 1991; **85**: 59–64.

11 Baughman RP, Teirstein AS, Judson MA *et al.* Clinical characteristics of patients in a case control study of sarcoidosis. *Am J Respir Crit Care Med* 2001; **164**: 1885–9.

12 Grutters JC, van den Bosch JMM. Corticosteroid treatment in sarcoidosis. *Eur Respir J* 2006; **28**: 627–36.

PROBLEM

18 Sarcoidosis (Radiographic Stages II and III)

Richard Leach

Case History

A 44-year-old black lady presented with an eight-month history of tiredness, rapidly progressive breathlessness and bilateral interstitial, perihilar shadowing on a chest radiograph (CXR). Non-caseating granulomas were detected in transbronchial biopsies consistent with a diagnosis of sarcoidosis. A computed tomography scan revealed extensive mid and upper zone intrapulmonary infiltration with confluent areas of fibrosis. Her forced expiratory volume in 1 second (FEV_1) was 2.39 l (82% predicted), forced vital capacity (FVC) 3.01 l (89% predicted), lung volumes normal and gas transfer (DLCO) 85% predicted. Liver function tests (LFT) were abnormal and serum angiotensin converting enzyme (ACE) was raised at 96 IU/l (normal 0–82 IU/l). Ophthalmology review was normal. She was treated with prednisolone 40 mg daily for three months with weekly bisphosphonate therapy for bone protection. At this time her breathlessness had resolved, repeat CXR showed clearing of the interstitial shadowing and FEV_1 was 2.90 l (94% predicted) and FVC 3.36 l (100% predicted). Both LFT and serum ACE were normal. She remained asymptomatic, with stable spirometry, as the steroid dose was tapered and stopped over twelve months.

Three months later the breathlessness, cough, reduced exercise tolerance and tiredness recurred. Perihilar interstitial shadowing reappeared on the CXR (Figure 18.1) and LFT and serum ACE had increased. The FEV_1 fell to 1.57 l (55% predicted) and FVC to 2.33 l (70% predicted). High-dose steroids were restarted with resolution of her symptoms, improved exercise tolerance and some improvement in spirometry; FEV_1 1.76 l (61% predicted) and FVC 2.59 l (78% predicted). Over the next six months, attempts to reduce the steroids below 20 mg daily resulted in symptoms, CXR relapse and further reductions in spirometry. The patient gained weight with significant steroid side effects. Spirometry on prednisolone 20 mg was FEV_1 1.55 l (54% predicted) and FVC 2.00 l (60% predicted).

How would you classify this patient's sarcoidosis and how often does relapse occur after steroid therapy?

What is the mechanism of action of steroids in sarcoidosis?

Do steroids prevent long-term pulmonary fibrosis?

Are inhaled steroids beneficial in pulmonary sarcoidosis?

What therapeutic options are available and how would you manage this patient now?

Is lung transplantation indicated in end-stage sarcoid-induced pulmonary fibrosis?

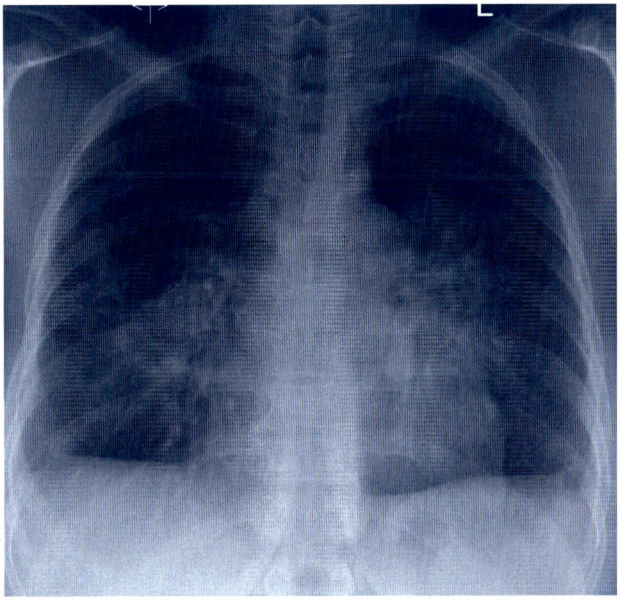

Figure 18.1 Chest radiograph.

Background

Sarcoidosis is a benign, multisystem inflammatory disorder of unknown cause that can affect most organs (e.g. eyes, liver) but most commonly affects the respiratory system (>90% of cases).[1–3] Pulmonary sarcoidosis may be asymptomatic (approximately 30% of cases) or cause non-productive cough, dyspnoea and chest discomfort (30%–50%). Constitutional symptoms including fever, malaise and weight loss occur in 30% and fatigue in 70% of cases. In contrast to idiopathic pulmonary fibrosis, physical findings are unusual. Clubbing is infrequent and crepitations occur in <20% of patients (despite extensive radiographic infiltrates).

Progressive, infiltrative lung disease is often asymptomatic. However, it may present with dyspnoea, dry cough, chest pain and constitutional symptoms and be associated with systemic disease. Pulmonary infiltrates are often present on CXR (Figure 18.1) and in some cases there may be bilateral hilar lymphadenopathy (BHL). Infiltrates may resolve or progress to fibrosis and respiratory failure. Lung function tests typically reveal a restrictive defect with reduced gas transfer but obstructive spirometry is not unusual. In the USA, 87% of sarcoidosis-related deaths are due to pulmonary involvement; in Japan cardiac complications account for 77% of deaths.

This patient has progressive pulmonary infiltrative sarcoidosis and is stage III on the standard radiographic classification (i.e bilateral infiltration without BHL; see Chapter 17). Although steroid treatment of patients with pulmonary infiltrates usually results in radiographic improvement and resolution of granulomas on repeat biopsy, recurrence of symptoms and radiographic infiltrates is common after discontinuation of therapy. Longitudinal studies have reported that more than one-third of patients relapse within two years in this subset of patients.[1–3]

Mechanism of action of steroid therapy in sarcoidosis

Glucocorticoids bind to cytosolic receptors and translocate to the cell nucleus where they directly or indirectly regulate up to 100 genes. Steroids suppress inflammatory genes (e.g. interleukin-1 [IL-1], tumour necrosis factor alpha [TNF-α]) and to a lesser extent activate anti-inflammatory genes (e.g. IL-1 receptor antagonist). They also reduce expression of nuclear factor-κB, elevated levels of which are linked to the pathogenesis of sarcoidosis by increasing production of TNF-α and interleukin-6 by macrophages and interferon gamma by T lymphocytes. Steroids have also been shown to restore the balance between type 1 and type 2 helper T-cell cytokines in sarcoidosis. Steroid-resistant sarcoidosis is characterized by exaggerated TNF-α release by alveolar macrophages.[4]

Do steroids prevent long-term pulmonary fibrosis?

Many uncontrolled studies have confirmed the efficacy of steroid therapy in pulmonary sarcoidosis.[4] The 2005 Cochrane review identified six randomized trials of steroid therapy in pulmonary sarcoidosis.[5] These are summarized in Table 18.1 and indicate that symptoms, biochemical markers, lung function and CXR all improved over 3–24 months, particularly in those with parenchymal disease on CXR (odds ratio of 2.54). Vital capacity (VC) increased by 4.2% of predicted values and carbon monoxide diffusing capacity (DLCO) by 5.7% of predicted values. However, these studies provide little indication of the value of long-term steroid therapy in chronic progressive parenchymal sarcoidosis, and it is unclear whether steroids can slow progression, prevent development of irreversible fibrosis or improve survival. Two studies with conflicting results have addressed this question:

- The British Thoracic Society investigated 149 sarcoid patients with parenchymal CXR abnormalities.[6] During six months of initial observation, 33 patients received steroid for symptoms and 58 showed spontaneous radiographic improvement. The remaining 58 patients were allocated to either 18 months of steroid therapy or observation; after five years, steroid-treated patients showed significant improvements in lung function compared to the observation group (approximately 10% difference in FEV_1 and VC). About 20% of the observation group progressed and eventually required steroid therapy.
- A Scandinavian meta-analysis of pulmonary sarcoidosis in referral versus population-based settings (e.g. government clinics) showed mortalities of 4.8% and 0.5%, respectively, and this disparity was unlikely to be caused by adverse selection (e.g. stage or ethnicity).[1,4] Patients in referral centres were seven times more likely

to receive steroid therapy, suggesting that excessive use of steroids might have an adverse influence on long-term outcome. However, there were major limitations in this study including the absence of specific mortality data on the steroid recipients in the two populations, making definite conclusions impossible.

Table 18.1 Randomized controlled trials of oral steroids in pulmonary sarcoidosis[5]

First author, date	Patient numbers on treatment or control	Follow-up (months)	Outcome
James DG, 1967	27 Pred 20 mg/day; 20 placebo	6	CXR improved at 6 months
Israel HL, 1973	41 Pred 15 mg/day; 42 placebo	3, 12–132	No difference
Roth I, 1975	54 Pred 40 mg/day; 38 no Rx	6, 12, 60–168	CXR improved at 12 months
Selroos O, 1979	19 Methylpred 32 mg/day; 18 no Rx	7, 48	CXR, VC, D_{LCO} improved at 7 months
Zaki MH, 1987	77 Pred 40→20 mg/day; 57 placebo	24, >36	No difference
Pietinalho A, 2002	91 Pred 20→10 mg/day; 94 placebo	3	CXR, serum ACE improved at 3 months and VC, DLCO at 18 and 60 months

ACE, angiotensin converting enzyme; CXR, chest radiograph; DLCO, carbon monoxide diffusing capacity; Pred, prednisolone; Rx, treatment; VC, vital capacity.

The American Thoracic Society/European Respiratory Society (ATS/ERS) criteria for steroid therapy in sarcoidosis are summarized in Table 18.2.[1] The optimal dose and duration of therapy have not been established and are often individualized. Initial high-dose prednisolone 0.5 mg/kg/day (20–40 mg/day) aims to control active pulmonary disease. The response is evaluated after 1–2 months. Failure to respond after three months is unlikely to be associated with a response to longer steroid courses and a cause for failure should be sought (e.g. non-compliance, fibrotic change or steroid resistance). In steroid responders the dose is reduced to 10–15 mg daily for approximately three months, then tapered and continued at 5–7.5 mg daily for 6–24 months before a trial of withdrawal. Patients should be monitored for relapse during and after withdrawal of therapy. Recurrent relapses occur in some patients and may require long-term low-dose therapy. Bisphosphonates should be considered during steroid therapy to prevent osteoporosis. Prophylactic agents to prevent gastric ulceration may be required in those at risk.

Table 18.2 ATS/ERS criteria for steroid therapy in sarcoidosis

- Progressive symptomatic pulmonary disease
- Asymptomatic pulmonary disease with persistent or progressive loss of lung function
- Cardiac disease
- Neurological disease
- Eye disease not responding to topical therapy
- Symptomatic hypercalcaemia
- Other symptomatic/progressive extrapulmonary disease

The use of inhaled steroids in pulmonary sarcoidosis

The pathological processes in pulmonary sarcoidosis are distributed along lymphatic pathways particularly around bronchovascular bundles, and steroid delivery by the inhaled route is an attractive concept. Initial uncontrolled trials suggested favourable outcomes. Subsequently there have been six small (n = 9–22 treatment/10–25 placebo) controlled trials of inhaled steroids (800–2000 μg daily) in sarcoidosis,[4] four of which showed no benefit (Table 18.3). In the largest trial there were significant improvements in symptom score and inspiratory vital capacity, but not in DLCO or CXR appearance. The remaining study demonstrated improvement in serum β_2-microglobulin and bronchoalveolar lavage (BAL) fluid lymphocytosis but no clinical benefit. These small studies cannot exclude the potential benefit of inhaled steroids in subgroups with sarcoidosis. For example, bronchial hyperresponsiveness and cough are common particularly when associated with sarcoid bronchial infiltration (see Chapter 17) and the role of inhaled steroids remains to be elucidated in this group.

Table 18.3 Randomized controlled trials of inhaled steroid in pulmonary sarcoidosis[4]

First author, date	Patient numbers on treatment or control	Rx + follow-up months	Outcome
Erkkila S, 1988	9 Bud 800 μg/day; 10 placebo	2–2.5, 0	β_2-microglobulin + BAL lymphocytes improved
Milman N, 1994	9 Bud 1200 μg/day; 12 placebo	12, 6	No difference (40% Rx oral steroids)
Alberts C, 1995	22 Bud 1200 μg/day; 25 placebo	6, 7–8	No difference (75% Rx oral steroids)
Du Bois RM, 1999	21 Flut 2000 μg/day; 22 placebo	6, 0	No difference
McGrath D, 2002	15 Beclo 1600 μg/day; 12 placebo	12, 0	No difference
Baughman R, 2002	10 Flut 1600 μg/day; 11placebo	6, 6	Improved symptoms and VCI

BAL, bronchoalveolar lavage; Beclo, beclomethasone; Bud, budesonide; Flut, fluticasone; Rx, treatment; VCI, inspiratory vital capacity.

Therapeutic management of progressive pulmonary sarcoidosis

In this case the patient is dependent on high-dose steroid therapy but has developed unacceptable side effects. A number of other immunosuppressive or immunomodulatory agents can be used in the treatment of pulmonary sarcoidosis and should be considered:

- In steroid-insensitive disease (i.e. progression despite >15 mg prednisolone daily for >3–12 months);
- As steroid sparing agents in patients who benefit from steroid therapy but cannot taper below 15 mg prednisolone daily;
- For patients with significant steroid side effects.

Methotrexate, azathioprine and hydroxychloroquine are the preferred agents on the basis of safety and efficacy data. A systemic Cochrane review examining immunosuppressive and cytotoxic therapy in pulmonary sarcoidosis found only four controlled trials comparing methotrexate, chloroquine and ciclosporin therapies.[1,4] However, data on symptoms, lung function and radiographic changes were largely inconclusive but demonstrated that some of these therapies were associated with severe side effects and that benefit should be assessed regularly to justify the associated risk.

Cytotoxic agents are usually combined with steroids, act as steroid sparing agents and are of particular value in patients who respond well to steroids but have associated side effects (i.e. as in this case).

- **Methotrexate** is used in many chronic inflammatory and autoimmune disorders (e.g. rheumatoid disease). Experience is limited but small series suggest benefit in

40%–60% of patients with pulmonary and/or extrapulmonary sarcoidosis. Results from a randomized trial in acute sarcoidosis[7] and a number of other trials suggest that methotrexate at a dose of 10–25 mg/week is significantly steroid sparing after six months. Relapses are frequent after discontinuation of therapy. The white cell count (WCC) and LFT should be monitored at monthly intervals. Hepatotoxicity with hepatic fibrosis occurs in 10% of cases when the total dose of methotrexate exceeds 5 g. Methotrexate-induced interstitial pneumonitis is heralded by non-productive cough, fever and breathlessness and starts within days to weeks of commencing therapy. Peripheral eosinophilia (50%), hilar lymphadenopathy (15%) and pleural effusion (10%) may also occur. Recovery usually occurs after withdrawal of the drug.

- **Azathioprine** is used as a steroid sparing agent rather than a standalone therapy. The response rate as a second-line agent varies from 20% to 80%.[3] It is a purine analogue which is converted to mercaptopurine and impairs RNA and DNA synthesis. Cellular rather than humoral immunity is affected. The enzyme thiopurine methyltransferase (TPMT) metabolizes azathioprine and should be measured before treatment as myelosuppression is greater in patients with low TPMT enzyme activity. The initial dose is 50 mg/day for two weeks, increasing by 25 mg/day every two weeks until the recommended dose of 2 mg/kg is achieved (usually 100–150 mg/day; maximum dose 150 mg/day). Benefit may not be detected for 3–6 months. Bone marrow suppression, gastrointestinal complaints (e.g. nausea, diarrhoea) and abnormal LFT (although severe hepatitis is rare) are the main side effects. The WCC should be maintained above 4×10^9/l. Azathioprine may be a teratogen and must be used with care in women of childbearing age. An increased risk of malignancy has been reported in renal transplant patients treated with azathioprine.
- **Other cytotoxic agents** include cyclophosphamide, either as a daily regime (<150 mg/day) or as pulsed therapy (0.5–1.0 g at 2–4-weekly intervals), which is used occasionally in pulmonary sarcoidosis and as a second-line drug in patients whose condition is deteriorating despite steroid therapy. Toxicity, in particular marrow suppression, cystitis, infertility, hepatotoxicity and teratogenicity, limits use. Chlorambucil has been used as a steroid sparing agent in sarcoidosis with reported benefit but is rarely used in non-neoplastic diseases because of the potential risk of malignancy (e.g. leukaemia). Ciclosporin is not associated with clinical improvement in pulmonary sarcoidosis.

Immunomodulators have been used successfully in selected patients with sarcoidosis. Many modulate the activity of TNF-α which has been implicated in granuloma formation.

- **Antimalarial drugs**, chloroquine and hydroxychloroquine, inhibit macrophage production of TNF-α. Chloroquine is often used in cutaneous sarcoid or neurosarcoid but also reduces disease activity in pulmonary sarcoidosis.[8] Unfortunately, benefit is not maintained after treatment is stopped and it can cause irreversible retinopathy and blindness. Treatment is best limited to six months. Hydroxychloroquine is preferred as it is less oculotoxic and can be used for long periods. A retrospective review suggests that hydroxychloroquine is less effective than azathioprine or methotrexate.[9]
- **Anti-TNF agents**. Infliximab is a murine monoclonal antibody that specifically blocks the effect of TNF-α. Limited data suggest benefit in the treatment of refrac-

tory pulmonary sarcoidosis,[10] but the associated breakdown in cell-mediated immunity risks reactivation of, or new infection with, tuberculosis. Etanercept blocks the TNF-α receptor but a preliminary trial in stage II and III pulmonary sarcoidosis was stopped after interval assessment due to treatment failure in 11 of 17 enrolled patients.

- **Pentoxifylline** (12.5 mg/kg twice daily), a xanthine useful in vascular insufficiency, also inhibits alveolar macrophage TNF-α synthesis. In a trial of 23 previously untreated patients with active sarcoidosis, 11 patients improved and the others remained stable.[11] Three previously refractory patients improved when pentoxifylline was added to the steroid regime. Gastrointestinal side effects prevented use in three patients.
- **Thalidomide** blocks release of alveolar macrophage TNF-α and is beneficial in chronic cutaneous sarcoidosis.[3] However, thalidomide enhances interferon gamma production, which is increased in active pulmonary sarcoidosis and may explain the lack of efficacy of thalidomide in pulmonary sarcoidosis.[12]

Lung transplantation in end-stage sarcoid-induced pulmonary fibrosis

Fortunately, mortality from severe pulmonary sarcoidosis has fallen with steroid therapy. However, lung transplantation offers the only hope of survival in the small number of patients with end-stage pulmonary fibrosis (stage IV disease). Pulmonary hypertension, oxygen dependence and African-American ethnicity are associated with increased surgical mortality, and extensive extrapulmonary disease (e.g. cardiac) may preclude transplantation. Although non-caseating granulomas may initially develop in the allografts of sarcoidosis patients, they disappear within a few months and significant organ dysfunction does not occur. Acute rejection episodes can be severe and lymphocytic bronchiolitis is more common following transplantation in sarcoid patients. The long-term outcome is unaffected despite the enhanced immune stimulation.

Conclusion

In this case the patient has been treated with prednisolone 7.5 mg/day and azathioprine 100 mg/day for the last four years, with regular blood checks and spirometry at eight-week intervals and CXR at six-month intervals. There has been no further deterioration in her spirometry or CXR. The DLCO has not deteriorated over this period.

Further Reading

1 Joint Statement of the American Thoracic Society (ATS), the European Respiratory Society (ERS) and the World Association of Sarcoidosis and Other Granulomatous Disorders (WASOG) adopted by the ATS Board of Directors and by the ERS Executive Committee, February 1999. Statement on sarcoidosis. *Am J Respir Crit Care Med* 1999; **160**: 736–55.

2 Wells AU, Hirani N. Interstitial lung disease guideline. British Thoracic Society in collaboration with Thoracic Society of Australia and New Zealand and the Irish Thoracic Society. *Thorax* 2008; **63**(Suppl 5): v1–v58.

3 Baughman RP, Lower EE, du Bois RM. Sarcoidosis. *Lancet* 2003; **361**: 1111–8.

4 Grutters JC, van den Bosch JMM. Corticosteroid treatment in sarcoidosis. *Eur Respir J* 2006; **28**: 627–36.

5 Paramothayan NS, Lasserson TJ, Jones PW. Corticosteroids for pulmonary sarcoidosis. *Cochrane Database Syst Rev* 2005; CD001114.

6 Gibson GJ, Prescott RJ, Muers MF *et al.* British Thoracic Society Sarcoidosis study: effects of long term corticosteroid treatment. *Thorax* 1996; **51**: 238–47.

7 Baughman RP, Winget DB, Lower EE. Methotrexate is steroid sparing in acute sarcoidosis: results of a double blind, randomized trial. *Sarcoidosis Vasc Diffuse Lung Dis* 2000; **17**: 60–6.

8 Baltzan M, Mehta S, Kirkham TH, Cosio MG. Randomized trial of prolonged chloroquine therapy in advanced pulmonary sarcoidosis. *Am J Respir Crit Care Med* 1999; **160**: 192–7.

9 Baughman RP, Lower EE. Alternatives to corticosteroids in the treatment of sarcoidosis. *Sarcoidosis Vasc Diffuse Lung Dis* 1997; **14**: 121–30.

10 Baughman RP, Lower EE. Infliximab for refractory sarcoidosis. *Sarcoidosis Vasc Diffuse Lung Dis* 2001; **18**: 70–4.

11 Zabel P, Entzian P, Dalhoff K, Schlaak M. Pentoxifylline in treatment of sarcoidosis. *Am J Respir Crit Care Med* 1997; **155**: 1655–69.

12 Baughman RP, Judson MA, Teirstein AS, Moller DR, Lower EE. Thalidomide for chronic sarcoidosis. *Chest* 2002; **122**: 227–32.

PROBLEM

19 Hypersensitivity Pneumonitis

Elizabeth Hadley, Boris Lams

Case History

A 49-year-old Cypriot woman was referred with a nine-month history of gradually increasing breathlessness and a dry cough. She was breathless at 100 yards. She had never smoked. She moved to England from Cyprus one year before presentation. She had no chest pain or fevers. In the preceding year she had lost 13 kg in weight. She had already seen a gastroenterologist because of the weight loss. At that time it was noted that she had an erythrocyte sedimentation rate (ESR) of 64 mm/hr and a normal gastroscopy, colonoscopy and abdominal ultrasound.

On examination she was thin. She was not clubbed. She had bilateral basal crepitations; the rest of the examination was normal. Her chest X-ray showed a subtle infiltrate predominantly in the lower zones of both lung fields. Lung function tests (Table 19.1) and a high-resolution computed tomography (HRCT) chest scan (Figure 19.1) were performed.

What is the diagnosis?

What is the pathophysiology of hypersensitivity pneumonitis?

What is acute, subacute and chronic hypersensitivity pneumonitis?

What is the management of hypersensitivity pneumonitis?

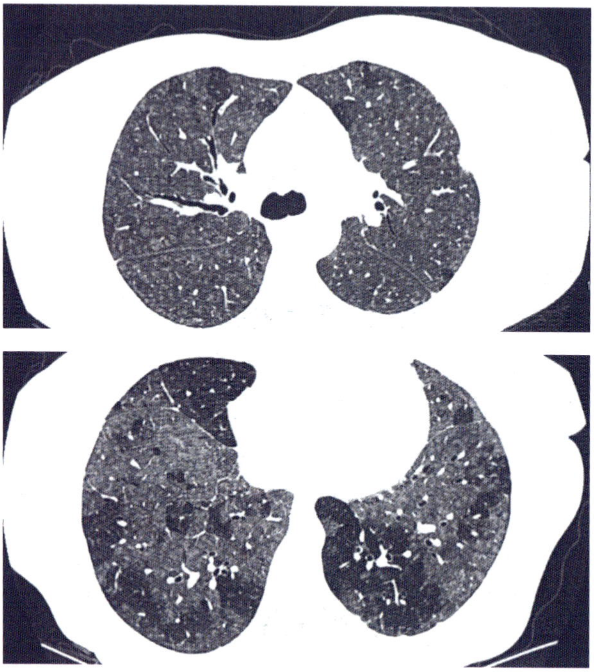

Figure 19.1 HRCT chest scan at presentation.

Background

Diagnosis

The spirometry shows evidence of restrictive lung disease with a reduced forced expiratory volume in 1 second (FEV_1) and reduced forced vital capacity (FVC) and an FEV_1/FVC ratio at the upper end of normal. The raised residual volume is suggestive of gas trapping. Her gas transfer (TLCO) is reduced suggesting she has either a reduction in alveolar capillary blood volume or a reduction of diffusion through the alveolar capillary membrane.

Table 19.1 Lung function at presentation and at one and two months after treatment

	At presentation		One month later (after giving up budgerigar)	Two months later (after 4 weeks of corticosteroids)
	Value	% Predicted	Value	Value
FEV_1	1.69	74	2.21	2.42
FVC	2.01	74	2.63	2.82
FEV_1/FVC	0.84	106	0.83	0.79
TLC	4.5	99		4.19
RV	2.46	150		1.22
RV/TLC	0.54	150		0.80
TLCO	2.93	39	4.28	4.90
VA	3.42	76	4.13	4.39
KCO	0.85	51	1.04	1.12

KCO, carbon monoxide gas transfer corrected for alveolar volume; RV, residual volume; TLC, total lung capacity; TLCO, carbon monoxide gas transfer; VA, alveolar volume.

The HRCT chest scan shows widespread ground glass shadowing preferentially affecting the upper zones. There are diffuse centrilobular nodules most striking in the upper zones and a mosaic pattern with areas of reduced attenuation in the lower zones consistent with air trapping. These three HRCT scan findings, of ground glass shadowing, centrilobular nodules and mosaic pattern, are characteristic of hypersensitivity pneumonitis (HP), also known as extrinsic allergic alveolitis.

A full exposure history was taken from the patient. She had kept a budgerigar at home for the past five years. A test for avian precipitins was sent and was weakly positive for pigeon and chicken, and strongly positive for budgerigar, parrot and cockatiel.

She agreed to a bronchoscopy and transbronchial biopsy. The bronchoalveolar lavage fluid contained a high number of lymphocytes, characteristic of hypersensitivity pneumonitis. The transbronchial biopsies revealed marked infiltration of alveolar spaces and alveolar walls by foamy macrophages. No granulomas were seen and there was no evidence of malignancy. The patient was diagnosed with subacute hypersensitivity pneumonitis (bird fancier's lung).

Pathophysiology

Hypersensitivity pneumonitis represents a complex immune-mediated pulmonary disorder of varying intensity and clinical presentation. It is characterized by a T-cell response of the lung parenchyma and airways following exposure to an organic antigen to which the patient has been previously sensitized. Over 300 of these organic antigens have been identified.[1–3]

Up to 15% of people who keep pigeons as a hobby will develop symptoms attributable to HP. The fact that the remainder do not suggests that individual host susceptibility factors play a role in pathogenesis. The majority of cases of HP occur in non-smokers, a fact that has been attributed to the immunosuppressive effect of tobacco smoke.[3]

Particularly interesting is the wide range of potential antigens. There are numerous inciting antigens including agricultural dusts, bioaerosols, microorganisms and chemicals. For example, farmer's lung can be due to a number of substances containing antigens such as mouldy hay (thermophilic actinomycetes), mouldy cheese (*Penicillium casei*, *Aspergillus clavatus*), tobacco plant (*Aspergillus* species), mushroom spores, mould on grapes (*Botrytis cinerea*), coffee bean dust and tea plants. The disease is constantly evolving with new antigens being reported every year. 'Hot tub lung' was first described in 2002 where the inciting antigen is *Mycobacterium avium* complex.[4] Since its first description it has rapidly become one of the most common documented causes of new cases of HP worldwide and may account for up to 20% of cases in some populations in the developed world.[5]

Several different classification schemes of HP exist but the simplest divides the disease into acute, subacute and chronic forms. There is considerable overlap between these forms of HP.[6]

Subacute hypersensitivity pneumonitis

As in the case presented here, subacute HP presents insidiously with a cough, dyspnoea, anorexia and weight loss. There may be a low-grade fever. Examination typically reveals tachypnoea and bilateral crepitations. Clubbing is rare. Chest X-ray appearances may be completely normal or show alveolar shadowing with a predominantly upper-zone distribution.

HRCT characteristically reveals ground glass shadowing usually with an upper-zone predominance, centrilobular nodules and evidence of air trapping. The ground glass shadowing is thought to represent underlying alveolar inflammation below the resolution of HRCT. A mosaic pattern is common in patients with HP; it was present in 19 out of 20 patients in one reported series.[7] Areas of increased lucency on the HRCT scan represent trapped air. Air trapping on the HRCT scan correlates with the raised residual volume seen on lung function tests. Centrilobular nodules characteristically spare the subpleural zone and do not affect interlobar fissures, in contrast to those in sarcoidosis. They are thought to represent the bronchiolitic component of the disease.[8,9]

Lung function can show a restrictive, obstructive or mixed pattern with the restrictive pattern being the correlate of the underlying alveolitis, and the obstructive that of the underlying air trapping related to bronchiolitis. TLCO is reduced. Exertional hypoxaemia is typically present, but resting hypoxaemia usually does not occur unless the patient has experienced a series of recurrent episodes over months to years. However, pulmonary function tests and arterial oxygen tension may be entirely normal between subacute episodes. Laboratory tests are typically normal, although lymphopenia may occur.

Bronchoalveolar lavage reveals a lymphocytosis with a characteristic raised CD8/CD4 ratio. Lung biopsy may reveal well-formed granulomas, evidence of a bronchiolitis and interstitial fibrosis.[1,10]

Transbronchial or lung biopsy should be considered in those people where the diagnosis of HP remains uncertain. It can be especially difficult to distinguish non-specific interstitial pneumonia from HP. Pathological features of HP include a lymphocytic infiltration in the alveolar walls, typically in a bronchocentric distribution. There may be small, poorly formed, non-caseating granulomas located around the bronchioles. Foamy macrophages may be seen within the alveolar spaces.

Serum precipitins are circulating serum immunoglobulin G antibodies against a specific antigen and indicate exposure to that antigen. They do not necessarily imply the existence of a resultant HP. As an example, 30% to 40% of farmers have positive serum precipitins to common causes of HP in the absence of clinical disease. The incidence of serum precipitins in asymptomatic bird breeders is even higher, probably due to more intense and prolonged exposure to inciting antigens.[11] Conversely, the absence of serum precipitins does not exclude HP because of the presence of false negatives. Although this is primarily because commercial assays test for only a small fraction of the potential causative antigens, the test may be non-reactive in some cases even if the correct antigen is included.

Skin-prick tests, which test for immediate type 1 hypersensitivity reactions, are not relevant to the diagnosis of HP. The strongest single predictor of HP is exposure to a known inciting antigen, which is present in most patients. Establishing a history of exposure is key to the diagnosis of HP.

Acute hypersensitivity pneumonitis

Acute HP is probably the most common form of HP but is under-recognized. It tends to start 4–8 hours after exposure to an antigen and typically resembles the early stages of influenza with fevers, chills and myalgia. Assuming that the exposure was a single event, the symptoms tend to resolve untreated over 1–2 days. In a similar fashion to people with peanut allergies, the symptoms tend to get worse with successive exposures until help is sought. It can therefore present as a severe acute respiratory illness.

In acute HP the chest X-ray typically shows bilateral pulmonary infiltrates, which resolve with time and/or treatment. Patients may have a neutrophilia and raised ESR and C-reactive protein. They may also be lymphopenic, and may have a positive rheumatoid factor. Serum immunoglobulin E is not normally raised. In between episodes the patient is usually well with a normal chest X-ray.

Chronic hypersensitivity pneumonitis

Chronic HP refers to the proportion of patients with HP – about 1 in 20 – that go on to develop chronic irreversible fibrotic pulmonary damage. This is seen in patients who present late and in those who are unwilling or unable to avoid antigen exposure over a prolonged period. The clinical appearance of such patients is of a breathless patient with a cough, often productive. They are often thin and may be clubbed. They have bilateral crackles on auscultation and are often hypoxic. HRCT findings are variable, but usually confirm areas of established fibrosis mixed with areas of ground glass shadowing, areas of lucency and centrilobular nodules.

It may be impossible to discern the offending antigen in chronic HP as serum precipitins are often undetectable and the exposure history is non-specific. Patients with chronic HP due to 'bird-fancier's lung' are at especially high risk of progressive pulmonary fibrosis and therefore carry a worse prognosis.[12–14]

Management

The primary treatment of HP is to avoid the offending inhaled antigen. Corticosteroids are also useful to assist in recovery. Difficulties can occur with patients who are unwilling or unable to stay away from the antigen causing their HP. This may be because of employment (e.g. farmers) or attachment to a hobby (e.g. pigeon fanciers).

In this case the patient removed the budgerigar and all associated equipment. One month later she returned saying that she felt better but admitted to some residual dyspnoea on exertion. Her repeat lung function tests revealed an improvement although her TLCO remained abnormal (Table 19.1). She was then started on prednisolone at 30 mg a day and a lung function test was performed a month later (Table 19.1). Her symptoms resolved. The corticosteroids were weaned and she has remained well.

Conclusion

Hypersensitivity pneumonitis is a fascinating and probably under-diagnosed condition. It is characterized by lung inflammation in response to organic antigens. Corticosteroids and avoidance of the offending antigen are effective treatment.

Further Reading

1 Selman M. Hypersensitivity pneumonitis: a multifaceted deceiving disorder. *Clin Chest Med* 2004; **25**: 531–47.

2 Agostini C, Trentin L, Facco M, Semenzato G. New aspects of hypersensitivity pneumonitis. *Curr Opin Pulm Med* 2004; **10**: 378–82.

3 Cormier Y, Lacasse Y. Keys to the diagnosis of hypersensitivity pneumonitis: the role of serum precipitins, lung biopsy, and high-resolution computed tomography. *Clin Pulm Med* 1996; **3**: 77.

4 Rickman OB, Ryu JH, Fidler ME, Kalra S. Hypersensitivity pneumonitis associated with *Mycobacterium avium* complex and hot tub use. *Mayo Clin Proc* 2002; **77**: 1233–7.

5 Hanak V, Golbin JM, Ryu J. Causes and presenting features in 85 consecutive patients with hypersensitivity pneumonitis. *Mayo Clin Proc* 2007; **82**: 812–6.

6 Richerson HB, Bernstein IL, Fink JN *et al.* Guidelines for the clinical evaluation of hypersensitivity pneumonitis. *J Allergy Clin Immunol* 1989; **84**: 839–44.

7 Hansell DM, Wells AU, Padley SP, Müller NL. Hypersensitivity pneumonitis: correlation of individual CT patterns with functional abnormalities. *Radiology* 1996; **199**: 123–8.

8 Glazer CS, Rose CS, Lynch DA. Clinical and radiologic manifestations of hypersensitivity pneumonitis. *J Thorac Imaging* 2002; **17**: 261–72.

9 Tateishi T, Ohtani Y, Takemura T *et al.* Serial high-resolution computed tomography findings of acute and chronic hypersensitivity pneumonitis induced by avian antigen. *J Comput Assist Tomogr* 2011; **35**: 272–9.

10 Reyes CN, Wenzel FJ, Lawton BR, Emanuel DA. The pulmonary pathology of farmer's lung disease. *Chest* 1982; **81**: 142–6.

11 King TE Jr. Diagnosis of hypersensitivity pneumonitis (extrinsic allergic alveolitis). UpToDate, 2009. www.uptodate.com (accessed 01 06 11).

12 Pérez-Padilla R, Salas J, Chapela R *et al.* Mortality in Mexican patients with chronic pigeon breeder's lung compared with those with usual interstitial pneumonia. *Am Rev Respir Dis* 1993; **148**: 29–53.

13 Lima MS, Coletta EN, Ferreira RG *et al.* Subacute and chronic hypersensitivity pneumonitis: histopathological patterns and survival. *Respir Med* 2009; **103**: 508–15.

14 Bang KM, Weissman DN, Pinheiro GA, Antao VC, Wood JM, Syamlal G. Twenty-three years of hypersensitivity pneumonitis mortality surveillance in the United States. *Am J Ind Med* 2006; **49**: 997–1004.

PROBLEM

20 Amiodarone Pulmonary Toxicity

Elizabeth Hadley, Boris Lams, Christopher Kosky

Case History

A 72-year-old woman presented to hospital with shortness of breath. Two years prior to presentation she had been commenced on amiodarone 200 mg a day for non-sustained ventricular tachycardia. One month prior, she developed shortness of breath, a cough and weight loss. Thyroid function tests at that time revealed she was thyrotoxic and the amiodarone was stopped. She was commenced on propylthiouracil and prednisolone for amiodarone-induced thyrotoxicosis and her symptoms resolved. Her prednisolone was tapered and stopped ten days prior to admission. Four days prior to admission, she noticed increasing shortness of breath.

On examination, her temperature was 36.7°C. Jugular venous pressure was not elevated. Heart sounds were normal with no third heart sound. She had bi-basal crepitations. Her oxygen saturation was 86% on room air. Arterial blood gas analysis revealed partial pressures of oxygen (PaO_2) 8.4 kPa and carbon dioxide ($PaCO_2$) 4.7 kPa and pH 7.36. Her full blood count revealed a haemoglobin level of 12.5 g/dl, white cell count of 14.7×10^9, neutrophil count of 14.0×10^9 and platelet count 307×10^9. Her C-reactive protein was 93 mg/l and renal function was normal. A chest radiograph (CXR) showed bilateral patchy mid and lower zone shadowing. The changes are new compared with a chest radiograph taken six months before presentation. A high-resolution computed tomography (HRCT) chest scan was performed (Figure 20.1).

What does the HRCT chest scan show and what is the diagnosis?

What are the risk factors associated with amiodarone pulmonary toxicity?

How can the diagnosis of amiodarone pulmonary toxicity be confirmed?

How is amiodarone pulmonary toxicity treated?

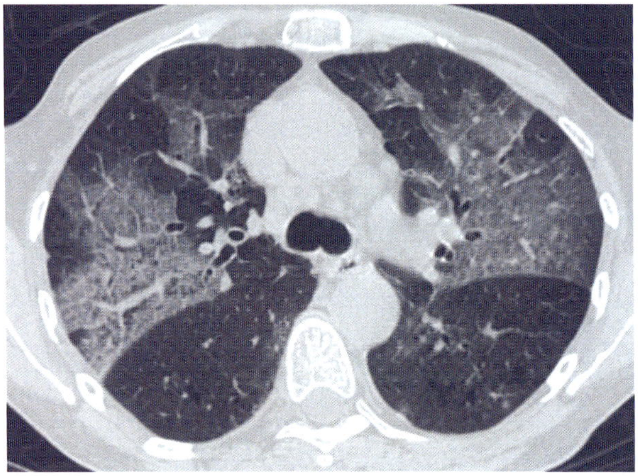

Figure 20.1 HRCT chest scan.

Background

In this case the HRCT shows widespread areas of demarcated ground glass shadowing throughout the lungs. The differential diagnosis of ground glass appearance includes pulmonary oedema, viral pneumonia, *Pneumocystis jirovecii* pneumonia, alveolar haemorrhage, acute interstitial pneumonia, early hypersensitivity pneumonitis, acute eosinophilic pneumonia and drug-induced lung disease. Amiodarone-induced pulmonary toxicity is the most likely diagnosis.

There are four patterns of amiodarone pulmonary toxicity. The commonest presentation is that of a chronic interstitial pneumonitis with progressive dyspnoea and cough, focal or diffuse interstitial changes on chest radiology and a fibrotic picture on biopsy. The second pattern, as in this case, is an acute organizing pneumonia. This presents with cough, fever and bilateral alveolar or ground glass opacities. Amiodarone pulmonary toxicity has also been reported to cause a solitary pulmonary opacity mimicking lung malignancy. Finally, amiodarone causes acute respiratory distress syndrome (ARDS). Case reports exist of amiodarone-induced alveolar haemorrhage and pleural effusions.[1–3]

Risk factors

The cumulative dose of amiodarone is an important risk factor for the development of amiodarone pulmonary toxicity. Toxicity typically occurs months to years after starting amiodarone. Daily doses of amiodarone above 400 mg/day are associated with 10%–15% incidence of pulmonary toxicity. However, there is also an appreciable incidence of lung disease with lower daily doses of amiodarone.[4–6]

Pre-existing lung disease may predispose to the development of amiodarone pulmonary toxicity. Surgery and pulmonary angiography have been reported to be risk factors for the development of the ARDS-type reaction in patients using amiodarone peri-operatively.

Early studies suggests dronedarone, an anti-arrhythmic related to amiodarone, does not cause pulmonary toxicity.[7]

Diagnosis

Proving the presence of amiodarone-induced lung disease can be difficult and to some extent the diagnosis is one of exclusion. Foamy macrophages in bronchoalveolar lavage (BAL) fluid are characteristically found in amiodarone pulmonary toxicity. The foamy appearance is due to macrophages accumulating phospholipids as a result of amiodarone causing inhibition of the enzyme phosphodiesterase A. The presence of foamy macrophages, in BAL fluid or biopsy specimens, does not in itself confirm the diagnosis as these cells are also seen in those exposed to amiodarone without lung disease. However, if foamy macrophages are not present amiodarone pulmonary toxicity is unlikely.

The BAL fluid in amiodarone-induced lung disease is also often found to contain neutrophils and CD8 lymphocytes, which is unusual in specimens from patients with an acute lung injury.

Transbronchial lung biopsy may reveal changes consistent with an underlying organizing pneumonia associated with amiodarone. Biopsy may not be helpful if the amiodarone-induced pathology is fibrotic, or there is non-specific interstitial pneumonitis or diffuse alveolar damage. Transbronchial lung biopsy may also be useful to exclude malignancy or infection. Open lung or video-assisted thoracoscopic surgical lung biopsy should be avoided because of the occurrence of ARDS after thoracic surgical procedures in patients with amiodarone pulmonary toxicity.[5,6,8]

Treatment

In patients with amiodarone pulmonary toxicity, amiodarone should be stopped immediately. However, amiodarone has a long half-life due to accumulation in fatty tissue, which can mean it continues to act for up to 45 days. Prednisolone 1 mg/kg tapered over two to six months is the usual treatment. Lung function usually returns to normal.[9] The mortality rate is low except for the amiodarone-induced ARDS reaction which carries a high mortality.

In this case, the patient described was commenced on prednisolone at a dose of 50 mg/day. Corticosteroids were gradually tapered over two months. There was resolution of her symptoms, hypoxia and radiological changes without recurrence of her pulmonary symptoms.

Conclusion

Amiodarone pulmonary toxicity is an under-recognized condition that will respond to treatment if caught at an early stage. Current recommendations are that a patient started on long-term amiodarone should have a CXR and baseline pulmonary function tests including transfer factor, and that these should be repeated at intervals of 3–6 months in the first two years of treatment.

Further Reading

1 Martin WJ, Rosenow EC. Amiodarone pulmonary toxicity. Recognition and pathogenesis (Part 1). *Chest* 1988; **93**: 1067–75.

2 Martin WJ, Rosenow EC. Amiodarone pulmonary toxicity. Recognition and pathogenesis (Part 2). *Chest* 1988; **93**: 1242–8.

3 Tanawuttiwat T, Harindhanavudhi T, Hanif S, Sahloul MZ. Amiodarone-induced alveolar haemorrhage: a rare complication of a common medication. *Heart Lung Circ* 2010; **19**: 435–7.

4 Vorperian VR, Havighurst TC, Miller S, January CT. Adverse effects of low dose amiodarone: a meta-analysis. *J Am Coll Cardiol* 1997; **30**: 791–8.

5 Schwaiblmair M, Berghaus T, Haeckel T, Wagner T, von Scheidt W. Amiodarone-induced pulmonary toxicity: an under-recognized and severe adverse effect? *Clin Res Cardiol* 2010; **99**: 693–700.

6 Papiris SA, Triantafillidou C, Kolilekas L, Markoulaki D, Manali ED. Amiodarone: review of pulmonary effects and toxicity. *Drug Saf* 2010; **33**: 539–58.

7 Singh D, Cingolani E, Diamond G, Kaul S. Dronedarone for atrial fibrillation: have we expanded the antiarrhythmic armamentarium? *J Am Coll Cardiol* 2010; **55**: 1569–76.

8 Greenspon AJ, Kidwell GA, Hurley W, Mannion J. Amiodarone-related postoperative adult respiratory distress syndrome. *Circulation* 1991; **84**(Suppl 3): 407–15.

9 The Drug-Induced Lung Diseases. www.pneumotox.com (accessed 06 05 11).

SECTION FOUR 04

Lung Cancer

PROBLEM

21 Small Cell Lung Cancer (SCLC)

Oni Choudhury, Richard Leach

Case History

A 62-year-old woman presented with a 2–3-month history of breathlessness, non-productive cough, weight loss, lethargy and ankle oedema. Her exercise tolerance was limited to 50 yards by breathlessness. Past medical history included osteoarthritis, eczema and oesophagitis. Her father had died from lung cancer aged 57 years old. She was a chronic smoker with a 50 pack-year history. On examination the patient's face and right arm were swollen. A 5 cm lymph node was palpable in the right supraclavicular fossa. Chest auscultation revealed reduced air entry at the right base. No organomegaly was detected on abdominal examination.

Routine blood tests were normal apart from hyponatraemia (sodium 129 mmol/l). The chest radiograph demonstrated a right hilar mass with some volume loss and associated elevation of the right diaphragm (Figure 21.1). A subsequent chest and abdominal computed tomography (CT) scan revealed a large pre-tracheal mass displacing the superior vena cava and a 1 cm nodule in the anterior segment of the right upper lobe. Bronchoscopy and bronchial biopsy confirmed a small cell lung cancer (SCLC).

How would you stage the SCLC in this patient?

What is the likely cause of the hyponatraemia?

What factors determine therapy and prognosis in SCLC?

How is SCLC treated?

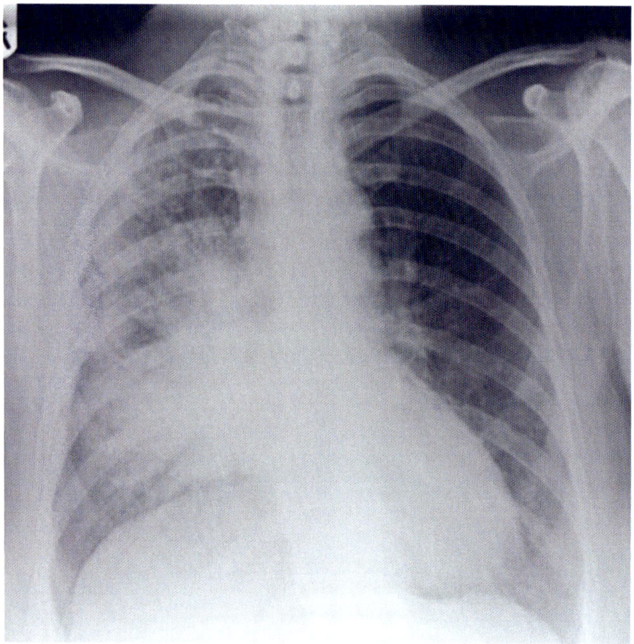

Figure 21.1 Chest radiograph.

Background

Small cell lung cancer (SCLC) causes 15%–25% of all lung cancers. They arise from neuroendocrine cells in the bronchial mucosa and typically present as a central mass with lymph node enlargement. They are aggressive tumours that invade blood vessels and lymphatics and at presentation 65%–70% have widespread metastases. Intrathoracic spread causes superior vena cava obstruction (SVCO) with facial and arm oedema (more often than in non-small cell lung cancer [NSCLC]), recurrent laryngeal palsy with hoarseness, phrenic nerve palsy with diaphragmatic paralysis, compression of the oesophagus with dysphagia and tracheal compression with stridor.

Untreated the median survival time is <4 months from diagnosis. Surgery is rarely appropriate and although SCLC is chemo- and radiosensitive, median survival time is only approximately twelve months in extensive disease (with a two-year survival rate of 4.6%) and 20 months in limited disease (with two- and five-year survival rates of 45% and 20%, respectively) using optimal therapy.[1,2]

Staging of SCLC

The purpose of staging is to determine management and prognosis. Following clinical, biochemical (e.g. liver function tests, calcium) and radiological (e.g. chest radiograph, CT scans of the chest, liver and adrenals, and selected imaging of symptomatic areas) evaluation for distant metastases, SCLC is staged as either:

- **Limited disease**, defined as a tumour that can be encompassed within one radiotherapy field. It includes patients with tumour confined to one hemithorax (including pleural effusion) and involving bilateral hilar and/or supraclavicular lymphadenopathy. About 40% of cases are classified as 'limited' at diagnosis. Untreated, median survival is 4–6 months.

- **Extensive disease** describes widespread disease beyond the definition of 'limited' disease and includes distant metastases (e.g. cerebral) and involvement of the contralateral lung. About 60% of cases are extensive at presentation and untreated median survival is approximately three months.

Paraneoplastic features of SCLC

Paraneoplastic syndromes are characteristic constellations of symptoms and signs associated with lung and other cancers but not directly related to the tumour or its metastases. They may precede clinical and radiographic tumour detection. Tumour hormone secretion or hormone/peptide-like substances, autoimmune phenomena including serum autoantibodies (e.g. anti-Hu; see below), growth factors or other factors may be responsible. They are often non-specific.

The syndrome of inappropriate antidiuretic hormone (SIADH) secretion occurs in 5%–10% of SCLC cases and 0.7% of NSCLC cases. Tumour release of antidiuretic hormone causes excessive water retention with associated hyponatraemia (<135 mmol/l) and serum hypo-osmolality. It presents with lethargy and confusion when serum sodium falls below 120–130 mmol/l. Diagnosis is confirmed by a low serum osmolality (<280 mOsm/kg) in the presence of a high urine osmolality (>100 mOsm/kg) and/or urinary sodium (>40 mmol/l) but normal acid-base balance and renal function. Patients are managed by restricting fluid intake (initially approximately 1 l/day). Demeclocycline (150–300 mg twice daily), a tetracycline derivative that blocks antidiuretic hormone action in distal renal tubules, is occasionally required. Use of hypertonic saline is best avoided as it may cause seizures and irreversible central pontine myelinolysis due to the associated rapid changes in serum osmolality. In SCLC, SIADH usually resolves a few weeks after chemotherapy.

Other endocrine paraneoplastic syndromes include ectopic adrenocorticotropic hormone syndrome which occurs in 5% of SCLC. Typically, it presents with hypokalaemia, alkalosis and mild hypertension. Hypercalcaemia occurs in 40% of cases, most commonly due to bone metastases, but it may also be the result of ectopic parathyroid hormone-related peptide production, especially in NSCLC. Ectopic melanocyte-stimulating hormone may cause hyperpigmentation. Thromboembolic events are also common in patients with lung cancer.

Other paraneoplastic features include fever, anorexia, cachexia, clubbing and hypertrophic pulmonary osteoarthropathy, acanthosis nigricans (hyperpigmentation in flexor areas) and dermatomyositis-polymyositis. Neurological syndromes are common and may be rapidly progressive. Type 1 anti-neuronal nuclear antibody (ANNA-1), also known as 'anti-Hu', is a marker of neurological autoimmunity and is strongly linked with SCLC (97%). Typical neurological syndromes include peripheral neuropathy (mainly sensory), cerebellar syndrome with progressive ataxia and limbic encephalitis. Eaton–Lambert syndrome (5%) is a myasthenia-like syndrome caused by ANNA-1 or immunoglobulin G autoantibodies and may pre-date detectable cancer by 2–4 years.

Factors that determine therapy and prognosis in SCLC

Selection of appropriate treatment and subsequent survival are not only determined by the extent of the disease (i.e. limited, extensive) but also by factors that indicate 'good' or 'poor' prognosis. Significant factors indicating poor prognosis are impaired performance status (i.e. patients who 'ambulate' for <50% of their waking hours), weight loss (>10% in six months), relapsed disease, elevated lactate dehydrogenase level, age and male sex.[1] However, even in good prognostic groups, median survival is only approximately 12–20 months.[1,2] It is important to establish treatment goals before initiating therapy.

Management of SCLC

Surgery is not suitable in most cases of SCLC as haematogenous spread will have occurred before diagnosis. Occasionally surgical resection is possible if bone and brain scanning show no evidence of metastasis. Nevertheless, post-operative chemotherapy is recommended for micrometastases.

Concurrent combination chemo-radiotherapy is the mainstay of treatment in both limited and extensive disease with an 80%–90% and 60%–80% response rate, respectively.[1–4] Even in patients with poor performance status, response is associated with quality of life benefits. Combination (as compared to single agent) chemotherapy is accepted widely as being associated with superior response rates and survival.[1,3]

SCLC responds rapidly to chemotherapy, with the risk of rapid tumour lysis and associated potentially life-threatening electrolyte abnormalities and renal impairment, especially in extensive disease. Prevention includes adequate hydration and, if possible, pre-medication with allopurinol. Unfortunately, relapse is usually rapid.

- **First-line induction chemotherapy** is usually with a platinum-based agent (e.g. cisplatin) and etoposide (or irinotecan) given every three weeks for 4–6 cycles (if the patient is well enough to tolerate the treatment).[1,3–5] The response rate is greater if etoposide is given over three days. In a randomized trial of 440 patients (of whom approximately half had limited-stage disease) combination chemotherapy with cisplatin and etoposide (PE) was superior to the previously preferred anthracycline-based (i.e. epirubicin) regime of epirubicin, cyclophosphamide and vincristine (ECV), with a mean survival time of 14.5 versus 9.7 months, two-year survival of 14% versus 6% and five-year survival of 5% versus 2%, respectively (P <0.0005).[3] Other regimes used in SCLC include the 'CAVE' regime (i.e. cyclophosphamide, doxorubicin, vincristine, etoposide), 'PEC' regime (paclitaxel, etoposide, carboplatin) and single agents (e.g. topotecan, which has a 50% response rate in previously untreated patients, or etoposide). In patients with impaired renal function, significant comorbidity or poor performance status, consider the use of carboplatin as part of a less intense regime but assess the response and toxicity before each cycle, especially in extensive disease.[1]
- **Second-line chemotherapy** may be considered if the patient relapses after first-line treatment and is able to tolerate further therapy.[1,5] If suitable, offer treatment with an anthracycline-containing or further platinum-based regime (maximum six cycles). If the relapse is >6 months after induction therapy, repeating the induction regime may be considered. Patients should be informed that there is limited evidence that second-line treatment will be beneficial if there was no response to first-line therapy. Second-line chemotherapy is generally most useful in patients who responded to first-line chemotherapy with a response that was sustained for at least three months and who have a reasonable performance status.[1,5,6] There is no convincing evidence to support one second-line regime over another.

Radiotherapy has an important role in treatment of SCLC.

- **Thoracic radiotherapy** is associated with a median survival benefit of about one month with a 6% improvement in two-year survival (i.e. chemotherapy alone 13% vs the addition of radiotherapy 19%).[1,5,7] Concurrent radiotherapy during chemotherapy, as compared with sequential (i.e. after completion of chemotherapy) radiotherapy, is associated with survival benefits in patients with 'limited' disease and a good performance status. Consequently, National Institute for Health and Clinical Excellence guidelines recommend that thoracic radiotherapy should start during the first or second chemotherapy cycles.[1,8] If the patient is unfit for concurrent chemoradiotherapy, and responded to chemotherapy, offer sequential radical radiotherapy within six weeks of completion of chemotherapy.

  In patients with extensive disease (e.g. cerebral metastases) consider thoracic radiation after chemotherapy if there has been a good response at distant sites and at least a good partial response in the thorax.

  Palliative radiotherapy is effective for symptoms related to the primary tumour or metastases (e.g. airway compression, haemoptysis, SVCO).
- **Prophylactic cranial irradiation (PCI)**. The brain is the primary site of extrathoracic recurrence as cytotoxic drugs traverse the blood–brain barrier poorly. PCI is advised on completion of chemotherapy to eradicate occult cerebral micrometastases in patients with a good performance status and a complete or good partial response to induction chemotherapy as there is a survival advantage in both limited and extensive disease.[1] In limited disease there is a 5% overall survival advantage.[9] In a recent study by the European Organisation for Research and Treatment of Cancer (EORTC) one-year survival was 27.1% with PCI versus 13.3% without PCI in patients with extensive disease who responded to initial chemotherapy.[10]

Supportive care is provided by multidisciplinary teams and specialist palliative care services.[1] Management should include symptom control (e.g. weight loss, depression, pain) and specific interventions (Table 21.1).

Table 21.1 Palliative symptom management

Symptoms	Management
Breathlessness	Local external beam radiotherapy, bronchoscopy procedures (e.g. de-bulking, photodynamic therapy, stents), pleural effusion drainage and talc pleurodesis
Cough, pain, haemoptysis	External beam radiotherapy
Superior vena cava obstruction	Chemo- and radiotherapy and occasionally stenting
Brain metastasis, spinal cord compression	Corticosteroids and radiotherapy ± surgery for spinal cord compression
Bone metastases	Analgesia ± radiotherapy

Conclusion

In this case the patient was assessed to have limited disease on the basis that the disease was confined to the right hemithorax with involvement of a right supraclavicular node that was encompassed in one radiotherapy field. In this case the lethargy, hyponatraemia and ankle oedema suggested the syndrome of inappropriate antidiuretic hormone secretion.

At presentation, this patient had limited disease, was relatively young and had a good performance status. Consequently, she entered a good prognostic group and the aim of treatment was to optimize survival. Had she fallen into a poor prognostic group the aim would have been palliation of symptoms with as little toxicity as possible.

The patient was treated with six cycles of chemotherapy using carboplatin and etoposide with concomitant radiotherapy, and reported an excellent symptomatic response with resolution of cough, increased appetite and improved exercise tolerance. The chemo-radiotherapy was well tolerated with her only toxicity being alopecia. Follow-up CT scans showed a good response. After completion of chemo-radiotherapy she underwent PCI.

Following a five-month disease-free period, a repeat CT scan (Figure 21.2) showed disease progression with a new right-sided upper lobe lesion (arrow in Figure 21.2) and an anterior jugular node. On examination she had developed a new 3 cm supraclavicular lymph node. Her performance status remained good and she underwent second-line therapy. Following three cycles, a further CT scan showed radiological progression in the supraclavicular fossa and lung. She subsequently underwent palliative radiotherapy for symptom relief and died 20 months after presentation.

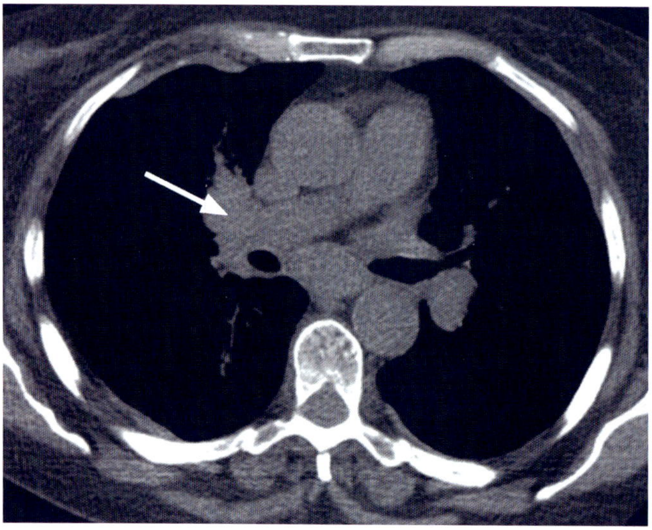

Figure 21.2 Repeat CT scan showing a new right-sided upper lobe lesion (arrow).

Further Reading

1 National Institute for Health and Clinical Excellence. Lung cancer: the diagnosis and treatment of lung cancer. Clinical guideline 121. London: NICE, 2011. www.nice.org.uk (accessed 01 07 11). (Update of NICE clinical guideline 24, 2005.)

2 American Cancer Society. Cancer facts and figures, 2010. www.cancer.org (accessed 01 07 11).

3 Sundstrøm S, Bremnes RM, Kaasa S *et al.* Cisplatin and etoposide regimen is superior to cyclophosphamide, epirubicin and vincristine regimen in small-cell lung cancer: results from a randomized phase III trial with 5 years' follow-up. *J Clin Oncol* 2002; **20**: 4665–72.

4 Amarasena IU, Walters JA, Wood-Baker R, Fong K. Platinum versus non-platinum chemotherapy regimens for small cell lung cancer. *Cochrane Database Syst Rev* 2008; CD006849.

5 Simon GR, Turrisi A. Management of small cell lung cancer: ACCP evidence-based clinical practice guidelines (2nd edition). *Chest* 2007; **132**(3 Suppl): 324S–39S.

6 Huisman C, Postmus PE, Giaccone G, Smit EF. Second-line chemotherapy and its evaluation in small cell lung cancer. *Cancer Treat Rev* 1999; **25**: 199–206.

7 Pignon JP, Arriagada R, Ihde DC *et al.* A meta-analysis of thoracic radiotherapy for small-cell lung cancer. *N Engl J Med* 1992; **327**: 1618–24.

8 Takada M, Fukuoka M, Kawahara M *et al.* Phase III study of concurrent versus sequential thoracic radiotherapy in combination with cisplatin and etoposide for limited-stage small-cell lung cancer: results of the Japan Clinical Oncology Group Study 9104. *J Clin Oncol* 2002; **20**: 3054–60.

9 Arriagada R, Le Chevalier T, Pignon JP *et al.* Initial chemotherapeutic doses and survival in patients with limited small-cell lung cancer. *N Engl J Med* 1993; **329**: 1848–52.

10 Slotman B, Faivre-Finn C, Kramer G *et al.* Prophylactic cranial irradiation in extensive small-cell lung cancer. *N Engl J Med* 2007; **357**: 664–72.

PROBLEM

22 Non-Small Cell Lung Cancer (NSCLC)

Suma Kumar, Richard Leach

Case History

A 68-year-old man presented with a four-week history of left-sided, dull, aching chest pain. He had known ischaemic heart disease, previous coronary artery bypass grafting, chronic obstructive pulmonary disease and treated duodenal ulceration. He smoked with a 20 pack-year history. Clinical examination was unremarkable. There was no clubbing or lymphadenopathy and the respiratory system examination was normal. Figure 22.1 illustrates the chest radiograph (CXR). This suggests a left upper lobe mass with mediastinal widening suspicious of lung cancer.

How would you investigate this patient?

How would you establish a histological diagnosis of lung cancer?

What genetic and environmental factors contribute to lung cancer?

How is lung cancer classified?

How is non-small cell lung cancer (NSCLC) staged and how does it affect therapy?

How would you manage this patient's NSCLC?

This patient would like to know his likely life expectancy.

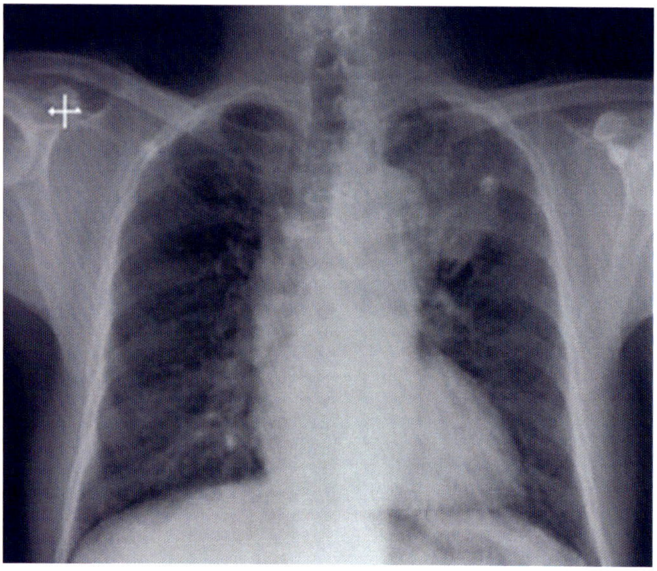

Figure 22.1 Chest radiograph.

Background

Lung cancer is the leading cause of cancer mortality in both men and women and is mainly due to cigarette smoking.[1–3] Non-small cell lung cancer (NSCLC) causes 85% of all lung cancers. Most are diagnosed at an advanced stage and subsequent prognosis is poor. Therapeutic decision-making is dependent on the size and spread of the tumour and patients with NSCLC need careful assessment and staging.[4]

Smokers with new chest symptoms (e.g. haemoptysis, cough, chest/shoulder pain, weight loss, hoarse voice or cervical lymphadenopathy) lasting longer than three weeks, and especially those >50 years old, require a CXR. About 7%–10% of NSCLC cases are asymptomatic at presentation and are diagnosed incidentally after a CXR performed for other reasons. In this case, the initial CXR was suspicious of lung cancer.

Baseline investigations should include:

- **Routine blood tests.** Abnormal liver function tests may suggest liver metastases and elevated calcium levels either metastatic bone disease or paraneoplastic production of parathyroid hormone-related peptide. A clotting profile is required if biopsies are planned. In this case baseline blood tests were normal.
- **Spirometry** should be performed before biopsy to establish histological type or surgery.
- **Pleural fluid aspiration** is required, if pleural fluid is present, for biochemical analysis, microbiology and cytology.
- **Computed tomography (CT) scans.** Early chest, liver and adrenal gland CT scans are essential to assess tumour size and site, local invasion and potential metastases (e.g. adrenal gland).[4] It also facilitates staging and histological diagnosis by identifying the lesion most amenable to biopsy. It does not accurately discriminate between enlarged lymph nodes that are reactive (i.e. infective) and those enlarged due to metastatic spread (specificity 78%, sensitivity 79%). A head CT scan is only required when neurological symptoms are present as cerebral metastases are rarely detected at presentation. However, it may also be considered for patients undergoing treatment with curative intent.
- **Sputum cytology**, although inexpensive, has a high false-negative rate and is only indicated in patients unfit for bronchoscopy or biopsy. Positive cytology is reported in approximately 40% of central tumours.

Further staging investigations include:

- **Positron emission tomography** (PET) utilizes uptake of labelled 18-fluorodeoxyglucose (^{18}FDG) by metabolically active malignant tissue to detect metastases. The combination of CT scanning and ^{18}FDG-PET has greater sensitivity (72%–100%) and specificity (67%–100%) than PET alone. However, ^{18}FDG uptake also occurs in non-malignant tissue including sarcoid, infective granulomas and benign pulmonary nodules. False negatives occur during hyperglycaemia, in bronchoalveolar carcinomas and with small nodules, as PET scanners can only detect tumours >8 mm. Every cancer network should have access to a CT-PET scan facility and all patients with potentially curable lung cancer should be offered CT-PET before treatment.[1]
- **Bone scans** are indicated when hypercalcaemia, bone pain or raised alkaline phosphatase suggest metastatic disease but should not be performed if PET scanning has not shown metastases.[1]
- **Magnetic resonance imaging** is used to assess brachial plexus involvement in apical lung cancer but has no role in nodule evaluation or routine staging of lung cancer.[1]
- **Ultrasound scans** aid assessment and biopsy of cervical lymph nodes or liver metastases.

Establishing a histological diagnosis

1. **Bronchoscopy**. Histological yield is highest with central tumours. Endobronchial biopsy of visible tumours has a sensitivity of 74%, brushings 59% and washings 48%. All three techniques combined increase detection to 88%. Brushings have the highest sensitivity in peripheral tumours beyond the visible segmental bronchi. Diagnostic yield is greatest if bronchoscopy is performed after a CT scan, as

abnormal areas can be targeted. Bronchoscopy also informs operative decisions. For example, tumour involvement of the main bronchi dictates a pneumonectomy and vocal cord palsy suggests inoperability due to malignant infiltration of the recurrent laryngeal nerve. Sensitivity of transcarinal and transtracheal lymph node aspirates is approximately 67% with a specificity of 96%. Endoscopic bronchial (or oesophageal) ultrasound (EBUS) with fine needle aspiration under conscious sedation is increasingly used to obtain histological diagnosis from enlarged hilar, paratracheal and/or mediastinal lymph nodes.

2. **Ultrasound-guided needle aspiration** of supraclavicular nodes (impalpable but >5 mm on ultrasound) is positive in 75% of cases and avoids invasive tests in 42%.[5]
3. **Mediastinoscopy/mediastinotomy** with biopsy of enlarged mediastinal lymph nodes can assist diagnosis (>90% sensitivity and specificity) and subsequent staging but has been largely superseded by EBUS.
4. **CT-guided lung biopsy** has >85% sensitivity in peripheral lung lesions >2 cm. Before biopsy, clotting should be checked. Spirometry must be performed to confirm the forced expiratory volume in 1 second (FEV_1) is >35% predicted as a pneumothorax occurs in approximately 10%–20% of cases and approximately 3% require a chest drain following biopsy. Haemoptysis occurs in approximately 5%.

Epidemiology of lung cancer

In the USA and Europe the incidence and mortality associated with lung cancer increased steadily from 1930 to 1995. Since 1995 it has decreased by 20%–30% in men and is stable in women due to reduced levels of tobacco smoking. However, it remains the commonest cause of cancer death in men and women in these countries causing 34 000 lung cancer deaths annually in the UK. It is the second commonest cancer after prostate cancer in men, causing approximately 22 000 new cases per year, and the third commonest cancer after breast and bowel cancer in women, causing approximately 16 000 new cases per year.[1,2,6]

Over 85% of lung cancer is related to tobacco smoking. Risk increases with earlier age of onset, number of cigarettes smoked daily, type of cigarette (i.e. unfiltered) and duration of smoking (i.e. 1 pack per day for 40 years is more hazardous than 2 packs per day for 20 years). The lifetime risk of developing lung cancer in a heavy smoker (i.e. >20 pack years) is 10%, about 10–30 times greater than for lifetime non-smokers (<0.3%).

Occupational exposure to many carcinogens (e.g. asbestos, arsenic, beryllium, cadmium, ether, polycyclic aromatic hydrocarbons, vinyl chloride) increases the risk of lung cancer, particularly in workers who also smoke.[7] Radon gas found naturally in rocks, soil and ground water also increases lung cancer risk in some areas. An association between chronic lung disease (e.g. idiopathic pulmonary fibrosis) and parenchymal scar tissue (e.g. pulmonary tuberculosis) and lung cancer is recognized.

Only 10%–15% of smokers develop lung cancer suggesting a genetic susceptibility. Polymorphisms in genes encoding enzymes important in metabolism of tobacco smoke-derived carcinogens and in DNA repair have been identified in patients with lung cancer, but sample sizes have been too small to demonstrate reproducibility at this stage.

Classification of lung cancer

The World Health Organization (WHO) classification (1999) identifies seven histological types of lung cancer (Table 22.1). For practical purposes lung cancer is divided into two groups, which influence prognosis, treatment and management:

1. **Non-small cell lung cancers (NSCLC)** account for 80%–85% of lung cancer.
   - *Squamous cell cancer (SCC)* is the commonest histological type (~30%–50%) and is strongly associated with smoking. These tumours develop in airway epithelium and therefore tend to be perihilar/central. SCC often presents as a mass on CXR, which may cavitate. Hypercalcaemia is most common in SCC.
   - *Adenocarcinoma (including bronchoalveolar carcinoma)* is increasing in prevalence, especially in women (~10%–30%). It is the commonest histological type in non-smokers and is almost as common as SCC in countries with a low incidence of smoking. Consequently, in the USA, adenocarcinoma is more common than SCC (33% vs 30%). It may be primary or metastatic and tends to occur in scar/fibrotic tissue. Tumours are often 'peripheral' (i.e. less accessible by bronchoscopy) and may involve the pleura causing secondary effusions. Bronchoalveolar carcinoma is rare and arises from type II pneumocytes that grow along alveolar septa. It is more common in women and non-smokers and can occasionally be associated with copious sputum production (bronchorrhoea). It usually presents as diffuse infiltration on CXR.
   - *Large cell carcinoma* (10%–15%) presents as central or peripheral masses with invasion of local structures.

2. **Small cell lung cancers (SCLC)** cause 15%–25% of lung cancer and arise from bronchial mucosa neuroendocrine cells. They typically present as a central mass with lymph node enlargement. Haematogenous spread leads to widespread metastasis before diagnosis. If untreated the prognosis is <6 months survival from the time of diagnosis. Surgery is rarely appropriate and although the tumour is chemo- and radiosensitive, survival time is usually only 12–14 months with therapy. The syndrome of inappropriate antidiuretic hormone secretion is common in SCLC.

Table 22.1 WHO classification of lung tumours (1999)
Squamous cell carcinoma
Small cell carcinoma
Adenocarcinoma
Large cell carcinoma
Adenosquamous carcinoma
Pleomorphic/sarcomatoid
Carcinoid tumour

Staging of NSCLC

Staging has therapeutic and prognostic implications and aims to establish whether NSCLC is surgically curable.[1,2,6,8,9] If not curable, it determines the most appropriate therapy (e.g. chemotherapy, radiotherapy, supportive care). It is based on the International Association for the Study of Lung Cancer (IASLC) classification which has been in routine use since 2009 (Table 22.2).[9] At diagnosis, stage I and II account for 20%, stage III 35% and stage IV 45% of cases. Five-year survival for each stage is reported in Table 22.2.

Staging may be clinical (c) – based on physical examination and radiology – or pathological (p) by examining tissue from lymph node biopsy, bronchoscopy and/or mediastinoscopy. In the most recent classification, T1 tumours have been subdivided into T1a <2 cm and T1b >2 cm but <3 cm. T2 tumours are subdivided into T2a >3 cm but <5 cm and T2b >5 cm but <7 cm. T3 tumours are >7 cm or have additional nodules in the same lobe as the primary tumour, and T4 tumours include nodules in an ipsilateral lobe. Nodal classification is unchanged; N0 = no nodes; N1 = ipsilateral hilar nodes; N2 = ipsilateral mediastinal or subcarinal nodes; and N3 = contralateral, scalene or supraclavicular nodes. Metastasis has been reclassified as M0 = no distant metastases; M1a = intrathoracic metastases including tumour nodules in the contralateral lung and pleural involvement; and M1b = distant metastases.

Table 22.2 NSCLC stage, terminology and treatment survival times from the IASLC clinical and pathological staging system (2009)

Stage	TNM	Terminology	Five-year survival with clinical (c) or pathological (p) staging
IA	T1, N0, M0	T1a <2 cm T1b Tumour size ≥2–<3 cm	c 50%; p 73%
IB	T2, N0, M0	T2a >3 cm–<5 cm	c 47%; p 58%
IIA	T1, N1, M0 T2a, N1, M0 T2b, N0, M0	T2b >5 cm–<7 cm N0 No regional nodes N1 Ipsilateral hilar nodes	c 36%; p 46%
IIB	T3, N0, M0	T3 >7 cm (± ipsilateral lung nodules)	c 26%; p 36%
IIIA	T1, N2, M0 T2, N2, M0 T3, N1–2, M0 T4, N0, M0 T4, N1, M0	N2 Ipsilateral mediastinal nodes N3 Contralateral hilar, mediastinal or any supraclavicular lymph node T4 Additional nodules in the same lobe as the primary tumour or mediastinal invasion	c 19%; p 24%
IIIB	T1–3, N3, M0 T4, N2, M0		c 19%; p 9%
IV	Any T or N, M1	M1a Intrathoracic metastases (+ pleural effusion/ involvement) M1b Distant metastasis	c 2%; p 13%

TNM, tumour, node, metastasis.

Patients judged suitable for surgery or radical radiotherapy on CT scan (and routine investigation) should have a PET scan to exclude intrathoracic lymph nodes or distant metastases as previous studies have demonstrated important treatment changes in approximately 50% of cases.

Management of NSCLC

Treatment of lung cancer is often complex and multimodal (i.e. involving a combination of surgery, chemotherapy and radiotherapy) and the management of all newly diagnosed lung cancer patients should be discussed with the local multidisciplinary lung cancer team, which should include an oncologist and thoracic surgeon.

In general, patients with NSCLC can be divided, at diagnosis, into three groups that reflect the extent of disease and treatment approach.

1. **Surgical group**. Stage I and II tumours are surgically removed by wedge resection or lobectomy if performance status and FEV_1 are adequate. More extensive surgery (e.g. pneumonectomy) should only be performed to ensure clear margins (i.e. complete tumour resection).[1,2,6] Mean five-year survival after surgery is 69% in stage

IA, falling to 33% in IIB. A few stage IIIA patients are considered for surgery but only 25% can be adequately resected and <25% will survive to five years. Adjuvant chemotherapy improves survival, compared to surgery alone, following macroscopically complete resection. The peri-operative mortality rate for pneumonectomy is 6%, lobectomy 3% and wedge resection 1%. Lymph node sampling for pathological staging or *en bloc* removal should occur during surgical resections undertaken with curative intent.[1] Endobronchial techniques (e.g. photodynamic therapy, neodymium-yttrium aluminium garnet [Nd-Yag] laser ablation, cryotherapy) are being evaluated for the treatment of *in situ* tumours and palliation.

2. **Radiotherapy and chemotherapy group**. Combination therapy (i.e. surgery, radiotherapy, chemotherapy) should be considered in patients treated with curative intent and combination chemo-radiotherapy for patients with stage II and III NSCLC who are not suitable for surgery.[1] The risks and benefits should be discussed with the patient and survival benefits balanced against the potential toxicity.
   - *Radiotherapy*. High-dose, 'curative', continuous hyperfractionated accelerated radiotherapy (CHART) is given to patients with resectable disease who have medical contraindications or decline surgery.[1,6,10] CHART is given as small doses three times a day for twelve days (total 54 Gy). Two-year survival is improved compared with conventional high-dose radiotherapy (29% vs 20%). Palliative radiotherapy is very effective in the management of haemoptysis, superior vena cava obstruction, painful lymphadenopathy, pain from bony metastases and airway obstruction.
   - *Chemotherapy*. About 80% of all patients with lung cancer are considered for chemotherapy at some point during the course of their illness. At present, chemotherapy alone has no role in potentially curative treatment for NSCLC, as these tumours are only moderately sensitive to chemotherapeutic drugs. However, many trials have demonstrated that combination chemotherapy is superior to a single-agent regime.

     Pre-operative (neo-adjuvant) and post-operative (adjuvant) chemotherapy improve survival in patients with good performance status and T1–3, N1–2, M0 tumours or T2–3, N0, M0 localized tumours >4 cm diameter.[1] In cases unsuitable for surgery with advanced tumours, chemotherapy improves symptoms and quality of life although survival gains are only 2–4 months compared with the best supportive care.
     - First-line chemotherapy combines a platinum drug (e.g. cisplatin) with a third-generation drug (e.g. gemcitabine) which avoids alopecia. Repeat CT scans establish response.
     - Second-line monotherapy (e.g. docetaxel, pemetrexed, paclitaxel) is used in relapse for patients with locally advanced or metastatic disease but causes alopecia.
     - Rescue chemotherapy and biological agents (e.g. gefitinib, bevacizumab) may be required (e.g. in tumours expressing epidermal growth factor receptors).
   - *Combined chemo-radiotherapy* is more effective when radiotherapy is concurrent (rather than sequential) with chemotherapy. Both quality of life and survival are improved but side effects increase.

3. **Supportive care**. Most patients with NSCLC present with advanced disease and only one-third of these are fit for palliative chemotherapy. Palliation of symptoms (e.g. pain, dyspnoea, depression) and complications (e.g. pleural effusions) is essential. Follow-up by a specialist multidisciplinary team in conjunction with the patient's family physician is important and ensures early recognition and management of symptoms.

Life expectancy

In the USA, the overall five-year survival rate for NSCLC is 14% but it is closer to 8% in Europe as approximately 75% of patients present with advanced disease.[1,2,9]

Conclusion

In this patient, the CT scan (Figure 22.2) demonstrated a 5 cm × 3 cm mass (indicated by the star in Figure 22.2) within the left upper lobe, in continuity with the chest wall (not shown), and extensive mediastinal adenopathy (indicated by the arrow in Figure 22.2). The lesion was not accessible by bronchoscopy and a CT-guided lung biopsy was performed.

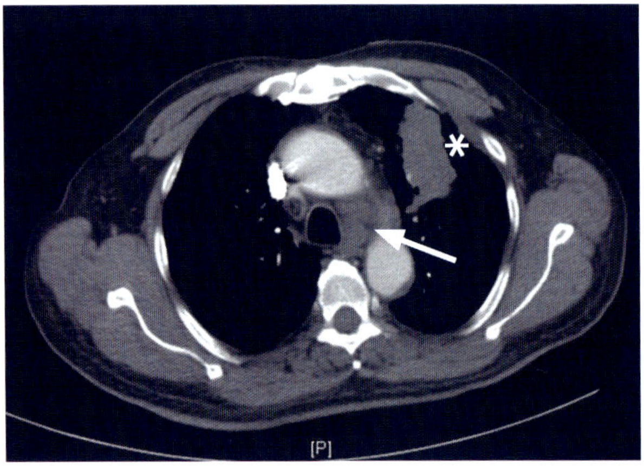

Figure 22.2 CT scan showing a 5 cm × 3 cm mass (star) within the left upper lobe and extensive mediastinal adenopathy (arrow).

Histology revealed infiltration by large atypical cells with pleomorphic nuclei, focal necrosis and surrounding acute inflammation. At immunohistochemistry the tumour cells were positive for thyroid transcription factor 1 (TTF-1), cytokeratin 7 (CK7) and pancytokeratin suggesting a poorly differentiated large cell carcinoma.

Following CT scan, the tumour was staged as IIIA (pT2a, N2, M0) but a subsequent CT-PET scan showed intense uptake in supraclavicular and contralateral paratracheal lymph nodes changing the staging from stage IIIA to IIIB (pT2a, N3, M0) and making him unsuitable for surgery or radical radiotherapy. In stage IIIB disease, five-year survival is approximately 10% with appropriate chemo-radiotherapy. At present this patient is under the care of the oncologists and receiving chemo-radiotherapy.

Further Reading

1 National Institute for Health and Clinical Excellence. Lung cancer: the diagnosis and treatment of lung cancer. Clinical guideline 121. London: NICE, 2011. www.nice.org.uk (accessed 01 07 11). (Update of NICE clinical guideline 24, 2005.)

2 American Cancer Society. Cancer facts and figures, 2010. www.cancer.org (accessed 01 07 11).

3 Doll R, Hill AB. Smoking and carcinoma of the lung; preliminary report. *Br Med J* 1950; **2**: 739–48.

4 Schreiber G, McCrory DC. Performance characteristics of different modalities for diagnosis of suspected lung cancer: summary of published evidence. *Chest* 2003; **123**(1 Suppl): 115S–128S.

5 Kumaran M, Benamore RE, Vaidhyanath R *et al.* Ultrasound guided cytological aspiration of supraclavicular lymph nodes in patients with suspected lung cancer. *Thorax* 2005; **60**: 229–33.

6 Tan WW, Farina GA, Huq S, Maghfoor I, Perry M, Ramnarine M. Non-small cell lung cancer. Medscape Reference, 2011. www.emedicine.medscape.com/article/279960-overview (accessed 01 07 11).

7 Hughes JM, Weill H. Asbestos and man-made fibers. In: Samet JM (ed). *Epidemiology of lung cancer*, pp 185–205. New York: Marcel Dekker, Inc., 1

8 Ries LAG, Melbert D, Krapcho M *et al.* (eds). SEER cancer statistics review, 1975–2005. Bethesda, MD: National Cancer Institute. http://seer.cancer.gov/csr/1975_2005/ (accessed 01 06 11).

9 Rami-Porta R, Crowley JJ, Goldstraw P. The revised TMN staging system for lung cancer. *Ann Thorac Cardiovasc Surg* 2009; **15**: 4–9.

10 Saunders M, Dische S, Barrett A, Harvey A, Gibson D, Parmar M. Continuous hyperfractionated accelerated radiotherapy (CHART) versus conventional radiotherapy in non-small-cell lung cancer: a randomised multicentre trial. *Lancet* 1997; **350**: 161–5.

PROBLEM

23 Pulmonary Nodules

Burhan Khan, Richard Leach

Case History

A 51-year-old man presented with a six-month history of paroxysmal cough following a viral upper respiratory tract infection. Apart from an episode of pneumonia as a child he had no other significant medical history, no allergies and he was on no medications. He was a lifelong non-smoker. Examination was unremarkable. The chest radiograph (CXR) was normal but a chest computed tomography (CT) scan (Figure 23.1) revealed two smooth-edged pulmonary nodules, the first 9 mm × 6 mm (indicated by the arrow in Figure 23.1) directly behind the sternum and the second 5 mm diameter in the posterior left lower lobe. Following treatment with inhaled steroid the cough resolved over three months.

What are the causes and significance of pulmonary nodules?

What features suggest a nodule is malignant or benign?

How would you manage this patient?

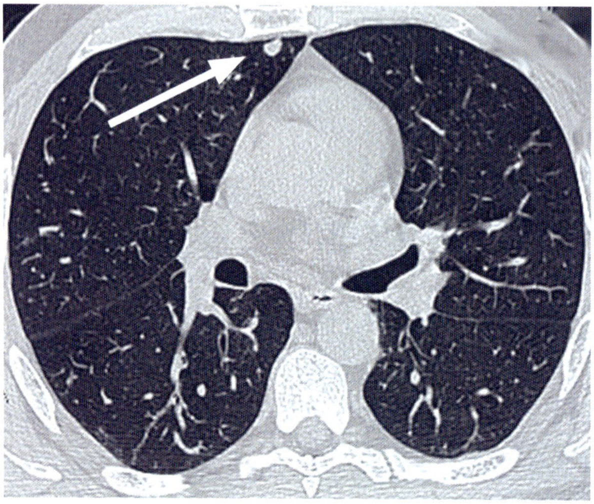

Figure 23.1 Chest CT scan revealing a pulmonary nodule (9 mm × 6 mm) directly behind the sternum (arrow).

Background

Pulmonary nodules (PNs) are focal or round areas of lung opacity measuring <3 cm in diameter. Although often identified on CXR, increased use of CT scans has resulted in more frequent detection of PNs, better evaluation and more precise location. Most PNs are benign (Table 23.1) but this depends on the type of population screened. A solitary PN is the presenting feature in 20%–30% of patients with lung cancer. In smokers with a normal CXR, about 1%–2.5% of PNs detected on a CT scan will be malignant.[1] The ability to identify small PNs improves with each new generation of CT scanners. Multidetector row CT scans can now detect PNs as small as 1–2 mm in diameter. Recent screening studies have found PNs in approximately 50% of smokers aged >50 years on an initial CT scan and a new PN developed during a one-year follow-up period in approximately 10% of cases.

The Early Lung Cancer Action Project – in which 1000 'healthy', symptom-free >60-year-old smokers (>10 pack-year history) underwent baseline CXR and CT scan –

Table 23.1 Causes of pulmonary nodules

Benign	Malignant
Bronchial adenoma	Primary lung cancer
Benign carcinoid tumour	Metastases
Infectious granulomas (e.g. tuberculosis)	
Non-infectious granulomas (e.g. sarcoidosis)	
Benign hamartoma	

detected non-calcified PNs in 7% of baseline CXRs and 23% of CT scans.[2] PNs <5 mm were followed-up and a repeat scan performed, PNs >6 mm were biopsied and those >11 mm received standard care. Of the PNs identified on CT scan that were subsequently biopsied about 11% were malignant.

A PN in a patient with extrathoracic malignancy could be a thoracic metastasis, new primary lung cancer or a benign nodule. This is partly dependent on the smoking history and histology of the extrathoracic malignancy. A primary lung tumour is more likely if the extrathoracic tumour is in the breast, oesophagus, stomach, prostate or bladder; a metastasis is more likely if the extrathoracic tumour is a sarcoma, melanoma or testicular tumour.[3]

Prognostic features of pulmonary nodules

The likelihood that a PN will be malignant increases with size such that less than 1% of PNs <5 mm are malignant, even in smokers, whereas 10%–20% of PNs ≥8 mm will eventually show malignant change. Cigarette smoking, increasing age (i.e. malignancy is rare in patients <35 years old) and specific PN features correlate with increased risk of lung cancer.

- **Features of malignant PNs** include size >0.8 cm, an irregular or 'spiculated' margin (although approximately 20% of malignant PNs have a smooth margin), contrast enhancement (i.e. increased vascularity), cavitation (with thick, irregular walls), rapid growth over time, and association with smoking especially in older age groups. 'Solid' rather than ground glass opacities are more likely to be malignant and have a more rapid growth rate.
- **Features of benign PNs** include size <0.5 cm, a smooth well-defined margin, calcification (which may be diffuse, laminated, central or 'popcorn-like'), stable or smaller with time, poor contrast enhancement, cavitation with thin, smooth walls, fat within the nodule (hamartoma), and association with young age and non-smokers.

Management

Investigation of a PN depends on the clinical presentation and CT features. Until recently it was recommended that all PNs were scanned at regular intervals for at least two years to monitor change in size over time. If the nodule increased in size or showed malignant features on repeat scans, a surgical biopsy or resection was recommended. However, this policy required large numbers of scans with the associated radiation exposure and the cost–benefit ratio was limited. Unfortunately, neither CT-guided biopsy nor positron emission tomography (PET) are reliable in lesions <7 mm in diameter.

The 2008 Fleischner Society PN recommendations suggest a graded approach to investigation and repeat CT scanning depending on PN size, clinical presentation, CT features and the potential for malignant change (Table 23.2).[4]

1. **Very small PN <4 mm**. In a non-smoker, no follow-up imaging is required. High-risk patients (i.e. older smokers) require a single follow-up CT at twelve months; if there is no change at one year no further imaging is required.
2. **Small PN 4–6 mm**. Low-risk patients require a CT at twelve months and if there is no change in the PN, no further imaging is required. High-risk patients require follow-up CT scans at 6–12 months and then at 18–24 months if no change is detected.
3. **Medium PN 6–8 mm**. Low-risk patients require follow-up CT scans at 6–12 months and then at 18–24 months if no change is detected. High-risk patients are followed-up at 3–6 months, then at 9–12 months and finally 24 months if no change.
4. **Large PN >8 mm** are followed-up with CT at 3, 9 and 24 months in either group. Patient choice is important as smokers may opt for excision biopsy rather than CT follow-up. CT-PET has a high false-negative rate for PNs <1 cm so cannot be used to avoid CT follow-up if negative, but is useful if positive.

Table 23.2 Follow-up and management of pulmonary nodules in patients aged >35 years old

Nodule size (mm)	Low-risk patients (non-smoker and no risk factors)	High-risk patients (smoker or other risk factors)
<4	No FU needed*	FU CT scan at 12 mo; if unchanged no further FU†
>4–6	FU CT scan at 12 mo; if unchanged no further FU	Initial FU CT scan at 6–12 mo, then at 18–24 mo if no change
>6–8	FU CT scan at 6–12 mo, then at 18–24 mo if no change	FU CT scan at 3–6 mo, then at 9–12 mo and 24 mo if no change
>8	FU CT scan at 3, 9, 24 mo, CT-PET scan (± biopsy)	Same as for low-risk patient

*Risk of malignancy <1%; †Non-solid (ground glass) or partly solid nodules may require longer follow-up to exclude indolent adenocarcinoma. FU, follow-up; mo, months.

An increase in size of a PN, especially in a smoker, should prompt excision biopsy if the patient is fit for surgery. When a diagnosis of malignancy has been established, treatment depends on histological type (e.g. adenocarcinoma) and whether the PN is a primary lung tumour or metastasis. Primary tumours are staged and treated as described for individual histological types (see Chapters 21 and 22). Metastatic nodules should be discussed in a multidisciplinary meeting to establish the appropriate therapy. All PNs should be followed-up by a specialist lung cancer multidisciplinary team.

Conclusion

In this case, the patient was followed-up with repeat CT scans at 3, 9 and 24 months as recommended by the Fleischner Society guidelines for a nodule >8 mm. During this time the nodules remained unchanged, consistent with a benign pathology (e.g. healed granulomatous disease) and the patient was subsequently discharged from the clinic.

Further Reading

1 National Institute for Health and Clinical Excellence. Lung cancer: the diagnosis and treatment of lung cancer. Clinical guideline 121. London: NICE, 2011. www.nice.org.uk (accessed 01 07 11). (Update of NICE clinical guideline 24, 2005.)

2 Henschke CI, McCauley DI, Yankelevitz DF *et al.* Early Lung Cancer Action Project: overall design and findings from baseline screening. *Lancet* 1999; **354**: 99–105.

3 Quint LE, Park CH, Iannettoni MD. Solitary pulmonary nodules in patients with extrapulmonary neoplasms. *Radiology* 2000; **217**: 257–61.

4 MacMahon H, Austin JHM, Gamsu G *et al.* Guidelines for management of small pulmonary nodules detected on CT scans: a statement from the Fleischner Society. *Radiology* 2005; **237**: 395–400.

PROBLEM

24 Mediastinal Mass: Bronchogenic Cyst

Elizabeth Hadley

Case History

A 24-year-old woman was seen in the chest clinic with an eight-week history of cough with occasional sputum, fever and malaise. She also described an occasional nagging pain under her sternum and palpitations. Her general practitioner had initially treated her for a lower respiratory tract infection with amoxicillin, followed by erythromycin, but after a brief improvement the symptoms had returned. She had no past medical history but was a smoker of ten cigarettes a day. She denied any long-distance travel or illicit drug use.

On examination she looked well; she was apyrexial and normotensive. Oxygen saturations and respiratory rate were normal. Her chest was clear on auscultation and she did not have a cardiac murmur. A chest X-ray showed clear lung fields; however, the mediastinal silhouette was abnormal with an abnormally wide vascular hilum. A computed tomography (CT) scan of the chest, blood tests and an echocardiogram were arranged. The chest CT scan is shown in Figure 24.1.

What does the chest CT show?

What causes a bronchogenic cyst?

Why should a bronchogenic cyst be surgically resected?

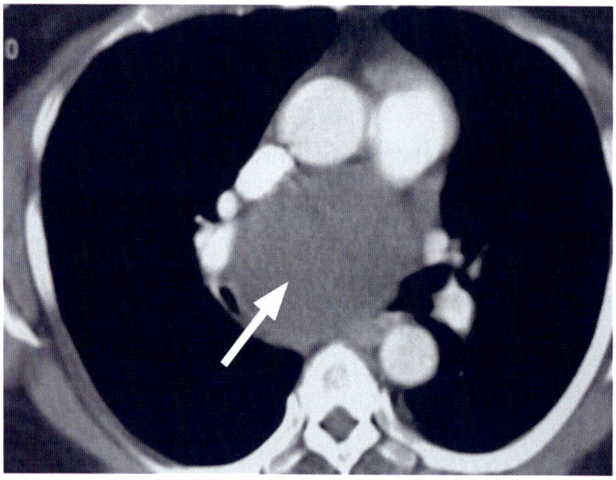

Figure 24.1 A chest CT scan showing a bronchogenic cyst in the posterior mediastinum (arrow).

Background

In this case the chest CT shows a mediastinal bronchogenic cyst located behind the aortic root and adjacent to the left atrium. Typically, bronchogenic cysts appear to be full of homogeneous fluid. The patient's symptoms were due to the bronchogenic cyst becoming infected. The average age of presentation is in the late teens, but the range is wide. The majority (>60%) of patients are symptomatic. Commonest symptoms in order of frequency are cough, dyspnoea, pain, fever, purulent sputum and haemoptysis, and dysphagia. In children, compressive symptoms, particularly of the oesophagus and trachea, are more common.[1]

Aetiology

Bronchogenic cysts are formed from the congenital remnants of the foregut. They are usually a single locule lined with respiratory epithelium including mucous-producing cells and are most commonly filled with clear fluid, although they can also be filled with air, mucous or blood. They can either be mediastinal (80%) or intrapulmonary (20%). They may occasionally be in communication with the lung parenchyma or bronchial tree, but are more often self-contained.[2]

Surgical resection

Complications of bronchogenic cysts are seen in half of patients; serious complications include rupture of infected cysts into the trachea, lung, pericardium or pleura. Pneumonia, haemoptysis, pneumothorax, empyema and pericarditis are reported. In a series collected over 25 years, 2.8% of cases presented with life-threatening symptoms. Those who already have a complication should always be considered for surgical resection, to treat the complication and to prevent future problems. The surgery should be done by an experienced thoracic surgeon who will remove the bronchogenic cyst intact to avoid soiling. Some cysts are also communicating with the bronchopulmonary tree needing complex dissection; incomplete resection may lead to a recurrence. Lobectomy is usually needed for an intrapulmonary cyst.[3–6]

For patients in whom surgical resection is contraindicated or in recurrent cysts where repeat surgery is not an option, there is a new technique of endobronchial ultrasound-guided drainage. This could be particularly useful for non-infected cysts which are causing compressive symptoms.[7,8] Recurrence is reported and may occur up to 25 years after the original resection.

Conclusion

The management of a bronchogenic cyst will depend on various factors; the age and health of the patient, the symptoms at presentation and the predicted future complications of either a conservative or interventional approach. Such cases are best discussed in a multidisciplinary setting which includes a thoracic surgeon.

Further Reading

1 Ribet ME, Copin MC, Gosselin B. Bronchogenic cysts of the lung. *Ann Thorac Surg* 1996; **61**: 1636–40.

2 Rappaport DC, Herman SJ, Weisbrod GL. Congential bronchopulmonary diseases in adults: CT findings. *AJR* 1994; **162**: 1295–9.

3 Kosar A, Tezel C, Orki A, Kiral H, Arman B. Bronchogenic cysts of the lung: report of 29 cases. *Heart Lung Circ* 2009; **18**: 214–8.

4 Liu HS, Li SQ, Cao ZL, Zhang ZY, Ren H. Clinical features and treatment of bronchogenic cyst in adults. *Chin Med Sci J* 2009; **24**: 60–3.

5 Limaïem F, Ayadi-Kaddour A, Djilani H, Kilani T, El Mezni F. Pulmonary and mediastinal bronchogenic cysts: a clinicopathologic study of 33 cases. *Lung* 2008; **186**: 55–61.

6 Calzada AP, Wu W, Salvado AR, Lai CK, Berke GS. Poorly differentiated adenocarcinoma arising from a cervical bronchial cyst. *Laryngoscope* 2011; **121**: 1446–8.

7 Galluccio G, Lucantoni G. Mediastinal bronchogenic cyst's recurrence treated with EBUS-FNA with a long-term follow-up. *Eur J Cardiothorac Surg* 2006; **29**: 627–9.

8 Imperatori A, Rotolo N, Nardecchia E, Mariscalco G, Spagnoletti M, Dominioni L. Bronchogenic cyst associated with pericardial defect: case report and review of the literature. *J Cardiothorac Surg* 2011; **6**: 85.

PROBLEM

25 Smoking Cessation

Suma Kumar, Richard Leach

Case History

The wife and daughter of a patient you are treating for lung cancer are concerned about their risk of developing cancer. The wife is an ex-smoker having stopped six months ago. The daughter has never smoked but has had lifelong passive cigarette-smoke exposure.

What are the risks of cigarette smoking?

Which age groups are most likely to smoke?

What are the effects of passive smoking on children?

Why is smoking addictive?

How can smoking cessation be achieved?

Background

Worldwide, over a billion people smoke and 5.4 million deaths occur annually due to smoking. Tobacco consumption accounts for 90% of lung cancer cases and approximately 30% of all cancer deaths in developed countries. It also causes cancer of the nasopharynx, larynx, oesophagus, stomach, pancreas, liver, urinary tract and uterine cervix and myeloid leukaemia. In the UK in 2005, 46 000 cancer deaths were attributed to smoking. It is recognized as the greatest single cause of other preventable illnesses including chronic obstructive pulmonary disease (COPD), stroke, coronary heart disease, peripheral vascular disease and peptic ulcer disease.[1]

In the UK, 6.3 million people died from smoking from 1950–2000. Currently 24% of UK adults smoke but the prevalence has been static for ten years. Every year there are 120 000 deaths, 365 000 hospital admissions, and 1.2 million general practitioner consultations; all related to tobacco. Smoking reduces a smoker's life expectancy by an average of ten years, or about twelve minutes for every cigarette smoked.[1–3]

In a long-term smoker the relative risk of developing lung cancer, compared to a lifelong non-smoker, is increased by 10–30 times. The risk is dependent on dose (determined by the number of cigarettes smoked daily, the depth of inhalation and number of years smoked), age of onset, the pattern of smoking (i.e. intermittent quit periods >3 months reduce subsequent risk) and race (e.g. African-Americans are at higher risk).[1–3]

Smoking prevalence

In the UK, young adults have the highest prevalence of smoking (32% in 20–24 year olds) in comparison to the national average of 24% for men and 23% for women.[1,4] Prevalence is also higher in manual occupations, socio-economically deprived people and men of South Asian descent. Chinese and Indian women are least likely to smoke.

In 2006, despite it being illegal to sell tobacco to young people under 18 years old, 24% of 15-year-old girls and 16% of boys were regular smokers consuming an average of 42 cigarettes weekly. In addition, 10% of 11–15-year-old girls and 7% of boys smoke more than one cigarette a week and 82% of smokers start as teenagers. Factors encouraging children to smoke include family members who smoke, one parent families, exposure to tobacco advertising and a poor academic record. Although it is often suggested that the appetite suppressant effects of smoking may be a factor in the high prevalence of smoking in young women trying to avoid weight gain, there is little or no evidence to support this.[4] However, the desire 'to be thin' is associated with an increased likelihood of smoking initiation. Smoking early in life increases lung cancer risk independently of the amount and duration of smoking.[1,2]

Passive smoking

Tobacco smoke is made up of 'sidestream smoke' from the tip of the cigarette and 'mainstream smoke' from the filter or mouth end. It is the 'sidestream smoke' that accounts for most (approximately 85%) of the environmental tobacco smoke (ETS) and contributes to passive (i.e. second-hand) smoking.[5] In a meta-analysis of 37 studies, non-smokers who lived with smokers had a 24% (95% confidence interval [CI] 13%–36%) increased incidence of lung cancer. The increased risk is 16%–19% in those exposed to ETS in the workplace. In the UK, it is estimated that there are 12 000 deaths each year that are attributable to ETS and 500 of these are due to ETS exposure in the workplace.

Passive smoking is harmful in children and increases respiratory disease, asthma attacks, middle ear infections and cot deaths. In the UK >30% of children live with an adult smoker and in low-income families this increases to 57%.

Smoking during pregnancy is associated with greater risk of spontaneous abortion, pre-term birth, stillbirth or low birth weight. In 2005, 32% of women smoked before or during pregnancy and 17% throughout pregnancy, increasing to 48% and 29%, respectively, in lower socio-economic groups.

Tobacco addiction

Tobacco contains nicotine, an alkaloid that mediates its addictive effects by the release of the reward neurotransmitter dopamine in the brain mesolimbic system. Cigarettes are popular because they rapidly achieve high brain nicotine levels, with a transit time from alveoli to brain via the bloodstream of 7–20 seconds. Repeated ingestion of nicotine alters the motivational system to create a 'drive', similar to hunger, for cigarettes. This drive is experienced as a 'need to smoke' and develops over the time since the last cigarette. Abstinence results in unpleasant withdrawal symptoms including depression.

Nicotine is the main barrier to smoking cessation due to the associated physical and psychological dependence. It exerts its effects through brain and muscle nicotinic acetylcholine receptors (nAchR). Stimulation of brain nAchR releases a variety of neurotransmitters: noradrenaline increases arousal and reduces appetite, vasopressin improves memory, serotonin regulates mood and beta-endorphin decreases anxiety.[4] Most importantly it activates dopamine-secreting neurones in the nucleus accumbens of the mesolimbic dopamine system (i.e. brain reward pathway) which elicit pleasurable sensations and leads to addictive behaviour. Repeated nicotine exposure gradually decreases nAchR sensitivity with a reduction in response and a fall in brain dopamine levels, despite a compensatory increase (~300%) in receptor numbers. Consequently, increased nicotine stimulation is required to achieve equivalent effects. These changes are the basis for the addictive effect of nicotine.

Nicotine substitution can relieve some of the 'need to smoke' by raising the tonic depression of nicotinic acetylcholine activity without being addictive and is the basis for nicotine replacement therapy in smoking cessation programmes.

Smoking cessation

Smoking cessation reduces the risk of lung cancer by up to 90% but the risk is always higher than in lifelong non-smokers. Risk reduction is dependent on the number of cigarettes previously smoked and age and time since smoking cessation.[2] The British doctors study reported a reduction in life expectancy of three months for every year smoking cessation was postponed after 40 years old.[3]

Most smokers would like to stop smoking, but only approximately 1% can stop without help. More than 70% have made at least one attempt. As little as 60 seconds advice about smoking cessation, from a health-care professional, triggers a 'quit attempt' in 40% of smokers and must be encouraged at every point of contact. All health-care workers should be able to offer accurate advice on all forms of assistance available, including availability of and referral to smoking cessation services, medications, help lines and self-help materials. Unfortunately, although 70% of smokers see a physician each year, <20% are encouraged to stop smoking.

Characteristics that predict success in smoking cessation must be recognized, as this helps match smokers with the most effective strategies and identifies those needing more intensive treatment (e.g. antidepressants, behavioural therapy). These characteristics include:

- **Gender**. Men have better long-term outcomes as they are less concerned about weight gain and are less likely to use smoking to deal with negative emotions.
- **Age at smoking initiation**. Early exposure (<14 years old) to tobacco leads to increased nicotine dependence and heavy smoking in later life.
- **Depression**. The association between nicotine dependence and affective disorders, especially depression, is well recognized but is not a barrier to smoking cessation. The presence of depression can be reliably ascertained by the simple question "Did you feel 'down' during most days of the past two weeks?"
- **Nicotine dependence** is inversely proportional to successful smoking cessation. It is usually assessed with the Fagerström Test for Nicotine Dependence (Table 25.1). The most important questions are time to first cigarette in the morning and number of cigarettes smoked daily. Those who smoke their first cigarette within one hour of waking and smoke >10–15 cigarettes per day are significantly addicted to nicotine.
- **Alcoholism** is a negative prognostic factor and stopping drinking is likely to increase successful smoking cessation.
- **Motivation** is assessed by asking "How important is it for you to give up smoking?" and perceived self-efficacy by asking "If you were to decide to stop smoking, how confident are you that you would succeed?" If readiness to quit is high but self-

efficacy low, treatment and support are critical for success. If self-efficacy is high, but willingness is low, effective health education is needed. If both variables are high, a quit date should be set imminently.
- **Previous cessation attempts** can predict smoking cessation success. Those with previous attempts lasting ≥5 days are more likely to succeed.
- **Social/family environment**. Occupational social class, number of smokers in the household, marital status and support from the family are important predictors.

Table 25.1 Fagerström Test for Nicotine Dependence

Question	Response	Score
1. How soon after you wake up do you smoke your first cigarette?	Within 5 min 6–30 min 31–60 min After 60 min	3 2 1 0
2. Do you find it difficult to refrain from smoking in places where it is forbidden?	Yes No	1 0
3. Which cigarette would you hate most to give up?	The first one in the morning Any other	1 0
4. How many cigarettes per day do you smoke?	≤10 11–20 21–30 ≥31	0 1 2 3
5. Do you smoke more frequently during the first hours after waking than during the rest of the day?	Yes No	1 0
6. Do you smoke if you are so ill that you are in bed most of the day?	Yes No	1 0
	Total score (0–10)	

A total score ≥7 indicates severe dependence.

Both behavioural and pharmacological therapies aid smoking cessation. Success rates are lower if smokers attempt to quit unaided, but doubled if they use a drug.

Behavioural strategy

Simple counselling stimulates patients to think about quitting although unassisted quit rates are only 1%–3% compared to controls. Counselling should include the 5As:

- Ask how much a person smokes and document pack years.
- Assess risk of continued smoking and inform the patient.
- Advise how to stop smoking and what help and treatment is available.
- Assist with behavioural support or replacement therapy.
- Arrange follow-up.

Individual or group counselling sessions and setting a 'quit date' result in about 20% abstinence at one-year follow-up. Telephone follow-up, Web-based support and multiple interviews can all improve cessation rates. Evidence for benefit with hypnosis or acupuncture is weak but these may be helpful following previous failed attempts.

Pharmacotherapy

Pharmacotherapy in conjunction with behavioural intervention is the cornerstone in the treatment of tobacco dependence and should be used in most patients attempting to quit smoking unless there are contraindications.

1. **Nicotine replacement therapy (NRT)** ameliorates the withdrawal symptoms of insomnia, irritability, anger, anxiety, poor concentration and increased appetite.[6,7] It is safe even in patients with cardiovascular disease. The Lung Health Study in COPD did not report an increased incidence in cardiovascular disease in smokers who had used nicotine gum for up to five years. In this study, intensive smoking cessation support combined with NRT achieved one-year abstinence rates of 35% versus 9% with usual care.[6] Nicotine is available as a transdermal patch, gum, sublingual tablet, nasal spray and inhaler. A 22 mg patch raises blood nicotine levels equivalent to that of one and a half packs of cigarettes. Meta-analysis has shown that all forms of NRT are equal (odds ratio [OR] of 1.77; 95% CI of 1.66–1.88). The National Institute for Health and Clinical Excellence guidelines recommend combined NRT, with a patch to maintain 'background' nicotine levels and a second NRT (e.g. gum, inhalator) to produce 'peaks of nicotine' to combat smoking urges.
2. **Antidepressants**. Smokers who are not depressed also benefit from this approach which corrects the low dopamine levels due to nicotine dependence.[8]
   - **Bupropion (Zyban®)**, a dopamine uptake inhibitor, is a non-competitive inhibitor of neuronal nAchR activity. It is started 1–2 weeks before stopping smoking and is given for eight weeks. Prolonged treatment may improve long-term success. In a meta-analysis of 31 studies, smoking cessation was doubled (OR 1.94, 95% CI 1.72–2.14). Combination with nicotine is not always beneficial. It is contraindicated in epilepsy and pregnancy.
   - **Nortriptyline**, a tricyclic antidepressant with noradrenergic properties, though not licensed for this indication, is an effective second-line agent.
   - **Selective serotonin reuptake inhibitors** have no long-term benefit.
3. **Varenicline** is a partial agonist at the $\alpha_4\beta_2$ subunit of the nAchR.[9] It reduces craving and withdrawal and as a partial agonist decreases the reward and reinforcement effects of smoking. A twelve-week course is recommended and it should be commenced 1–2 weeks before the 'quit date'. Studies show that it is more effective than placebo (OR 3.22), bupropion and probably nicotine replacement. Twelve-week quit rates in two major studies comparing varenicline, bupropion and placebo were 45%, 30% and 18%, respectively, and at twelve months were 23%, 16% and 9%, respectively.[9] All studies combined behavioural therapy with varenicline and this may be the best appropriate approach for smoking cessation.

Relapse is common with all drugs and longer courses of NRT, bupropion and varenicline should be considered. An additional twelve-week course of varenicline reduced smoking relapse by 30%, six months after the end of all treatment, compared to placebo.

Conclusion

In this scenario, the wife's risk of developing lung cancer will be reduced by over 90% if she remains an ex-smoker for a number of years. However, she will always have a higher risk than a lifelong non-smoker and this risk will be dependent on the number of cigarettes she has previously smoked and her age and the time since she stopped smoking. Statistically, the daughter who has been exposed to prolonged passive smoke inhalation has a 24% increase in the risk of developing lung cancer (whilst she remains exposed) compared to a non-smoker.

Further Reading

1 Cancer Research UK. Statistical Information Team. Cancer Stats Mortality, UK. 2007. http://info.cancerresearchuk.org/cancerstats (accessed 01 06 11).

2 Peto R, Darby S, Deo H, Silcocks P, Whitley E, Doll R. Smoking, smoking cessation, and lung cancer in the UK since 1950: combination of national statistics with two case-control studies. *BMJ* 2000; **321**: 323–9.

3 Doll R, Peto R, Boreham J. Sutherland I. Mortality in relation of smoking: 50 years' observations on male British doctors. *BMJ* 2004; **328**: 1519.

4 Nichter M, Nichter M, Vuckovic N, Tesler L, Adrian S, Ritenbaugh C. Smoking as a weight-control strategy among adolescent girls and young women: a reconsideration. *Med Anthropol Q* 2004; **18**: 305–24.

5 Hackshaw AK, Law MR, Wald NJ. The accumulated evidence on lung cancer and environmental tobacco smoke. *BMJ* 1997; **315**: 980–8.

6 Anthonisen NR, Connett JE, Kiley JP *et al.* Effects of smoking intervention and the use of an inhaled anticholinergic bronchodilator on the rate of decline of FEV1. The Lung Health Study. *JAMA* 1994; **272**: 1497–505.

7 Silagy C, Lancaster T, Stead L, Mant D, Fowler G. Nicotine replacement therapy for smoking cessation. *Cochrane Database Syst Rev* 2004; CD000146.

8 Hughes JR, Stead LF, Lancaster T. Antidepressants for smoking cessation. *Cochrane Database Syst Rev* 2007; CD000031.

9 Cahill K, Stead LF, Lancaster T. Nicotine receptor partial agonists for smoking cessation. *Cochrane Database Syst Rev* 2007; CD006103.

SECTION FIVE 05

Pulmonary Vascular: Including PE and AVM

PROBLEM

26 Pulmonary Hypertension

Bethia Bradley, Richard Leach

Case History

A 26-year-old woman presented to the chest clinic with a two-year history of slowly progressive exertional dyspnoea. At presentation she was experiencing difficulty walking up inclines, keeping up with friends when walking on the flat, climbing two flights of stairs and cleaning the house. She reported occasional palpitations, ankle oedema and dizziness on standing and when exercising. There was no wheeze, cough, pleuritic pain or haemoptysis. The past medical history was unremarkable. In particular there was no history suggestive of vasculitis, connective tissue disease (CTD) or previous respiratory disease. She was on no medication apart from the oral contraceptive pill. There was no occupational dust, avian or animal exposure and she was a lifelong non-smoker.

On examination she appeared well with no cyanosis (oxygen saturation [SaO_2] 93%), anaemia, clubbing or lymphadenopathy. The cardiovascular system was normal apart from a soft systolic murmur and a slightly elevated jugular venous pulse. Blood pressure was 110/60 mmHg. There was no peripheral oedema. Chest examination was unremarkable with no wheeze or crepitations. Abdominal examination was normal. Routine blood tests and spirometry (forced expiratory volume in 1 second [FEV_1] 3.2 l [98% predicted], forced vital capacity [FVC] 3.65 l [94% predicted], peak expiratory flow rate 489 l/min) were normal. Chest radiography (CXR) demonstrated normal lung fields with a cardiothoracic ratio at the upper limit of normal and some hilar prominence.

How is pulmonary hypertension defined and classified?

How is the diagnosis established?

What is the pathogenesis of pulmonary hypertension?

How would you manage pulmonary arterial hypertension and what new pharmacological therapies are available?

Background

The 2009 Dana Point Consensus Conference defined pulmonary hypertension (PHT) as a mean pulmonary artery pressure (PAP) ≥25 mmHg at rest as assessed by right heart catheterization (RHC).[1] In a normal subject, mean PAP is 14 ± 3 mmHg with an upper limit of normal of approximately 20 mmHg. The definition of PHT on exercise as a mean PAP >30 mmHg (as assessed by RHC) is not supported by published data. Increased PAP may be due to increased pulmonary vascular resistance (e.g. hypoxia, pulmonary embolism), an increase in pulmonary blood flow (e.g. atrial septal defect) or a rise in pulmonary venous pressure (e.g. left heart failure).

In pre-capillary PHT the pulmonary capillary wedge pressure (PCWP) is ≤15 mmHg, whereas in post-capillary PHT PCWP is ≥15 mmHg. Cardiac output is normal or reduced in both pre- and post-capillary PHT. Pulmonary vascular resistance grading is not specified as a requirement in the most recent definition but was >240 dynes/s/cm^2 (>3 mmHg/l/min [Wood units]) in the previous Venice classification of 2003.

The 2009 'Dana Point' classification (Table 26.1) has replaced the 'Venice' (2003) and 'Evian' (1998) PHT classifications.[1–5] Both the 2003 and 2009 classifications abandoned the concept of primary pulmonary hypertension, favouring the term 'pulmonary arterial

Table 26.1 Dana Point clinical classification of PHT (2009)

1	**Pulmonary arterial hypertension (PAH)**
1.1	Idiopathic (IPAH)
1.2	Heritable (HPAH); *BMPR2, ALK-1, endoglin*
1.3	Drug and toxin induced
1.4	Associated with (APAH) CTD, HIV infection, portal hypertension (cirrhosis), CHD, schistosomiasis, chronic haemolytic anaemia
1.5	Persistent PHT in the newborn (PPHN)
2	**Pulmonary veno-occlusive disease and/or pulmonary capillary haemangiomatosis**
3	**PHT due to left heart disease** including systolic or diastolic dysfunction or valvular disease
4	**PHT due to lung diseases (± hypoxia)** including COPD, ILD, sleep disordered breathing, alveolar hypoventilation, chronic high altitude exposure and developmental abnormalities
5	**PHT due to chronic thromboembolism**
6	**PHT with unclear (± multifactorial) mechanisms** including haematological disorders, systemic disorders (e.g. sarcoidosis, Langerhans cell histiocytosis, lymphangiomatosis), metabolic disorders (e.g. thyroid, GSD) and other causes (e.g. tumour obstruction, dialysis)

CHD, congenital heart disease; COPD, chronic obstructive pulmonary disease; CTD, connective tissue disease; GSD, glycogen storage disease; HIV, human immunodeficiency virus; ILD, interstitial lung disease; PHT, pulmonary hypertension.

hypertension' (PAH). PAH is a clinical condition characterized by pre-capillary PHT in the absence of other causes for pre-capillary PHT such as lung, thromboembolic or other rare diseases (Table 26.1). The risk factors for PAH (e.g. anorexigenic drugs) and associated conditions in PAH are reported in Table 26.2. Functional status of PHT patients is based on the New York Health Association (NYHA)/World Health Organization (WHO) functional class (WHO-FC; Table 26.3). In Europe and the USA, PAH prevalence is in the range of 15–30 per 10^6 population with approximately 40% due to idiopathic PAH (IPAH) and 4% heritable PAH (HPAH). Mean age at diagnosis is 36 years old and the female to male ratio is 2:1. Although rare, diagnosis of PAH is important, as it affects young people and has a poor prognosis without treatment.

Establishing the diagnosis of pulmonary hypertension

An electrocardiogram (ECG) and transthoracic Doppler echocardiography (TTE) are performed as these are abnormal in 80%–90% of suspected cases of PHT. The ECG shows right ventricular hypertrophy in 87% and right axis deviation in 79% of patients with IPAH. However, the ECG is a poor screening tool for PHT with low sensitivity (55%) and specificity (70%). TTE usually shows right heart chamber enlargement, abnormal motion of the interventricular septum and tricuspid insufficiency. The pulmo-

Table 26.2 Risk factors and associated conditions in the development of PAH

1 Drugs and toxins
- 1.1 Definite: anorexigens (e.g. fenfluramine), toxic rapeseed oil
- 1.2 Very likely: amphetamines, L-tryptophan
- 1.3 Possible: cocaine, chemotherapeutic agents
- 1.4 Unlikely: OC, antidepressants, cigarette smoking

2 Demographic and medical conditions
- 2.1 Definite: gender (females > males)
- 2.2 Possible: pregnancy, systemic hypertension
- 2.3 Unlikely: obesity

3 Diseases
- 3.1 Definite: HIV infection
- 3.2 Likely: portal hypertension, liver disease, CTD, cardiac shunts
- 3.3 Possible: thyroid disorders, haematological (e.g. splenectomy, SCD, thalassaemia, chronic myeloproliferative disorders), rare genetic/metabolic disorders (e.g. GSD, Gaucher's disease, HHT)

CTD, connective tissue disease; GSD, glycogen storage disease; HHT, hereditary haemorrhagic telangiectasia; HIV, human immunodeficiency virus; OC, oral contraceptives; PAH, pulmonary arterial hypertension; SCD, sickle cell disease.

Table 26.3 NYHA/WHO classification of functional status in PHT

Class	
I	Patients with PH in whom there is no limitation of usual physical activity
II	Patients with PH who have mild limitation of physical activity. There is no discomfort at rest, but normal physical activity causes dyspnoea, fatigue, chest pain or pre-syncope
III	Patients with PH who have marked limitation of physical activity. There is no discomfort at rest, but less than ordinary activity causes dyspnoea, fatigue, chest pain or pre-syncope
IV	Patients with PH who are unable to perform any physical activity and who may have signs of right heart failure at rest. Dyspnoea and/or fatigue may be present at rest and symptoms are increased by almost any physical activity

nary artery systolic pressure (PASP) can be estimated using Doppler TTE techniques and is <40 mmHg in 95% of normal subjects. It is equivalent to the right ventricular systolic pressure (RVSP) in the absence of pulmonary outflow obstruction. The RVSP is determined from the systolic regurgitant tricuspid flow velocity (v) and an estimate of the right atrial pressure (RAP) applied to the formula $RVSP = 4v^2 + RAP$; where RAP is estimated from the inferior vena cava characteristics or jugular venous distension. Tricuspid regurgitant jets can be assessed in 74% of patients with PHT. PASP estimated with TTE correlates well with measurements using right heart catheterization. In studies of healthy controls, normal RVSP is reported to be 28 ± 5 mmHg.[1–5]

Guidelines recommend a stepwise approach to diagnosis of PHT.[1]

1 Symptoms (± signs) raise clinical suspicion.
2 Detection or confirmation is achieved with ECG, CXR and TTE.
3 Classification requires pulmonary function tests, arterial blood gases, ventilation-perfusion (V/Q) scan, contrast-enhanced or high-resolution spiral computed tomography (CT) scans or pulmonary angiography. Consider referral to a specialist centre if investigation suggests PHT is not due to a cardiac or respiratory cause.
4 Evaluation includes blood tests, immunology, human immunodeficiency virus (HIV) test, abdominal ultrasound scan and six-minute walking tests. Cardiopulmonary exercise testing measures exercise tolerance and peak oxygen consumption (peak VO_2), and RHC and vasoreactivity testing assess haemodynamics.

Routine blood tests include a thrombophilia screen (e.g. anti-phospholipid antibodies), autoantibodies (e.g. anti-nuclear antibody) to exclude CTD, and HIV serology. Abdominal ultrasound scan excludes liver cirrhosis and portal hypertension as a cause. Six-minute walks (6MW) are an inexpensive test to evaluate severity and response to treatment and may predict survival. In IPAH a 10% fall in saturation during 6MW increased mortality risk by 2.9 over 26 months.

Spirometry excludes chronic lung disease as a cause but gas transfer (TLCO) is often slightly reduced in PAH (40%–80% predicted). V/Q scans detect chronic thromboembolic pulmonary hypertension (CTEPH), which causes segmental perfusion defects, and distinguish between IPAH and CTEPH with a sensitivity of 90%–100% and specificity of 94%–100%. A high-resolution CT scan excludes obstructive airways and interstitial lung disease. Pulmonary venous occlusive disease is associated with diffuse central ground glass opacification. Contrast-enhanced CT scans exclude pulmonary emboli but pulmonary angiography identifies distal obstruction better and is still required to help identify those patients with small distal emboli and those requiring endarterectomy.

RHC confirms the diagnosis of PAH and tests the vasoreactivity of the pulmonary circulation. RHC is recommended in symptomatic patients (NYHA/WHO class II, III, IV) detected by Doppler TTE and is best performed following early referral to a specialist centre. It has prognostic significance, with raised RAP and PAP and reduced cardiac output and central venous saturation identifying IPAH patients with the worst prognosis. PCWP distinguishes between arterial and venous hypertension in left heart disease.

Acute vasodilator testing using short-acting pulmonary vasodilators (e.g. adenosine, prostacyclin or inhaled nitric oxide) identifies patients who may benefit from long-term calcium channel blocker (CCB) therapy. A positive response with a reduction in PAP of >10 mmHg to a mean of <40 mmHg is detected in about 10%–15% of IPAH patients.

Long-term CCB therapy can only safely be used in positive responders and is beneficial in about 50% in the long term.

Pathogenesis of pulmonary hypertension

Recent research and histopathological features suggest that endothelial injury, potassium channel dysfunction and proliferative stimuli are fundamental processes in the pathogenesis, although the exact mechanisms have not been established. Mutations of the bone morphogenetic protein receptor 2 (*BMPR2*), a member of the transforming growth factor β superfamily, are present in most cases of familial PAH.[1,3] However, fewer than 20% of individuals with *BMPR2* mutation develop PAH, suggesting other gene mutations and environmental factors are involved. For example, mutations of activin receptor-like kinase 1 (*ALK-1*) and endoglin genes are associated with PAH in patients with hereditary haemorrhagic telangiectasia.

Management and new pharmacological therapies for pulmonary arterial hypertension

Only patients in Group 1 of the Dana Point classification (Table 26.1; i.e. IPAH, HPAH and associated PAH [APAH]) should receive specific treatment for PHT. However, when an underlying cause for PHT is established (e.g. pulmonary embolism) this must be treated.

The past decade has witnessed major advances in the treatment of PAH. At least four medical therapies that target specific pathogenic pathways have received worldwide regulatory approval and several new therapies are under assessment.[1–5] Figure 26.1 summarizes the management of PAH. Patients in whom the diagnosis is unclear or those with PAH, CTEPH or severe PHT (PASP >60 mmHg) should be managed in specialist centres.

- **General management**. The cause should be treated (e.g. chronic obstructive pulmonary disease) and supportive therapies addressed (e.g. immunization, exercise, pulmonary rehabilitation). Pregnancy is associated with a high maternal mortality (>30%) and contraceptive advice is essential. Early termination may be required. Supplemental oxygen should be used to maintain SaO_2 >90%, because hypoxaemia is a pulmonary vasoconstrictor. Digoxin is occasionally used in refractory right ventricular failure (RVF) and for rate control of the atrial dysrhythmias that frequently complicate severe PAH with RVF.[1–5]
- **Anticoagulation** with warfarin (international normalized ratio 1.5–2.5) is recommended in IPAH and CTEPH. Prevention of microscopic thrombosis improves survival in IPAH, HPAH and PAH due to anorexigens.[1] In PAH due to other aetiologies (e.g. scleroderma) anticoagulation is controversial, although during therapy with intravenous epoprostenol, anticoagulation is recommended to reduce the risk associated with catheter-associated thrombosis.[1–5]
- **Diuretics** may be required for RVF but their use risks systemic hypotension due to hypovolaemia, renal insufficiency and electrolyte abnormalities.
- **Calcium channel blockers**. Of the 10%–15% of IPAH patients who respond to acute vasodilators (e.g. adenosine) only about 50% have sustained vasodilation and improved long-term survival with the use of high-dose CCB. Typically, nifedipine 120–240 mg/day is used in patients with relative bradycardia, and diltiazem 240–720 mg/day in patients with relative tachycardia. Treatment should be started at low dose with careful monitoring for systemic hypotension and peripheral oedema.

CCB therapy in those patients without an acute vasodilator response (and in untested patients) is potentially dangerous due to the associated side effects (i.e. right heart failure, hypotension) and is not recommended.

- **Phosphodiesterase-5 inhibitors**. Sildenafil (20–80 mg tds) is an orally active, potent inhibitor of cyclic guanosine monophosphate (cGMP)-specific phosphodiesterase type 5 which increases cGMP, augmenting relaxation and reducing proliferation in lung vascular smooth muscle. In a recent large, randomized controlled trial it improved exercise capacity, functional class and haemodynamics in PAH patients (WHO-FC II and III).[6] Tadalafil is a once-daily alternative.
- **Endothelin receptor antagonists**. Endothelin-1 (ET-1) is a potent vasoconstrictor and smooth muscle mitogen. ET-1 expression, production and levels are increased in PAH and correlate with disease severity. Bosentan, a dual ETA and ETB receptor antagonist, improved exercise tolerance, symptoms, haemodynamics and functional class in the large Bosentan Randomized trial of Endothelin Antagonist Therapy of pulmonary Hypertension (BREATH-1) study and previous smaller studies.[7,8] Bosentan is licensed for WHO-FC II and III PAH. Therapy is started at 62.5 mg twice daily for four weeks increasing to 125 mg twice daily thereafter. Liver function tests should be monitored due to the risk of hepatic toxicity. Bosentan may also cause anaemia, oedema, testicular atropy, male infertility and teratogenicity. The selective ETA receptor antagonist ambrisentan (5–10 mg daily) has been demonstrated to be effective in WHO-FC II and III patients with IPAH and APAH. Sitaxentan, another selective ETA receptor antagonist, which had been demonstrated to be clinically effective in a similar group of patients, was withdrawn from use in December 2010 due to potential liver toxicity.
- **Prostanoids**. Prostacyclin is a metabolite of arachidonic acid produced in vascular endothelium. It is a potent pulmonary (and systemic) vasodilator, has antiplatelet effects and is relatively deficient in PAH.
  1. Epoprostenol by continuous intravenous infusions improves haemodynamics, exercise capacity (6MW) and survival compared to normal therapy (e.g. diuretics, anticoagulants) in IPAH and scleroderma-like diseases.[1,2,9] Therapeutic difficulties relate to the short half-life, rebound hypertension during treatment breaks and side effects associated with the central venous infusion (e.g. infection). Side effects include headache, rash, musculoskeletal pain, nausea, jaw pain, hypotension and diarrhoea. It is licensed for WHO-FC III and IV PAH but is generally reserved for patients with disease refractory to oral therapies. Benefit can be maintained for many years.[10]
  2. Treprostinil has a longer half-life (three hours) than epoprostenol. Subcutaneous infusion produces modest improvements in 6MW and haemodynamic parameters when compared to placebo. It is licensed for subcutaneous and intravenous use in WHO-FC II–IV PAH.[1–5]
  3. Iloprost has a half-life of 20 minutes and inhalation 6–9 times daily improves haemodynamics, functional class and 6MW.[1–5] Side effects include flushing, headache and cough. It is licensed for WHO-FC III PAH and may be a useful adjunct to oral therapy.
- **Combination pharmacological therapy** is common in many centres and may be associated with improved outcomes, although long-term safety and efficacy have not been established.

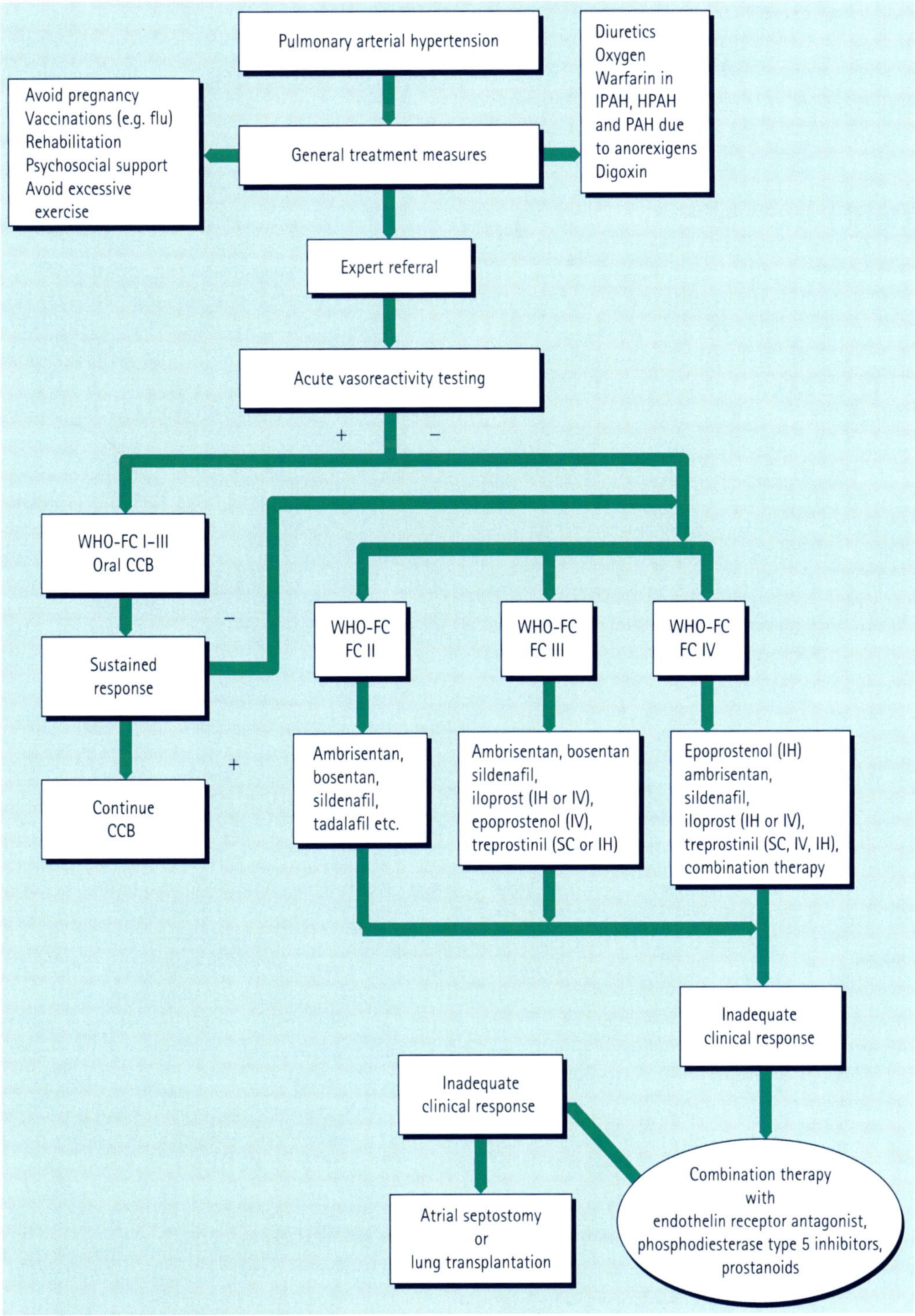

Figure 26.1 Treatment algorithm for PAH. CCB, calcium channel blockers; FC, NYHA/WHO functional class; IH, inhaled; IV, intravenous; SC, subcutaneous.

- **Interventional/surgical therapies**. Atrial septostomy creates a right-to-left shunt and decompresses the failing right heart. It is a largely palliative procedure or bridge to lung transplantation. Patient selection, timing and septostomy size are vital.[1] Lung transplantation (preferably bilateral) is reserved for failed medical therapy and one-year survival is approximately 65%–75%.[11]

Conclusion

This patient was confirmed to have IPAH following investigation. Her mean PAP was 32 mmHg but she did not have an acute vasodilator response to adenosine. She has been anticoagulated and referred to a specialist centre for ongoing treatment. Recent advances in the therapeutic options available for treatment of this rare condition have considerably improved her long-term prognosis.

Further Reading

1 Galiè N, Hoeper MM, Humbert M *et al.* ESC/ERS Guidelines for the diagnosis and treatment of pulmonary hypertension. *Eur Respir J* 2009; **34**: 1219–63.

2 Rubin LJ. Pulmonary arterial hypertension. *Proc Am Thorac Soc* 2006; **3**: 111–5.

3 Simonneau G, Galiè N, Rubin LJ *et al.* Clinical classification of pulmonary hypertension. *J Am Coll Cardiol* 2004; **43**(Suppl S): 5S–12S.

4 Galiè N, Seeger W, Naeije R, Simonneau G, Rubin LJ. Comparative analysis of clinical trials and evidence-based treatment algorithm in pulmonary arterial hypertension. *J Am Coll Cardiol* 2004; **43**(Suppl S): 81S–88S.

5 Consensus statement on the management of pulmonary hypertension in clinical practice in the UK and Ireland. National pulmonary hypertension centres of the UK and Ireland. *Thorax* 2008; **63**(Suppl 2): ii1–ii41 or *Heart* 2008; **94**(Suppl 1): i1–41.

6 Galiè N, Ghofrani H, Torbicki A *et al.* Sildenafil citrate therapy for pulmonary arterial hypertension. *N Engl J Med* 2005; **353**: 2148–57.

7 Rubin LJ, Badesch DB, Barst RJ *et al.* Bosentan therapy for pulmonary arterial hypertension. *N Engl J Med* 2002; **346**: 896–903.

8 Channick RN, Simonneau G, Sitbon O *et al.* Effects of the dual endothelin-receptor antagonist bosentan in patients with pulmonary arterial hypertension: a randomised, placebo-controlled trial. *Lancet* 2001; **358**: 1119–23.

9 Badesch DB, Tapson VF, McGoon MD *et al.* Continuous intravenous epoprostenol for pulmonary hypertension due to the scleroderma spectrum of disease. A randomized, controlled trial. *Ann Intern Med* 2000; **132**: 425–34.

10 McLaughlin VV, Shillington A, Rich S. Survival in primary pulmonary hypertension: the impact of epoprostenol therapy. *Circulation* 2002; **106**: 1477–82.

11 Doyle RL, McCrory D, Channick RN, Simonneau G, Conte J. Surgical treatments/interventions for pulmonary arterial hypertension: ACCP evidence-based clinical practice guidelines. *Chest* 2004; **126**(1 Suppl): 63S–71S.

PROBLEM

27 Massive Pulmonary Embolism

Elizabeth Hadley, Christopher Kosky

Case History

A 46-year-old Afro-Caribbean man presented to hospital after he collapsed with brief loss of consciousness. He was short of breath at rest and felt as if he couldn't take a breath in. He felt dizzy on standing. He did not have chest pain. He had no significant past medical history. He had never smoked.

On examination he was overweight, sweaty and tachypnoeic. His systolic blood pressure was 88 mmHg and heart rate was 120 beats/min. He was afebrile. Jugular venous pulse was at 7 cm. Auscultation of his chest revealed normal breath sounds with no added sounds. Oxygen saturation was 94% on 10 l/min of oxygen. Arterial blood gas analysis, on oxygen, revealed a pH 7.46, and partial pressure of oxygen (PaO_2) of 9.5 kPa and carbon dioxide ($PaCO_2$) of 3.9 kPa. His chest radiograph was unremarkable. A twelve-lead electrocardiogram (ECG) showed borderline ST elevation in the chest leads and T wave inversion in lead V. D-dimer and troponin were positive. An urgent computed tomography pulmonary angiogram (CTPA) was performed (Figure 27.1).

What do you see on the CTPA?

How do you explain the results of the d-dimer, troponin and ECG?

How would you manage this patient?

Background

In this case the CTPA shows a large saddle embolus in the pulmonary artery; further cuts showed scattered thrombus in the proximal pulmonary arteries bilaterally. The patient was diagnosed with a massive pulmonary embolism (PE).

Massive PE is characterized by persistent hypotension, usually defined as a systolic blood pressure <90 mmHg. A fall in systolic blood pressure of at least 40 mmHg for greater than 15 minutes is also significant. Typically the patient is shocked with a clear chest and raised jugular pressure. It is important to exclude an acute myocardial infarction and tension pneumothorax. Massive PE can lead to acute right heart failure; death is usually within 1–2 hours of the embolism.

Investigations

In this case PE was diagnosed on a CTPA. A CTPA has been shown to be an accurate diagnostic tool for pulmonary thromboembolic disease, with higher interobserver con-

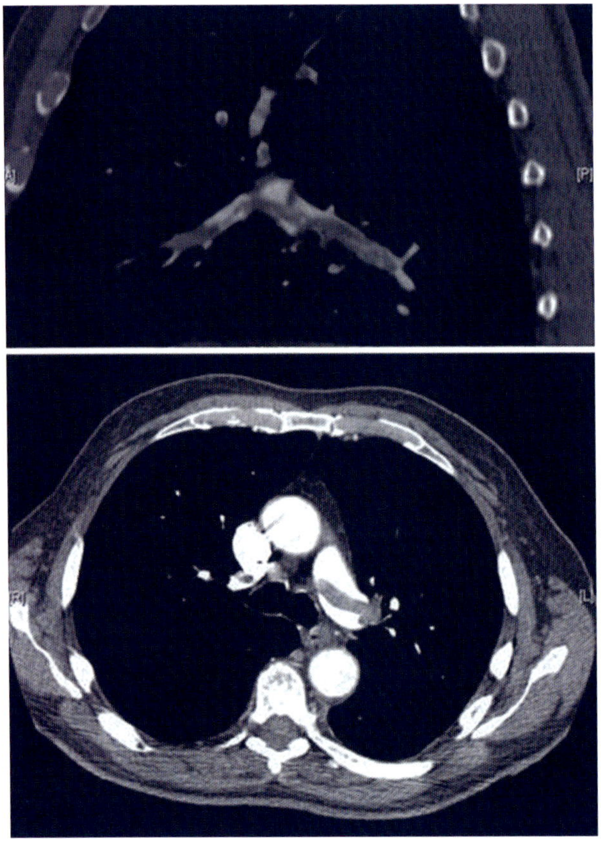

Figure 27.1 Computed tomography pulmonary angiogram.

cordance than ventilation-perfusion (V/Q) scanning. Evidence shows that sensitivity and specificity with CTPA are higher than V/Q scanning, and that a negative CTPA is as good as a negative or low-probability V/Q scan to rule out PE.[1,2] There is a debate over whether some smaller subsegmental pulmonary emboli that are found on a CTPA actually require treatment. Magnetic resonance imaging has not yet been found to be any more useful than traditional imaging.[3]

Bedside echocardiography can be useful to assist in the diagnosis of PE when the patient is too unwell to undergo a CTPA. A real-time echocardiogram may show right ventricular dysfunction, tricuspid valve regurgitation and possibly thrombus in the right ventricle.

The d-dimer is a non-specific indicator of the presence of thromboembolic disease. It measures the by-product of intravascular fibrinolysis. A positive d-dimer result informs you that the process of clot formation and degradation may be taking place, but does not tell you where or in what circumstances. As a test for PE or deep vein thrombosis (DVT) the d-dimer is only really useful when negative. A positive d-dimer test has a high sensitivity for thromboembolic disease; however, its positive predictive value is low, with many positive results in the absence of proven PE or DVT.[4,5]

The Wells' score is a clinical probability score useful for excluding PE and DVT without further investigations (Table 27.1).[6] A PE can usually be excluded if the patient has a low clinical probability score and a negative d-dimer test. However, in cases of moderate to high clinical probability, a negative d-dimer result cannot be relied upon to exclude PE. Clinical probability scoring is now commonplace as part of the work-up for PE. The Wells' score is not intended to be used in post-operative and long-term inpatients.[7]

Table 27.1 Wells' criteria for assessment of pre-test probability for pulmonary embolism

Criteria	Points
Suspected DVT	3.0
An alternative diagnosis is less likely than PE	3.0
Heart rate >100 beats per minute	1.5
Immobilization or surgery in the previous four weeks	1.5
Previous DVT or PE	1.5
Haemoptysis	1.0
Malignancy (on treatment, treated in the last 6 months or palliative)	1.0

Score range	Mean probability of PE %	Risk of pulmonary embolism
<2 points	3.6	Low
2–6 points	20.5	Moderate
>6 points	66.7	High

Cardiac troponin as evidence of myocardial damage is a strong prognostic marker in acute PE. An elevated serum troponin correlates with right ventricular dysfunction on a 'same-time' echocardiogram; higher troponin rises are also predictive of increased in-hospital mortality, post-PE complications and recurrent PE.[8,9] In this case the troponin rise suggested that this patient was at greater risk of cardiovascular instability in the acute setting and that he might be at risk of future thromboembolic disease. Brain natriuretic peptide (BNP) is a useful but less commonly utilized marker of cardiomyocyte stretch and shear stress in acute PE.[10]

Duplex venous ultrasound of the lower limb may assist in the diagnosis of PE. Residual lower limb DVT can be seen in 30%–50% of patients with a PE.[11]

Treatment of pulmonary embolism

The majority of patients with a proven PE are anticoagulated, usually with low molecular weight heparin whilst being loaded and stabilized on warfarin. In the presence of a known temporary trigger, such as a long bone fracture, anticoagulation for PE can be discontinued after 4–6 weeks. For an idiopathic PE in the absence of any known ongoing risk factors anticoagulation is usually continued for between three and six months.[12]

Thrombolysis for massive PE is recommended when there is evidence of arterial hypotension, cardiogenic shock, hypoxia with a metabolic acidosis, a reduced conscious level or oliguria.[11] Early mortality in patients with massive PE is at least 15%, and in these patients the bleeding risks associated with thrombolysis are acceptable. The Cochrane Collaboration found that thrombolysis improved haemodynamic outcomes and post-PE imaging appearances, but had no appreciable benefit in death rate or recurrence; there was no significant difference in minor or major bleeding events. Patients should be managed in a high-dependency setting as they are at increased risk of death for 24–72 hours.

There are a few patients worldwide each year that undergo emergency open pulmonary thromboembolectomy for acute massive PE; a further group have this procedure electively as a treatment for chronic post-PE pulmonary hypertension. It is a high-risk operative procedure; however, in a specialist centre with appropriate clinical support it has been shown to have comparable mortality to thrombolysis in the acute setting.[11]

Prognosis

Current guidance on treatment of PE in the absence of ongoing risk factors is to anticoagulate for three to six months.[11] Lifelong anticoagulation should be considered in patients with recurrent PE or DVT. Most patients make a complete recovery after a PE. However, a minority (1%–3%) develop chronic thromboembolic pulmonary hypertension. PE should be suspected in patients with continued dyspnoea, signs of pulmonary hypertension and/or echocardiographic evidence of right ventricular dysfunction. Massive PE is a risk factor for the development of chronic thromboembolic pulmonary hypertension. A positive troponin or BNP at six months has been shown to indicate continued right ventricular dysfunction.[13] Patients with chronic thromboembolic pulmonary hypertension should receive lifelong warfarin and be referred for consideration of pulmonary thromboembolectomy.

Conclusion

Massive PE is life threatening and should be a potential differential diagnosis for all acutely unwell patients. If PE is suspected, imaging to confirm the diagnosis should be arranged immediately and thrombolysis should be considered within an hour of presentation.

Further Reading

1 Mayo JR, Remy-Jardin M, Müller NL *et al.* Pulmonary embolism: prospective comparison of spiral CT with ventilation-perfusion scintigraphy. *Radiology* 1997; **205**: 447–52.

2 Rubins JB. The current approach to the diagnosis of pulmonary embolism: lessons from PIOPED II. *Postgrad Med* 2008; **120**: 1–7.

3 Sostman DH, Jablonski KA, Woodard PK *et al.* Factors in the technical quality of gadolinium enhanced magnetic resonance angiography for pulmonary embolism in PIOPED III. *Int J Cardiovasc Imaging* 2011. DOI: 10.1007/s10554-011-9820-7. www.springerlink.com/journals (accessed 01 07 11).

4 de Moerloose P, Palareti G, Aguilar C, Legnani C, Reber G, Peetz D. A multicenter evaluation of a new quantitative highly sensitive D-dimer assay for exclusion of venous thromboembolism. *Thromb Haemost* 2008; **100**: 505–12.

5 Perrier A, Desmarais S, Miron M-J *et al.* Non-invasive diagnosis of venous thromboembolism in outpatients. *Lancet* 1999; **353**: 190–5.

6 Wells PS, Anderson DR, Rodger M *et al.* Derivation of a simple clinical model to categorize patients probability of pulmonary embolism: increasing the models utility with the SimpliRED D-dimer. *Thromb Haemost* 2000; **83**: 416–20.

7 Kruip MJHA, Slob MJ, Schijen JHEM, van der Heul C, Büller HR. Use of a clinical decision rule in combination with d-dimer concentration in diagnostic workup of patients with suspected pulmonary embolism: a prospective management study. *Arch Intern Med* 2002; **162**: 1631–5.

8 Palmieri V, Gallotta G, Rendina D *et al.* Troponin I and right ventricular dysfunction for risk assessment in patients with nonmassive pulmonary embolism in the Emergency Department in combination with clinically based risk score. *Intern Emerg Med* 2008; **3**: 131–8.

9 Mehta NJ, Jani K, Khan IA. Clinical usefulness and prognostic value of elevated cardiac troponin I levels in acute pulmonary embolism. *Am Heart J* 2003; **145**: 821–5.

10 Kucher N, Printzen G, Goldhaber SZ. Prognostic role of brain natriuretic peptide in acute pulmonary embolism. *Circulation* 2003; **107**: 2545–7.

11 The PIOPED Investigators. Value of the ventilation/perfusion scan in acute pulmonary embolism. Results of the prospective investigation of pulmonary embolism diagnosis (PIOPED). *JAMA* 1990; **263**: 2753–9.

12 British Thoracic Society Standards of Care Committee Pulmonary Embolism Guideline Development Group. British Thoracic Society guidelines for the management of suspected acute pulmonary embolism. *Thorax* 2003; **58**: 470–83.

13 Kline JA, Zeitouni R, Marchick MR, Hernandez-Nino J, Rose GA. Comparison of 8 biomarkers for prediction of right ventricular hypokinesis 6 months after submassive pulmonary embolism. *Am Heart J* 2008; **156**: 308–14.

PROBLEM

28 Sickle Cell Lung Disease

Elizabeth Hadley, Boris Lams, Christopher Kosky

Case History

A 40-year-old man with known homozygous (HbSS) sickle cell disease (SCD) presented to the emergency department with a three-day history of cough, fever and sweats. He denied any chest pain. Seven days prior he had had a painful crisis affecting both his knees which had resolved with oral analgesia and oral fluids. He was not taking penicillin prophylaxis. On examination he had a temperature of 39.8°C, a pulse of 120 beats/min and a blood pressure of 135/68 mmHg. His respiratory rate was 32 breaths/min and he appeared anxious. His extremities were warm. Auscultation of his chest revealed a few crackles anteriorly on the right.

Investigations revealed a haemoglobin level of 7.6 g/dl, white cell count of 47.7×10^9, neutrophil count of 45.3×10^9, platelet count 307×10^9 and reticulocyte count of 134×10^9. The C-reactive protein was 275 mg/l. A renal profile showed a urea of 2.9 mmol/l and a creatinine of 74 μmol/l. A liver profile revealed a bilirubin of 209 g/l, alkaline phosphatase of 109 IU/l and alanine aminotransferase of 40 IU/l. His chest radiograph is shown in Figure 28.1. Over the ensuing three days he did not improve with intravenous cefuroxime and clarithromycin. He remained persistently febrile up to 39°C and his C-reactive protein and neutrophil count failed to decrease. A second chest radiograph was taken (Figure 28.2).

What is the initial diagnosis?

Why is the neutrophil count raised?

What complication may have occurred during his admission?

What further investigation would you perform?

How would you manage the patient in the high-dependency unit?

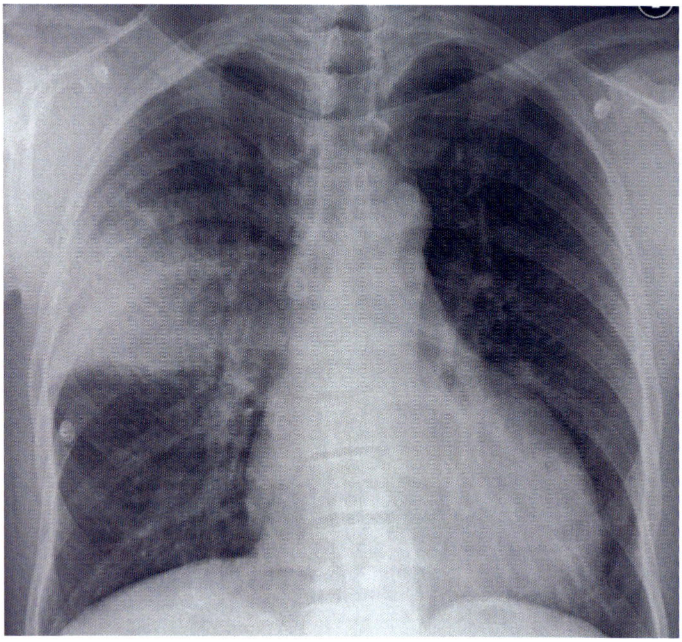

Figure 28.1 Chest radiograph at presentation.

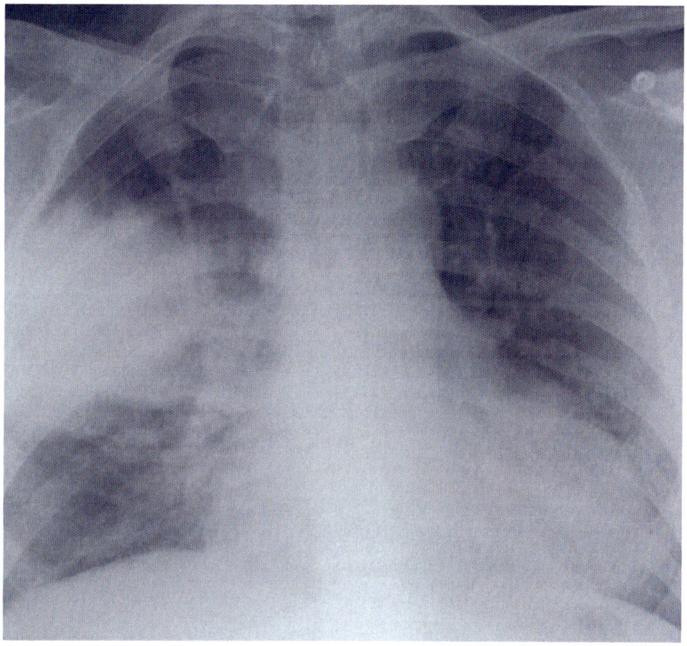

Figure 28.2 Chest radiograph 24 hours after presentation.

Background

In this case, the differential diagnosis includes pneumonia or an acute chest syndrome.

The acute chest syndrome is a frequent cause of hospitalization and the leading cause of mortality in patients with SCD.[1] In SCD the replacement of a valine for a glutamic acid in the beta haemoglobin chain leads to a haemoglobin molecule that is poorly soluble when deoxygenated. The deoxygenated haemoglobin polymerizes and distorts the erythrocyte into the characteristic sickle shape. This sickle-shaped erythrocyte has a tendency to obstruct and occlude small blood vessels. Acute chest syndrome is thought to be due to vaso-occlusion of the pulmonary microvasculature due to *in situ* thrombosis from intravascular sickling. Hypoxia during an acute chest syndrome can also be caused by fat embolism from bone marrow infarction. Painful rib infarcts and opiates can cause hypoventilation.[2]

Acute chest syndrome in SCD is loosely defined as a new pulmonary infiltrate on chest X-ray accompanied by respiratory symptoms such as chest pain, fever, dyspnoea and cough. Examination may reveal tenderness over the ribs or sternum and signs of pulmonary consolidation. Laboratory findings include those of erythyrocyte haemolysis, with elevated lactate dehyrogenase and bilirubin accompanied by falling haemoglobin. Leukocytosis is also common. In adults with acute chest syndrome, radiographic infiltrates almost always involve the lower lobes and are bilateral in a third of patients. In children, an upper lobe infiltrate normally predominates.

Although the acute chest syndrome is often a self-limiting illness it may also lead to life-threatening respiratory insufficiency, particularly in adults for which it has a mortality rate of 4.3%, which is three times that in children.[3]

Patients with SCD are at increased risk of developing bacterial pneumonia because of autosplenectomy. Although commonly thought to be pneumococcal in origin, other organisms have been identified as causing pneumonia or leading to an acute chest syndrome, including *Haemophilus influenzae*, *Mycoplasma pneumoniae* and *Chlamydia pneumoniae*.

Raised neutrophil count

In SCD there is a raised number of circulating nucleated red blood cells and the erythrocytes are resistant to standard lysing reagents. Automated systems for leukocyte counting and differentiation can falsely include these erythrocytes in the white cell count. In this case the elevated neutrophil count was confirmed by a blood film and manual differentiation. Neutrophilia in this case may be due to acute bacterial infection, pulmonary infarction or pulmonary inflammation.

Pulmonary gangrene

In this case, the second chest radiograph (Figure 28.2), taken after admission, reveals that the area of consolidation has increased in size and the minor fissure appears to be bulging inferiorly, a radiographic finding associated with pulmonary gangrene.[4] This rare condition, also known as massive sequestration, occurs in the setting of a severe bacterial pneumonia, with the intense inflammatory response leading to arterial thrombosis within the affected parenchyma and subsequent necrosis and cavity formation. Consideration should be given to performing a lobectomy in those who are failing to improve or who suffer massive haemoptysis. The failure of the C-reactive protein to fall by 50% within the first four days of commencing antibiotics has been shown to be a marker of treatment failure in pneumonia.

Investigation

This patient underwent a computed tomography (CT) chest scan 72 hours after presentation (Figure 28.3). The CT chest scan shows cavitation related to the pulmonary gangrene, widespread air bronchograms and lower lobe infiltrates. The patient was transferred to the high-dependency unit.

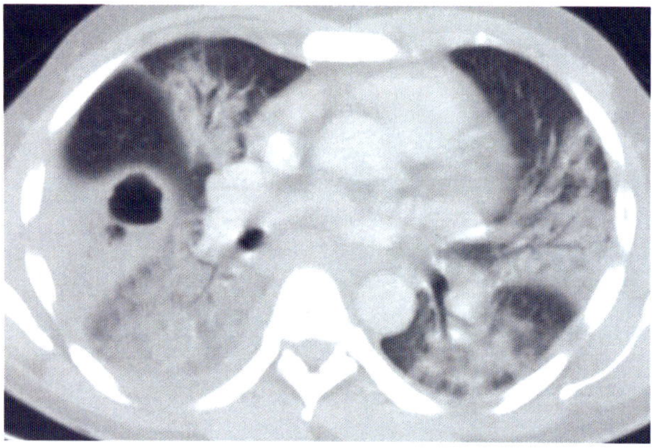

Figure 28.3 Chest CT scan 72 hours after presentation showing cavitating pulmonary consolidation in the right upper lobe consistent with pulmonary gangrene and bilateral pulmonary infiltrates.

Treatment

In the high-dependency unit, the patient was treated for both pulmonary gangrene and acute chest syndrome. Acute chest syndrome can be precipitated by a severe pulmonary infection.

Therapy for the acute chest syndrome relies on careful attention to fluid balance, analgesia and oxygenation.[5] Oxygen should be given to maintain a partial pressure of arterial oxygen between 10 and 12 kPa. Hypoxia will trigger the formation of sickle cells. Management of hydration in the patient with the acute chest syndrome must balance between volume depletion, which can lead to further erythrocyte sickling, and volume overload resulting in pulmonary oedema. Careful use of opiate analgesia is required in the presence of chest pain secondary to rib infarction. Uncontrolled pain leads to regional hypoventilation, atelectasis, ventilation-perfusion mismatch and further sickling. Hypercapnia reported in 46% of 107 patients with an acute chest syndrome was thought to be due to hypoventilation from rib pain rather than opiates. However, care must be taken to avoid opiate-induced respiratory depression. Incentive spirometry has been shown to be beneficial in avoiding progression to acute chest syndrome in those with painful crises affecting the thorax. Anticoagulation is normally avoided because of the risks of cerebral and renal bleeding in those with SCD.

In acute chest syndrome, progressive pulmonary infiltrates or worsening hypoxia are an indication for exchange transfusion. The patient is venesected and then transfused via either central or peripheral access. Exchange transfusion rapidly replaces sickling cells with normal erythrocytes. There is also emerging evidence for the use of inhaled nitric oxide as an adjunct to exchange transfusion.[6]

In this case, the patient had exchange transfusion of six units of blood, which reduced his sickle percentage to below 30%. In the days following the exchange transfusion, his symptoms and fever resolved and his white cell count and C-reactive protein fell to normal values. His chest radiograph cleared leaving a right upper lobe cavity (Figure 28.4).

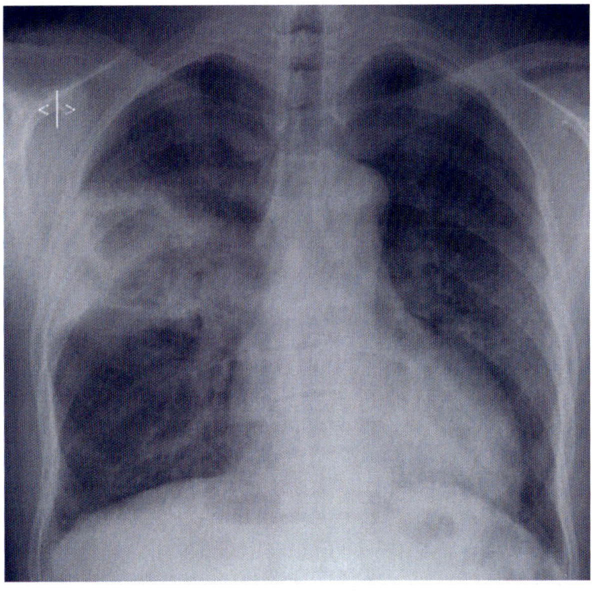

Figure 28.4 Chest radiograph ten days after presentation.

Conclusion

The key to management of the patient with sickle lung is early recognition. Morbidity and mortality are substantially reduced if appropriate intervention is made promptly. These patients should be managed by a multidisciplinary team with a low threshold for high-dependency unit care.

Further Reading

1 Vij R, Machado RF. Pulmonary complications of hemoglobinopathies. *Chest* 2010; **138**: 973–83.

2 Stuart MJ, Setty BN. Acute chest syndrome of sickle cell disease: new light on an old problem. *Curr Opin Hematol* 2001; **8**: 111–122.

3 Vichinsky EP, Styles LA, Colangelo LH, Wright EC, Castro O, Nickerson B. Acute chest syndrome in sickle cell disease: clinical presentation and course. Cooperative Study of Sickle Cell Disease. *Blood* 1997; **89**: 1787–92.

4 Hammond JM, Lyddell C, Potgieter PD, Odell J. Severe pneumococcal pneumonia complicated by massive pulmonary gangrene. *Chest* 1993; **104**; 1610–2.

5 Maitre B, Habibi A, Roudot-Thoraval F *et al.* Acute chest syndrome in adults with sickle cell disease. Therapeutic approach, outcome, and results of BAL in a monocentric series of 107 episodes. *Chest* 2000; **117**: 1386–92.

6 Laurie GA. Acute chest syndrome in sickle cell disease. *Intern Med J* 2010; **40**: 372–6.

PROBLEM

29 Pulmonary Arteriovenous Malformation

Elizabeth Hadley

Case History

A 45-year-old lady was referred to the chest clinic because of dyspnoea. She had gradually become more breathless over two years and was now breathless at rest. The patient mentioned that she felt less breathless at night when she was lying flat. She had no cough, but did admit to a single episode of haemoptysis six weeks earlier that had been during a 'cold'. She had no known past medical history apart from frequent nosebleeds.

On examination she had multiple small red lesions around her lips which blanched on pressure. She was not cyanotic. She had early clubbing. Her chest was clear on auscultation. She did not have signs of liver disease. Her oxygen saturations were 90% on air. Her oxygen saturations rose to 93% when she lay flat. Oxygen saturations fell to 87% on exercise. Blood tests revealed normal clotting and polycythaemia. A chest radiograph was normal. A chest computed tomography (CT) scan was performed (Figure 29.1)

What does the chest CT scan show?

What is the diagnosis?

How can pulmonary shunt be confirmed?

What is the treatment of an arteriovenous malformation?

What is the prognosis for this patient following bronchial artery embolization?

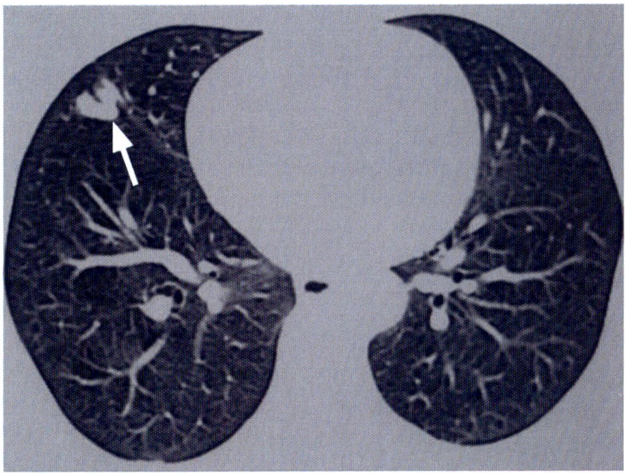

Figure 29.1 CT scan demonstrating pulmonary arteriovenous malformation (arrow) in the right lung.

Background

In this case the chest CT scan showed a contrast-enhancing lesion in the lung parenchyma with a vascular appearance. The diagnosis was of a pulmonary arteriovenous malformation (AVM) on a background of previously unrecognized hereditary haemorrhagic telangiectasia.

The breathlessness and hypoxia associated with a pulmonary AVM are due to a right-to-left shunt of a significant amount of deoxygenated blood, which passes through the pulmonary circulation back to the left atrium without being reoxygenated. This deoxygenated blood mixes in the left atrium with oxygenated blood. The overall hypoxia of the patient is determined by the size of the shunt. During exercise the effect of the shunt increases leading to exercise desaturation. As demonstrated in this case, pulmonary shunt can cause platypnoea (dyspnoea relieved by lying down) and orthodeoxia (deoxygenation accompanying a change to sitting or standing from a recumbent position). Platypnoea and orthodeoxia are due to changes in ventilation-perfusion matching with position, which may in turn reduce the impact of a pulmonary shunt.

Bubble echocardiogram

Pulmonary shunt can be confirmed by bubble echocardiogram or calculating the shunt fraction. A bubble echocardiogram involves injecting a small amount of agitated saline with microbubbles into a peripheral vein whilst a transthoracic echocardiogram is performed. In patients with no right-to-left shunting the bright bubbles are seen in the right atrium only, as the bubbles are filtered out as the blood travels through the lungs. In those with an intracardiac right-to-left shunt, the bubbles are seen in the right atrium and then on the left-hand side of the heart within 3–5 cardiac cycles (about 4 seconds).This is because the blood flowing through the shunt has bypassed the lungs. In patients with a clinically significant intrapulmonary shunt (i.e. a pulmonary AVM) the bubbles are seen in the right atrium first, then appear on the left-hand side of the heart after a delay of between three and eight minutes. This is a highly sensitive test, and can be used to screen for suspected pulmonary AVM in symptomatic cases.[1,2]

The amount of blood travelling through the shunt or shunt fraction can be calculated using the 100% oxygen method. This involves measurement of oxygen partial pressure (PaO_2) and saturation (SaO_2) after breathing 100% oxygen for 15 to 20 minutes and using the right-to-left shunt calculation.[3] A shunt fraction of greater than 5% is abnormal. In this case the patient's shunt fraction was 8%.

Radionucleotide perfusion lung scanning is another method to detect AVMs and calculate shunt fraction. Using this method, technetium-99m (99mTc)-pertechnetate-labelled albumin is injected into a peripheral vein. In normal subjects, most of the radiolabelled albumin is caught in the small capillaries of the lungs. If an intrapulmonary shunt exists this will allow radiolabelled albumin to collect in the capillary beds of the kidneys and brain. The amount that collects in the brain and kidneys depends on the size of the shunt.[4]

Bronchial artery embolization

Untreated pulmonary AVMs have a significant mortality due to stroke, cerebral abscess, haemoptysis and haemothorax. The treatment of pulmonary AVM is bronchial artery embolization or surgical resection.

Bronchial artery embolization was first performed in 1977. Prior to that, surgical resection of pulmonary AVMs was the only curative option. Bronchial artery embolization is now performed worldwide, but is still usually restricted to specialist centres where radiologists have the most experience and best facilities available. During the procedure, which is performed under conscious sedation, the bronchial artery is catheterized via a peripheral vein. The feeding artery of the AVM is then selectively catheterized under radiological screening; the artery is embolized using a heated steel coil. This can be repeated in several selected places in one session. Intra-operative complications of the procedure include problems with bleeding, damage or occlusion of other vessels. Arrhythmias are often seen, and one in twenty patients may suffer an air embolism which can cause angina or stroke-like effects; fortunately these are mostly transient. Rarely there can be device migration.

Following the procedure, the commonest complication is pleuritic chest pain. This is reported in up to 12% of patients, and in a quarter of these it is possible to see radiographical evidence of pulmonary infarction distal to the embolized segments. This is observed less in patients with well-developed collaterals. A further reported complication seen when big AVMs are embolized is post-procedure pulmonary hypertension. This is due to a sudden redirection of a large volume of the circulation through the pulmonary bed. For this reason larger AVMs or very complex AVMs might be best considered for surgical resection via a lobectomy, for example.[5]

Prognosis

Patients followed-up over eight years following coil embolization have demonstrated up to a 12% rate of representation with recurrence of the AVM or growth of a new clinically significant AVM. Patients with hereditary haemorrhagic telangiectasia and cystic fibrosis are most at risk of recurrence, the latter due to ongoing chronic infection and new vessel growth. It is recommended that patients with known pulmonary AVMs are offered prophylactic antibiotics for invasive procedures.[6]

Conclusion

Physicians should be alert for refractory hypoxia and look for clues to the diagnosis of pulmonary AVM. Once suspected, the correct investigations should be simple to arrange and diagnosis straightforward. Modern interventional radiology techniques allow treatment with significantly improved morbidity and mortality for all but the most complex patients.[7]

Further Reading

1 van Gent MW, Post MC, Snijder RJ *et al.* Grading of pulmonary right-to-left shunt with transthoracic contrast echocardiography: does it predict the indication for embolotherapy? *Chest* 2009; **135**: 1288–92.

2 Gazzaniga P, Buscarini E, Leandro G *et al.* Contrast echocardiography for pulmonary arteriovenous malformations screening: does any bubble matter? *Eur J Echocardiogr* 2009; **10**: 513–8.

3 Chiang ST. A nomogram for venous shunt (Qs-Qt) calculation. *Thorax* 1968; **23**: 563–5.

4 Gossage JR, Kanj G. Pulmonary ateriovenous malformations. A state of the art review. *Am J Respir Crit Care Med* 1998; **158**: 643–61.

5 Pick A, Deschamps C, Stanson AW. Pulmonary arteriovenous fistula: presentation, diagnosis, and treatment. *World J Surg* 1999; **23**: 1118–22.

6 Pollak JS, Saluja S, Thabet A, Henderson KJ, Denbow N, White RI Jr. Clinical and anatomic outcomes after embolotherapy of pulmonary arteriovenous malformations. *J Vasc Interv Radiol* 2006; **17**: 35–44.

7 Hsu CC, Kwan GN, Thompson SA, van Driel ML. Embolisation therapy for pulmonary arteriovenous malformations. *Cochrane Database Syst Rev* 2010; CD008017.

SECTION SIX 06

Vasculitis/Rare Diseases

PROBLEM

30 Wegener's Granulomatosis and the Small Vessel Pulmonary Vasculitides

Elizabeth Hadley, Richard Leach

Case History

A 41-year-old Asian salesman presented following an episode of haemoptysis in which he expectorated a teaspoonful of fresh blood. For several weeks he had been experiencing influenza-like symptoms with lethargy, low-grade fever, arthralgia, breathlessness on climbing stairs and weight loss. In addition he described long-standing intermittent sinusitis, blocked nose, snoring at night and occasional nose bleeds. There was no history of hayfever, allergy, travel abroad or tuberculosis contact. He was a non-smoker with no pet, bird, industrial dust or allergen contact.

Examination was unremarkable apart from a constant 'sniff'. Investigation demonstrated a normochromic, normocytic anaemia, an elevated erythrocyte sedimentation rate (ESR) and a raised white cell and platelet count. Serum urea was elevated and the creatinine was three times the upper limit of normal. The chest radiograph (CXR) shows diffuse, bilateral, mid-zone, alveolar shadowing, worse on the left (Figure 30.1). The apices and lung bases are clear. The hila are normal and distinct from the alveolar shadowing. *Aspergillus* serology, anti-nuclear antibody and sputum examination for acid-fast bacilli and cytology were negative. Anti-neutrophil cytoplasmic antibody (ANCA) was positive with a diffusely cytoplasmic pattern.

High-resolution computed tomography (HRCT) showed bilateral alveolar shadowing which crossed segmental borders suggesting pulmonary infiltrates or haemorrhage (Figure 30.2). Bronchoscopy was complicated by epistaxis and although the bronchial mucosa was inflamed, no lesions suitable for biopsy were detected. Blood-stained bronchoalveolar lavage fluid demonstrated an inflammatory infiltrate with a high proportion of neutrophils (40%) and eosinophils (4%). There were large numbers of damaged leukocytes and leukocyte remnants. The lavage fluid was ANCA positive.[1] Transbronchial biopsies were not performed as the oxygen saturation was <89% on air. A renal biopsy was performed and demonstrated segmental necrotizing glomerulonephritis.

How are the vasculitides classified?

What is the significance of ANCA?

What is the likely diagnosis in this case and how is it confirmed?

What is the pathogenesis in this condition?

Are lung function tests useful?

How would you treat this patient?

This patient is keen to know his prognosis.

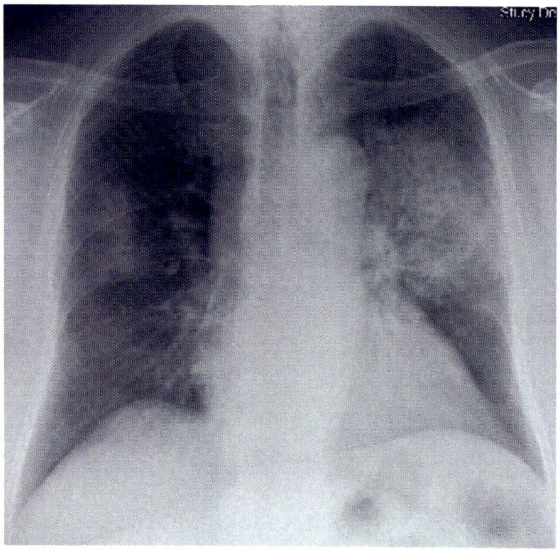

Figure 30.1 Chest radiograph.

Background

The vasculitides are rare conditions with a high untreated mortality.[2] They are non-specific and mimic many other diseases. Typical systemic features include low-grade fever, weight loss, haematuria, proteinuria, renal impairment, raised ESR and auto-antibodies. Pulmonary involvement usually occurs as part of a systemic vasculitis. The primary pathology is inflammation and necrosis of blood vessels. The Chapel Hill International Consensus Classification (1992) is illustrated in Table 30.1.

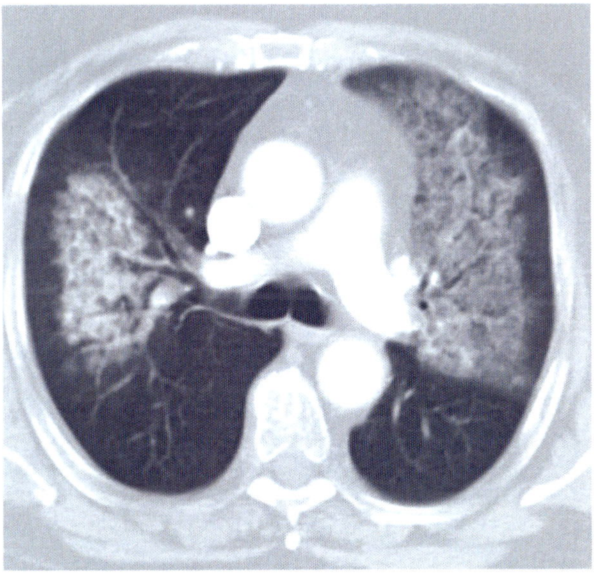

Figure 30.2 HRCT scan.

Table 30.1 Classification of vasculitis and pulmonary involvement

Primary vasculitis	Pulmonary involvement	ANCA
Small vessel vasculitides		
Wegener's granulomatosis	Often	c-ANCA 75%+ p-ANCA 15%
Churg–Strauss syndrome	Often	p-ANCA 70%
Microscopic polyangiitis	Often	c/p-ANCA >70%
Goodpasture's syndrome	Often	p-ANCA 10%–20%
Medium-sized arteritis		
Polyarteritis nodosa	Infrequent	Negative
Large vessel vasculitides		
Giant cell arteritis	Infrequent	Negative
Takayasu arteritis	Often	Negative

Small vessel vasculitides affect arterioles, capillaries or venules in lung interstitium. Neutrophil infiltration and fibrinoid necrosis cause damage to vessel walls. Capillary rupture results in red cells entering the alveolus and alveolar haemorrhage. Typical chest symptoms and signs which may not have responded to recent treatment include dyspnoea, wheeze, hypoxia, haemoptysis, sinus disease, CXR infiltrates and abnormal gas transfer (KCO).

In this case the constellation of haemoptysis, sinusitis, alveolar shadowing, raised ESR and renal impairment suggests a differential diagnosis of systemic vasculitis, autoimmune connective tissue disease or Goodpasture's syndrome. Malignancy and infective causes, including tuberculosis and aspergillosis, appear less likely.

Anti-neutrophil cytoplasmic antibodies

Anti-neutrophil cytoplasmic antibodies are markers of pulmonary vasculitides and may have a direct role in disease pathogenesis.[2,3] Using indirect immunofluorescence techniques, ANCA are demonstrated to react with cytoplasmic granule enzymes in neutrophils. The resulting staining pattern is either diffusely cytoplasmic (c-ANCA) or perinuclear (p-ANCA).

Modern enzyme-linked immunosorbent assay (ELISA) testing identifies ANCA as specific antibodies that target proteinase 3 (anti-PR3 antibodies) and myeloperoxidase (anti-MPO antibodies).

- The c-ANCA pattern is associated with anti-PR3 antibodies which occur in 75% of cases of Wegener's granulomatosis and about 45% of cases with microscopic polyangiitis. The c-ANCA level correlates with disease activity.
- The p-ANCA pattern is associated with anti-MPO antibodies. It is associated with a wider range of diseases including other vasculitides, autoimmune disease, pulmonary fibrosis, human immunodeficiency virus infection, lung cancer and pulmonary emboli.

Wegener's granulomatosis

This patient has Wegener's granulomatosis; a necrotizing systemic, 'granuloma-forming' vasculitis which presents with a combination of upper and lower respiratory tract disease and renal impairment. It is classified with microscopic polyangiitis (MPA) and Churg–Strauss syndrome. It affects mainly medium and small arteries, although it can also involve venules, arterioles and occasionally large arteries.

It is rare, without sex predominance, affecting all ages but mainly those between 40 and 55 years old.[3] It occurs in 3 per 100 000 people, mostly Caucasians, although 10% of cases occur in other ethnic groups. At presentation the disease is usually 'generalized' involving many systems although 25% of cases, typically young women, are 'limited' to the upper and lower airways. Nevertheless, 80% of 'limited' cases will develop renal involvement and a more generalized picture including cardiac, skin and central nervous system (CNS) involvement.

Wegener's granulomatosis can present as the classical triad of sinusitis, pulmonary symptoms and renal insufficiency, although non-specific upper airway, joint, skin and eye symptoms usually precede the diagnosis by several months. Acute cases occasionally present with pulmonary distress secondary to infiltrates and alveolar haemorrhage, acute renal failure and overwhelming systemic vasculitis. Some clinical manifestations only present in the remission phase, such as subglottic tracheal stenosis.

Tests that suggest the diagnosis include normocytic, normochromic anaemia, raised ESR, leukocytosis and thrombocytosis. Abnormal renal function, especially with proteinuria and/or haematuria, should prompt urgent urine cytology to detect dysmorphic red blood cells and casts suggestive of glomerular disease. HRCT lung scans may show pulmonary infiltrates, haemorrhage or bilateral multifocal subpleural nodules. Nodules are 0.5–10 cm in size, with cavitation in 20%–50% of those >2 cm in size. Feeding vessels are present in 88%. Pleurally based lesions may mimic infarcts.[4]

Circulating ANCA (75%–90% anti-PR3; the remainder anti-MPO antibodies) occurs in about 90% of patients with active generalized Wegener's granulomatosis. Dual positivity can occur, but raises the possibility of other disorders like systemic lupus erythematosus (SLE). However, in patients with disease limited to the upper respiratory tract, as many as 40% are ANCA negative and biopsy is essential for diagnosis. A positive PR3-ANCA helps differentiate between alveolar haemorrhage due to Wegener's granulomatosis and other causes including Goodpasture's syndrome, idiopathic pulmonary haemosiderosis, SLE and polyarteritis nodosa. In renal limited disease ANCA is 75%–80% MPO-ANCA.

In general, biopsy confirmation is essential before initiating prolonged immunosuppressant and/or cytotoxic therapy, although this requirement is occasionally waived in extremely ill (e.g. intensive care) patients who require immediate therapy. If the upper airway or skin are involved, biopsy is simple and non-invasive. Transbronchial biopsy may be diagnostic but even with HRCT guidance yield is low (<10%) and it risks complications.[5] Open lung biopsy is occasionally required in localized lung disease. Renal biopsy risks haemorrhage, which can be substantial, and may not differentiate histologically between MPA and Wegener's granulomatosis, although clinically the distinction is not that important.[6]

Pathogenesis of Wegener's granulomatosis

Wegener's granulomatosis may involve an abnormal host immune process triggered by environmental factors. Following adhesion to ANCA-positive tissues, activated polymorphonuclear neutrophils and endothelial cells cause necrotizing inflammation of blood vessel walls.[7] Granuloma formation is closely associated with CD4-positive T cells which occur in large numbers alongside macrophages in granuloma-containing biopsies. These T cells express helper T cell type 1 (Th1) phenotypes suggesting cell-mediated immunity and a potential infectious origin (e.g. mycobacteria), although no studies have detected infectious agents.[8] Recent work focusing on other potential environmental triggers (e.g. hobbies, vocations) concluded that heavy metal exposure and a prior history of allergy may play a role in pathogenesis.[9]

Lung function tests in Wegener's granulomatosis

Both restrictive and obstructive patterns are reported.[10,11] A reduced diffusing capacity (DLCO) is seen with interstitial involvement, although it may be paradoxically raised in alveolar haemorrhage. Airflow obstruction is seen in tracheal stenosis and should prompt review of the flow-loop and further imaging. A restrictive defect may be seen with interstitial disease.

Management of Wegener's granulomatosis

Untreated, 80%–90% of patients with extensive Wegener's granulomatosis will die within two years. Early diagnosis and treatment are essential to prevent end-organ damage and improve prognosis. Management should involve a multidisciplinary team including chest, renal and other specialists.

- The standard regime to induce remission in progressive pulmonary, renal or CNS disease combines oral prednisolone (1 mg/kg/day, for one month, tapered over 6–12 months) and oral cyclophosphamide (2 mg/kg/day or maximum 200 mg daily for 6–12 months). Typically 90% of cases respond within 3–6 months although recovery may take up to a year. The regime is repeated in relapse, which occurs in 50% of patients. Large ongoing studies are comparing variations of this treatment.[12,13] No difference was found between daily oral cyclophosphamide and monthly intravenous cyclophosphamide.[14] Low-dose methotrexate is used in patients with mild disease who cannot tolerate cyclophosphamide.

- Ongoing maintenance immunosuppressive therapy with methotrexate, azathioprine or low-dose steroid is recommended for at least a year as relapses are common. Cyclophosphamide may be substituted for an alternative immunosuppressant after the induction phase as it has been demonstrated that azathioprine is as effective as cyclophosphamide for maintaining early remission but less toxic in the long term.[15] *Pneumocystis* pneumonia prophylaxis (co-trimoxazole 960 mg × 3 weekly) and a bisphosphonate to protect against steroid-induced osteoporosis are also recommended. Sinusitis is treated with antibiotics and nasal steroids.
- Acutely ill patients with rapidly progressive renal failure or pulmonary haemorrhage are treated with pulsed methylprednisolone (0.5–1.0 g/day for three days) and intravenous cyclophosphamide (600 mg/m^2). However, plasma exchange/plasmapheresis may be more effective and preferable in severe cases when rapid induction of remission is required. Unfortunately, relapses are common and initial remission should be consolidated with standard therapy.[16]
- Therapeutic strategies that act to inhibit ANCA-driven processes and prevent vasculitic and granulomatous damage to small vessels are the focus of current studies. Rituximab in combination with glucocorticoids is now established as an effective agent for inducing remission in ANCA-positive vasculitides, and is likely to be less toxic than cyclophosphamide-containing regimes. Its use as maintenance therapy is in current trials, whilst other agents such as infliximab are under review.[17,18]

Prognosis

The treated prognosis in Wegener's granulomatosis has improved. Survival is 72%–80% at five years and 65% at ten years. Even so, sufferers have a mortality ratio of 2.9 times an age/sex-matched population. The main causes of death within the first year after diagnosis are infection and active vasculitis.[19] Outcome is dependent on early treatment as end-organ damage is often irreversible (e.g. renal impairment). Optimizing induction and maintaining remission with the minimum of drug-related adverse effects is vital. However, the consequences of prolonged therapy with immunosuppressant and cytotoxic drugs must not be underestimated. There is a strong association with malignancy following prolonged cyclophosphamide treatment including bladder cancer, myelodysplasia and lymphoma.[20] Skin cancer is also increased with immunosuppression and patients should take appropriate precautions.

Conclusion

Wegener's granulomatosis and other similar pulmonary vasculitides are diagnosed infrequently outside specialist clinics. Because of this there is often a delay in diagnosis which may impact on prognosis. This case demonstrates how patients may present acutely. However, recognition with appropriate diagnostics and referral to pulmonary and renal physicians at any stage is the gold standard of care.

Further Reading

1 Hoffman GS, Sechler JM, Gallin JI *et al.* Bronchoalveolar lavage analysis in Wegener's granulomatosis. A method to study disease pathogenesis. *Am Rev Respir Dis* 1991; **143**: 401–7.

2 Schwarz M, Brown K. Small vessel vasculitis of the lung. *Thorax* 2000; **55**: 502–10.

3 Langford C, Hoffman G. Wegener's granulomatosis. *Thorax* 1999; **54**: 629–37.

4 Karthikeyan D. *High-resolution Computed Tomography of the Lungs. A Pattern Approach.* London: Hodder Arnold, 2005.

5 Schnabel A, Holl-Ulrich K, Dalhoff K, Reuter M, Gross WL. Efficacy of transbronchial biopsy in pulmonary vaculitides. *Eur Respir J* 1997; **10**: 2738–43.

6 Lane SE, Watts RA, Shepstone L, Scott DG. Primary systemic vasculitis: clinical features and mortality. *QJM* 2005; **98**: 97–111.

7 Kallenberg CG. Pathogenesis of ANCA-associated vasculitides. *Ann Rheum Dis* 2011; **70**(Suppl 1): i59–63.

8 Gross WL, Trabandt A, Csernok E. Pathogenesis of Wegener's granulomatosis. *Ann Med Interne (Paris)* 1998; **149**: 280–6.

9 Albert D, Clarkin C, Komoroski J, Brensinger CM, Berlin JA. Wegener's granulomatosis: possible role of environmental agents in its pathogenesis. *Arthritis Rheum* 2004; **51**: 656–64.

10 Hoffman GS, Kerr GS, Leavitt RY *et al.* Wegener's granulomatosis: an analysis of 158 patients. *Ann Intern Med* 1992; **116**: 488–98.

11 Rosenberg DM, Weinberger SE, Fulmer JD, Flye MW, Fauci AS, Crystal RG. Functional correlates of lung involvement in Wegener's granulomatosis. Use of pulmonary function tests in staging and follow-up. *Am J Med* 1980; **69**: 387–94.

12 Guillevin L, Cordier JF, Lhote F *et al.* A prospective, multicenter, randomized trial comparing steroids and pulse cyclophosphamide versus steroids and oral cyclophosphamide in the treatment of generalized Wegener's granulomatosis. *Arthritis Rheum* 1997; **40**: 2187–98.

13 Adu D, Pall A, Luqmani RA *et al.* Controlled trial of pulse versus continuous prednisolone and cyclophosphamide in the treatment of systemic vasculitis. *QJM* 1997; **90**: 401–9.

14 Booth AD, Pusey CD, Jayne DR. Renal vasculitis – an update in 2004. *Nephrol Dial Transplant* 2004; **19**: 1964–8.

15 Jayne D, Rasmussen N, Andrassy K *et al.* A randomized trial of maintenance therapy for vasculitis associated with antineutrophil cytoplasmic autoantibodies. *N Engl J Med* 2003; **349**: 36–44.

16 Schoenfeld Y, Sherer Y, Langevitz P, Levy Y. Treatment of 13 patients with vasculitis and other autoimmune diseases with intravenous immunoglobulin. *Clin Exp Immunol* 2000; **120**(Suppl 1): 12–13.

17 Stone JH, Merkel PA, Spiera R *et al.* Rituximab versus cyclophosphamide for ANCA-associated vasculitis. *N Engl J Med* 2010; **363**: 221–32.

18 Lee RW, D'Cruz DP. Novel therapies for anti-neutrophil cytoplasmic antibody-associated vasculitis. *Drugs* 2008; **68**: 747–70.

19 Flossmann O, Berden A, de Groot K *et al.* Long-term patient survival in ANCA-associated vasculitis. *Ann Rheum Dis* 2011; **70**: 488–94.

20 Knight A, Askling J, Ekbom A. Cancer incidence in a population-based cohort of patients with Wegener's granulomatosis. *Int J Cancer* 2002; **100**: 82–5.

PROBLEM

31 Diffuse Alveolar Haemorrhage

Christopher Kosky

Case History

A 29-year-old Ghanaian woman presented to the emergency department with a 24-hour history of haemoptysis and shortness of breath. She also had a four-month history of widespread arthralgia involving both large (knees and hips) and small (hands and feet) joints. For the previous three years she had been receiving propylthiouracil for the treatment of Graves' disease. A total thyroidectomy had been scheduled. Her other medication was naproxen and omeprazole. There was no personal or contact history of tuberculosis. She had never smoked. She had not travelled outside the UK during the preceding twelve months.

On examination she was unwell with a respiratory rate of 32 breaths/min. Her pulse was 115 beats/min and her blood pressure was 142/92 mmHg. Her oxygen saturation was 89% on room air. She had widespread crackles throughout both lung fields. She had a diffuse non-tender fleshy goitre. Blood tests showed a normocytic anaemia (haemoglobin 7.8 g/dl) and a raised C-reactive protein (123 mg/l). Urine analysis showed the presence of protein and blood but no casts or dysmorphic red cells. Renal function was normal. A chest radiograph was performed (Figure 31.1).

What is the diagnosis?

What is the likely cause of diffuse alveolar haemorrhage?

What investigations should be done?

How is diffuse alveolar haemorrhage managed?

Background

Differential diagnosis

In this case, the chest radiograph shows bilateral alveolar infiltrates with sparing of the peripheral lung fields. The differential diagnosis includes pulmonary oedema or diffuse alveolar haemorrhage. There are no other radiological features to support the diagnosis of pulmonary oedema such as pleural effusions, fluid in the horizontal fissure, upper lobe blood diversion or Kerley B lines. With the history of haemoptysis, the most likely diagnosis is diffuse alveolar haemorrhage.

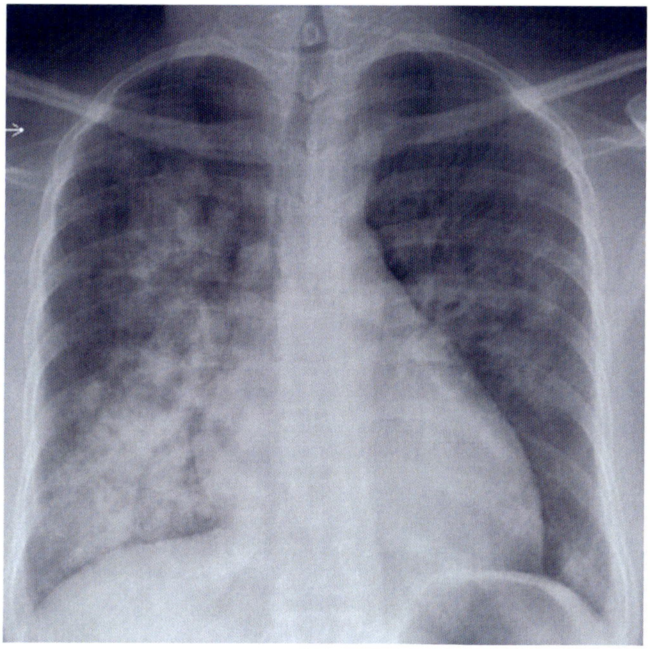

Figure 31.1 Chest radiograph at presentation.

Diffuse alveolar haemorrhage

Diffuse alveolar haemorrhage is characterized by bleeding into the alveolar space. It is due to disruption of the alveolar–capillary basement membrane of the pulmonary blood vessels or capillaries. It can be rapidly fatal and it is important that the cause is identified quickly. Causes of diffuse alveolar haemorrhage include connective tissue disorders, systemic vasculitis, infections and drugs (see Table 31.1).[1,2] In this case, the most likely cause for diffuse alveolar haemorrhage was the propylthiouracil therapy.

Diffuse alveolar haemorrhage usually presents abruptly with cough, haemoptysis and dyspnoea. There may be symptoms and signs of an underlying connective tissue disease or vasculitis. Haemoptysis may be absent in a third of patients. The only clue to alveolar haemorrhage in these patients may be a falling haemoglobin level, raised transfer factor on lung function tests or increasingly blood-stained fluid on sequential bronchoalveolar lavage. A computed tomography chest scan usually shows non-specific bilateral airspace or ground glass opacities.

Investigations

A urine analysis is essential in the investigation of diffuse alveolar haemorrhage. Urinary red blood cells, protein, casts and/or dysmorphic erythrocytes may indicate a pulmonary renal syndrome (such as Goodpasture's syndrome) or glomerulonephritis (Wegener's granulomatosis).

Urgent blood tests for vasculitis and connective tissue diseases should be sent. Blood tests should include anti-neutrophil cytoplasmic antibodies (Wegener's granulomatosis), anti-nuclear antibodies (lupus, mixed connective tissue disease), anti-DNA antibodies

Table 31.1 Causes of diffuse alveolar haemorrhage

Connective tissue diseases	Goodpasture's syndrome Mixed connective tissue disease Polymyositis Rheumatoid arthritis Systemic lupus erythematosis Systemic sclerosis
Systemic vasculitis	Behçet's syndrome Cryoglobulinaemia Henoch–Schönlein purpura IgA nephropathy Wegener's granulomatosis
Infection	Any infection causing ARDS Infective endocarditis Leptospirosis Viruses
Drugs	Anticoagulants Amiodarone Bleomycin Crack cocaine Diphenylhydantoin Nitrofurantoin Penicillamine Propylthiouracil Retinoic acid Sirolimus
Other	ARDS Antiphospholipid syndrome Idiopathic pulmonary haemosiderosis Lung or bone marrow transplant Mitral valve disease Pulmonary infarction Pulmonary veno-occlusive disease Trimellitic anhydride Tuberous sclerosis

ARDS, acute respiratory distress syndrome; IgA, immunoglobulin A.

(lupus), anti-basement membrane antibodies (Goodpasture's syndrome), anti-cardiolipin antibodies (antiphospholipid syndrome), creatinine kinase (polymyositis) and rheumatoid factor (rheumatoid arthritis).

In this case, the titre of anti-neutrophil cytoplasmic antibody (ANCA) against myeloperoxidase (MPO) was 495 units/ml (normal 0–10). All other antibody markers for causes of alveolar haemorrhage were normal. ANCA-associated vasculitides are a rare complication of thionamide (propylthiouracil and methimazole) therapy.[3]

Treatment

Untreated, diffuse alveolar haemorrhage is often fatal. Key to managing diffuse alveolar haemorrhage is to identify and treat the underlying cause before irreversible renal or respiratory failure ensues. A co-ordinated multidisciplinary approach with input from respiratory, renal, rheumatology and immunology specialists and intensivists is often required. Ventilation and/or dialysis in a high-dependency setting may be needed whilst a cause is sought. Any offending drugs should be stopped immediately. Patients with alveolar haemorrhage due to connective tissue disease or vasculitis often require immunosuppression with methylprednisolone and cyclophosphamide.

In this case, propylthiouracil was stopped and replaced with carbimazole. The patient continued to deteriorate and was treated with intravenous methylprednisolone and cyclophosphamide. She rapidly improved and was discharged home two weeks after admission. She required maintenance corticosteroids and immunosuppressive agents as her ANCA titre slowly normalized over two years.

Conclusion

Diffuse alveolar haemorrhage should be suspected in patients presenting with haemoptysis and diffuse pulmonary infiltrates on chest radiograph. Common causes include connective tissue disease, vasculitis and drugs.

Further Reading

1 Collard HR, Schwarz MI. Diffuse alveolar hemorrhage. *Clin Chest Med* 2004; **25**: 583–92.

2 Franks TJ, Koss MN. Pulmonary capillaritis. *Curr Opin Pulm Med* 2000; **6**: 430–5.

3 Stankus SJ, Johnson NT. Propylthiouracil-induced hypersensitivity vasculitis presenting as respiratory failure. *Chest* 1992; **102**: 1595–6.

SECTION SEVEN 07

Ventilatory Failure/Sleep

PROBLEM

32 Obesity Hypoventilation Syndrome

Christopher Kosky, Boris Lams

Case History

A 42-year-old man presents to your clinic because of paroxysmal nocturnal dyspnoea. For the last two years he wakes from sleep gasping for air. He describes morning headaches. He admits to falling asleep during the day if sitting quietly. His wife reports loud snoring. She has also witnessed long pauses in his breathing whilst he is asleep. He is dyspnoeic after walking 200 metres on flat ground. He is an ex-smoker of 30 pack years. He works as a minibus driver with disabled children.

On examination his body mass index (BMI) is 64.7 kg/m^2. He has a hypercapnic flap. He has a large tongue and you are unable to visualize his oropharynx. Chest examination is normal. His jugular venous pressure is elevated and he has pitting oedema to his mid shin. A chest radiograph is normal. Oxygen saturations are 85% on air. Spirometry reveals a moderate restrictive pattern. An arterial blood gas analysis on room air reveals pH 7.38, partial pressures of carbon dioxide ($PaCO_2$) 7.2 kPa and oxygen (PaO_2) 7.8 kPa, bicarbonate (HCO_3) 31 mmol/l and base excess 5.

What do the blood gases show?

What is the A–a gradient?

What is the likely cause of the ventilatory failure?

What would be your next investigation?

How should the patient be managed?

What advice would you give this patient about driving?

Background

In this case the patient has chronic hypercapnic respiratory failure as evidenced by raised $PaCO_2$ (>6.0 kPa) with a normal pH and raised bicarbonate. Hypercapnia can be due to alveolar hypoventilation which may be due to poor drive to ventilate (e.g. brainstem lesion, opiates), respiratory muscle weakness (e.g. myasthenia gravis, phrenic nerve palsy), chest wall abnormalities (e.g. obesity, kyphoscoliosis) or severe parenchymal lung disease.

He also has a significant hypoxia. There are five causes of hypoxia: hypoventilation; ventilation-perfusion (V/Q) mismatch; shunt; impaired diffusion; and low inspired oxygen (altitude).

A-a gradient

Calculation of the A-a gradient is useful in determining the cause of hypoxia. The A-a gradient distinguishes extrapulmonary hypoxia (hypoventilation) from intrapulmonary hypoxia (V/Q mismatch, shunt or impaired diffusion). An abnormal A-a gradient suggests the hypoxia is intrapulmonary from V/Q mismatch, shunt or impaired diffusion. In contrast, a normal A-a gradient suggests the cause of hypoxia is hypoventilation. The A-a gradient is the partial pressure of oxygen in the alveolus (PAO_2) compared to that in the artery (PaO_2). The PaO_2 is measured by the blood gas sample. The PAO_2 (alveolar oxygen pressure) is calculated as follows.

Calculating the PAO_2

$$PAO_2 = PiO_2 - PaCO_2/0.8$$

PiO_2 = partial pressure of oxygen in airways
= FiO_2 × (barometric pressure – partial pressure of water vapour)
$= 0.21 \times (101 - 6.3)$
= 19.9 kPa

$PAO_2 = 19.9 - 7.2/0.8$
= 10.9 kPa

Calculating the A-a gradient

$PAO_2 - PaO_2 = 10.9 - 7.8$
= 3.1 kPa

The A-a gradient is only slightly raised at 3.1 kPa (normal <3 kPa) suggesting that the predominant cause of hypoxia is hypoventilation. For simplicity the PAO_2 can be calculated by substituting inspired oxygen concentration (FiO_2; as a percentage) for PiO_2 in the equation, although this will overestimate the A-a gradient by approximately 1 kPa.

Obesity hypoventilation syndrome

In this case, the most likely diagnosis is obesity hypoventilation syndrome (OHS), also called Pickwickian syndrome. This is likely a consequence of obstructive sleep apnoea/hypopnoea syndrome, smoking-related lung disease and lung restriction due to obesity. OHS is defined as a combination of obesity (BMI >30 kg/m^2) together with daytime hypercapnia ($PaCO_2$ >6 kPa) in the absence of other known causes of hypoventilation.[1]

It is likely that this man has obstructive sleep apnoea in view of his snoring, paroxysmal nocturnal dyspnoea, the witnessed apnoeas and excessive daytime sleepiness. In addition it is highly probable that he has a degree of nocturnal hypoventilation related to his obesity to explain his hypercapnia during the day.

Morning headache and hypercapnic flap suggest hypercapnic respiratory failure, which is unusual to be caused by obstructive sleep apnoea alone. Breathlessness on exertion is common in patients with OHS, but uncommon in patients with obstructive sleep apnoea alone.[2]

Typically, OHS can be thought of as a spectrum of sleep-disordered breathing from snoring and obstructive sleep apnoea and finally to the development of hypoventilation in sleep. Rarely, hypoventilation in sleep from obesity can also occur in isolation without upper airway obstruction.

In OHS, hypercapnia first appears in rapid eye movement (REM) sleep. In REM sleep the only active muscles are diaphragm and occular muscles. Other muscles, including accessory muscles of the chest, are atonic. Muscle atonia is probably to prevent dream enactment. If an excessive load, such as abdominal obesity, is placed on the diaphragm then this can lead to hypoventilation in REM sleep and hypercapnia. It is hypothesized that hypercapnia during REM sleep leads to ventilatory failure in non-REM sleep and then later in wakefulness. In non-REM sleep the stimulus to breathe is mediated through chemoreceptor response to the level of arterial carbon dioxide. Hypercapnia in REM sleeps may result in adaptation of these chemoreceptors to tolerate higher levels of arterial carbon dioxide in non-REM sleep and wakefulness. With the reduced stimulus to breathe resulting there is hypoventilation and hypercapnic respiratory failure.

Investigation

The most appropriate investigation would be to perform a sleep study. Ideally this would be a polysomnography with transcutaneous capnography. However, in this case, a limited study using oximetry and pulse rate provided sufficient information (Figure 32.1).

Transcutaneous capnography was also performed (not shown) and this confirmed raised $PaCO_2$ levels throughout the night, at approximately 8 kPa.

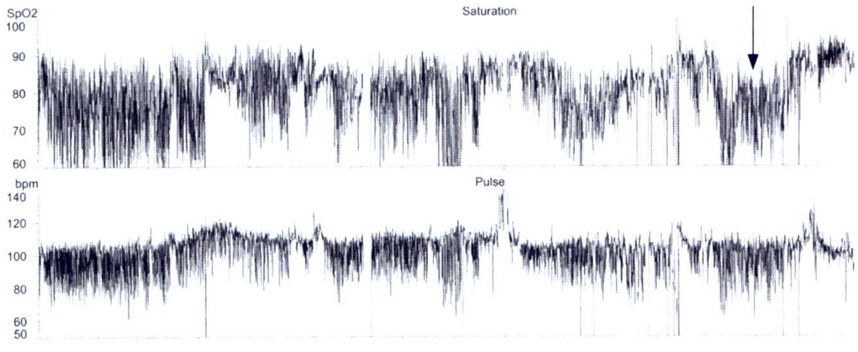

Figure 32.1 Baseline overnight oxygen saturation (upper panel) and pulse recording (lower panel) on room air showing repetitive oxygen desaturations with associated heart rate variability. The arrow indicates a period at the end of the study of prolonged desaturation where the resaturations fail to return to baseline, consistent with REM hypoventilation.

Treatment

In this case, the patient has hypercapnic respiratory failure due to nocturnal hypoventilation and OHS. Continuous positive airway pressure (CPAP) is the most effective treatment for obstructive sleep apnoea/hypopnoea syndrome.[3] However, CPAP will not improve nocturnal hypoventilation. Hypercapnic respiratory failure is an indication for bi-level ventilation during sleep.

The patient was started on nocturnal bi-level ventilation. A moderate inspiratory positive airway pressure (IPAP) was required to overcome the reduced chest wall compliance from obesity. A high expiratory positive airway pressure (EPAP) was needed to treat the upper airways resistance. Entrained oxygen into the bi-level ventilator was required to establish adequate saturations.

For morbidly obese patients, bariatric surgery is an emerging treatment for sleep-disordered breathing.[4] Patients need to be assessed for sleep-disordered breathing and established on ventilatory support prior to surgery.

Driving

Patients with obstructive sleep apnoea/hypopnoea syndrome have a higher incidence of motor vehicle accidents probably due to excessive sleepiness. Recommendations regarding driving with sleep apnoea vary between countries. In the United Kingdom, patients with obstructive sleep apnoea/hypopnoea syndrome should not drive until excessive sleepiness is controlled. Drivers are also required to inform the Driver and Vehicle Licensing Agency of the diagnosis. In the case of drivers of heavy goods vehicles or people-carrying vehicles, compliance and control of sleep apnoea needs to be confirmed by a specialist.[5]

In this patient, the ventilator usage was recorded by the technicians and it was confirmed that he was using the bi-level ventilator for an average six hours per night. Repeat blood gases on air and overnight oximetry on bi-level ventilation were much improved.

Conclusion

Obesity hypoventilation syndrome is characterized by sleep-disordered breathing and chronic hypercapnic respiratory failure. Nocturnal non-invasive ventilation and weight loss are the primary treatments.

Further Reading

1 Olson AL, Zwillich C. The obesity hypoventilation syndrome. *Am J Med* 2005; **118**: 948–56.

2 Nowbar S, Burkart KM, Gonzales R *et al.* Obesity-associated hypoventilation in hospitalized patients: prevalence, effects, and outcome. *Am J Med* 2004; **116**: 1–7.

3 National Institute for Health and Clinical Excellence. Continuous positive airway pressure for the treatment of obstructive sleep apnoea/hypopnoea syndrome. Technology appraisal guidance 139. London: NICE, 2011. www.nice.org.uk (accessed 01 06 11).

4 Buchwald H, Avidor Y, Braunwald E *et al.* Bariatric surgery: a systematic review and meta-analysis. *JAMA* 2004; **292**: 1724–37.

5 Drivers Medical Group. Driver and Vehicle Licensing Agency. At a glance guide to the current medical standards of fitness to drive. Driver and Vehicle Licensing Agency, 2011. www.dft.gov.uk/dvla/medical/ataglance.aspx (accessed 01 06 11).

PROBLEM

33 Guillain-Barré Syndrome

Nicholas Hopkinson, Christopher Kosky

Case History

A 34-year-old male civil servant presented to the emergency department with a three-day history of malaise and tingling in his hands and feet. He described weakness such that he was unable to get out of the bath unaided. Four weeks previously he had had a brief episode of diarrhoea and abdominal pain, which had resolved spontaneously. He had no headache or fever, and reported no recent foreign travel. He was alert and oriented, a non-smoker, denied any recreational drug use and had no family history of note.

The patient was observed to have symmetrical weakness, more pronounced in his arms than his legs. He was unable to walk unaided. His reflexes were absent. No sensory deficit was noted nor any cranial nerve abnormalities. His muscles were not tender and no fasciculation was noted. He was apyrexial and no other abnormalities were apparent on examination. Spirometry was performed and indicated forced expiratory volume in 1 second (FEV_1) was 3.0 l with a forced vital capacity (FVC) of 3.6 l. Oxygen saturations were 96% on air.

The patient was admitted to a general ward and started on treatment with intravenous immunoglobulin. The following day he was noted to have become drowsy and weaker. His oxygen saturations were 91%. His FVC had fallen to 1.46 l. Arterial blood gas analysis revealed pH 7.25 and partial pressures of carbon dioxide ($PaCO_2$) 7.9 kPa and oxygen (PaO_2) 9.4 kPa.

What is the initial diagnosis?

Which investigations should be performed?

What complication has occurred following admission?

What is the treatment of Guillain-Barré syndrome?

Background

This patient has a progressive symmetrical weakness consistent with Guillain-Barré syndrome (GBS), which typically occurs a few weeks following an apparently minor respiratory or gastrointestinal infection. Historically, the most important differential diagnosis would have been polio. In an intravenous drug user, botulism should be considered, particularly in association with 'skin popping'. Other causes of peripheral weakness that can be excluded are myasthenia gravis and transverse myelitis. Myasthenia gravis is unlikely in the absence of cranial nerve features and fatigability. Transverse myelitis is unlikely in the absence of sensory signs.

Investigations for Guillain-Barré syndrome

Investigations should include a lumbar puncture, nerve conduction studies and a test for antibodies to *Campylobacter jejuni*.

A lumbar puncture was performed immediately in this patient. It revealed an opening pressure of 12 cmH_2O. The cerebrospinal fluid (CSF) revealed a normal lymphocyte count of 3 per mm^3 and glucose 3.6 mmol/l with an elevated protein level of 0.64 g/l. This 'typical' CSF pattern in GBS may not be present within the first seven days of presentation.

Antibodies to *Campylobacter jejuni* may be useful in the diagnosis of GBS, though clinicians do not usually have the results immediately. In one study, antibodies to *Campylobacter jejuni* were found in 26% of patients presenting with GBS.[1] The presence of antibodies to *Campylobacter jejuni* was associated with a worse prognosis. GBS also occurs in the context of other infections including human immunodeficiency virus, cytomegalovirus, *Mycoplasma* and Lyme disease. An association with influenza vaccination has also been reported.

Respiratory failure

In this case the patient has developed acute hypercapnic respiratory failure from respiratory muscle weakness. The major concern in GBS is the development of respiratory failure, which can occur rapidly, with 20%–30% of patients in published series requiring ventilatory support.

There are several ways of predicting acute respiratory failure in GBS. The '20/30/40 rule' derives from the observation that patients with a vital capacity (VC) <20 ml/kg, a maximum inspiratory pressure of less than 30 cmH_2O and a maximum expiratory pressure <40 cmH_2O are likely to require intubation.[2] Measurement of mouth pressures may not be readily available in the emergency department but most intensive care units should have a mouth pressure meter available.

More recently, a study of 722 patients admitted to neurological units in France identified a number of factors as predicting the need for intubation. These included a time from onset to admission of less than seven days, the inability to cough, the inability to stand independently, being unable to lift elbows or head and an increase in liver enzymes. Where VC had been measured, VC <60% predicted, rapid onset and inability to lift the head were independent predictors. The presence of bulbar features is also a marker of increased risk.[3]

Autonomic dysfunction is common, occurring in up to half of patients. Autonomic neuropathy can manifest as arrhythmias, postural hypotension, ileus and urinary retention. Patients should therefore have monitoring of electrocardiogram and blood pressure. Patients should be watched for urinary retention and constipation.

Treatment

Specific treatment for GBS is plasma exchange or intravenous immunoglobulin. The efficacy of plasma exchange compared to placebo is supported by a meta-analysis of six randomized controlled trials.[4] A further systematic review found no difference in efficacy between plasma exchange and intravenous immunoglobulin.[5] Combined treatment does not appear to be more effective.[6] However, in practice, where one treatment has not produced a satisfactory response it is common to try the other.

In this case, the patient was transferred to an intensive therapy unit and electively intubated and treatment with intravenous immunoglobulin continued. On day ten, because of persistent weakness, a percutaneous tracheostomy was inserted. He subsequently developed ventilator-acquired pneumonia. Because of his initial slow progress he was subsequently treated with plasma exchange. His strength gradually recovered and he was successfully weaned onto non-invasive ventilation on day 46 and then off ventilatory support entirely by day 66. He was discharged home, able to walk independently, on day 86.

Conclusion

Factors that predict respiratory failure in Guillain-Barré syndrome include rapid disease onset, a vital capacity less than 60% predicted and an inability to lift the head.

Further Reading

1 Rees JH, Soudain SE, Gregson NA, Hughes RA. *Campylobacter jejuni* infection and Guillain-Barré syndrome. *N Engl J Med* 1995; **333**: 1374–9.

2 Lawn ND, Fletcher DD, Henderson RD, Wolter TD, Wijdicks EF. Anticipating mechanical ventilation in Guillain-Barré syndrome. *Arch Neurol* 2001; **58**: 893–8.

3 Sharshar T, Chevret S. Bourdain F, Raphaël JC. Early predictors of mechanical ventilation in Guillain-Barré syndrome. *Crit Care Med* 2003; **31**: 278–83.

4 Raphaël JC, Chevret S, Hughes RA, Annane D. Plasma exchange for Guillain-Barré syndrome. *Cochrane Database Syst Rev* 2001; CD001798.

5 Fergusson D, Hutton B, Sharma A *et al.* Use of intravenous immunoglobulin for treatment of neurologic conditions: a systematic review. *Transfusion* 2005; **45**: 1640–57.

6 Plasma Exchange/Sandoglobulin Guillain-Barré Syndrome Trial Group. Randomised trial of plasma exchange, intravenous immunoglobulin, and combined treatments in Guillain-Barré syndrome. *Lancet* 1997; **349**: 225–30.

SECTION EIGHT 08

Immunocompromised/HIV

PROBLEM

34 *Pneumocystis jirovecii* Pneumonia

Elizabeth Hadley, Boris Lams

Case History

A 39-year-old African man presented with a one-week history of cough, fever and increasing breathlessness. He had recently arrived from the Ivory Coast. On examination he was febrile at 39°C and he had bilateral crackles on auscultation of his chest. The remainder of his examination was normal. His oxygen saturations on air were 87% increasing to 96% on a non-rebreathing reservoir bag mask with 15 l/min of oxygen. His arterial blood gases on high-flow oxygen showed partial pressures of oxygen (PaO_2) 11.2 kPa and carbon dioxide ($PaCO_2$) 3.7 kPa, pH 7.37 and base excess of −3.5. A chest radiograph was performed (Figure 34.1). His blood tests showed a white cell count 17.7×10^9/l (neutrophils 15.4×10^9/l), haemoglobin 13.6 g/dl and platelet count 297×10^9/l. He had normal renal function and electrolytes, and his albumin was low at 30 g/l with a normal total protein. His C-reactive protein was 86 mg/l and lactate dehydrogenase (LDH) was 1835 IU/l.

He was started on intravenous cefuroxime and clarithromycin, and intravenous fluids at 125 ml/hour. The next morning he had an ongoing fever and oxygen saturations of 96% on 15 l/min of oxygen. His C-reactive protein had risen to 186 mg/l.

What is the differential diagnosis?

What are the next steps in this patient's management?

What is *Pneumocystis jirovecii* pneumonia (PJP)?

What is the treatment of PJP?

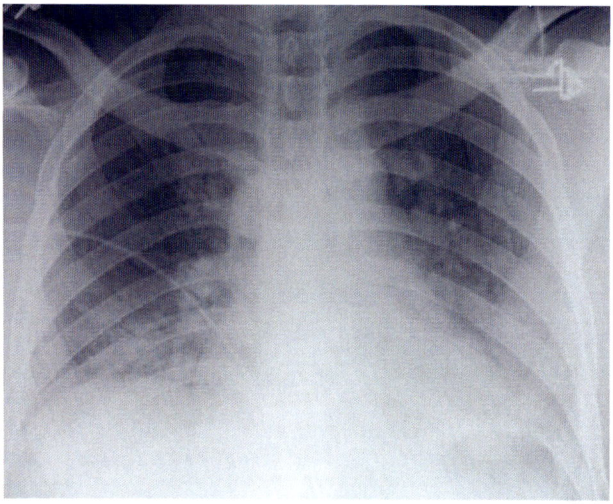

Figure 34.1 Chest radiograph at presentation.

Background

Differential diagnosis

In this case, the chest radiograph shows bilateral alveolar shadowing most prominent in the lower and mid zones. Although it is possible that this might represent early acute lung injury secondary to a severe pneumonia, this pattern is also consistent with PJP on a background of human immunodeficiency virus (HIV) infection. PJP was previously called *Pneumocystis carinii* pneumonia. The taxonomy of *Pneumocystis* was revised in 2002 and renamed from *carinii* to *jirovecii*, referring to the scientist who described the unicellular fungus as a human pathogen rather than to the original description in rats.[1]

Investigations and management

This patient consented to HIV testing and a bronchoscopy. Given the likelihood that this presentation represented *P. jirovecii* infection he was started on treatment with high-dose intravenous co-trimoxazole and oral prednisolone 40 mg bd. A positive HIV result was confirmed later that day. A bronchoalveolar lavage (BAL) sample taken during the bronchoscopy confirmed PJP.

Pneumocystis jirovecii pneumonia

Pneumonia caused by the respiratory commensal *Pneumocystis carinii/jirovecii* is an opportunistic infection typically associated with HIV infection. However, it was originally described many years ago in severely malnourished individuals during World War Two. In recent times, PJP became strongly associated with HIV infection, especially from 1983 onwards.[2,3] There was a peak in PJP–acquired immune deficiency syndrome in the late 1980s and early 1990s, which subsided with the introduction of highly active antiretroviral therapy (HAART) after 1997.

Patients with *Pneumocystis* pneumonia may complain of exertional breathlessness, a fever and dry cough. They may also have chest pain and other constitutional symptoms such as rapid weight loss. On examination the patient may be febrile, tachycardic and tachypnoeic. They may be hypoxic at rest or only desaturate on exercise. This sign, which is anecdotally linked to PJP, has evidence of sensitivity but is not always practical to perform.[4]

Lymphopenia is common in *Pneumocystis* pneumonia, even in non-HIV-related cases, and often precedes the acute clinical illness. Other clues to PJP infection include elevated serum LDH.

Although the chest radiograph is usually sufficient in suspected cases, occasionally a high-resolution computed tomography scan of the chest can add further information, particularly in those patients with a normal chest radiograph. Some centres also use gallium scanning which may reveal alveolar 'leakiness' suggestive of PJP in a patient with a normal chest radiograph.

Definitive diagnosis of the disease requires detection of the organisms in respiratory secretions (either BAL fluid or induced sputum) via immunofluorescence techniques such as the modified 'Grocott' stain or by immunocytology. *Pneumocystis* cannot be cultured, but DNA detection methods are showing promise. BAL alone has a diagnostic yield of between 30% and 90% in HIV-infected patients. Transbronchial biopsy should be considered alongside BAL when possible and is thought to increase yield, sensitivity and specificity, although there is no consensus.[5,6] Site-directed lavage, which involves sampling the most heavily involved lobes on chest radiograph, can also increase the yield in patients with focal infiltrates.[7] Results may be affected by pre-test treatment in sick patients, particularly in patients using aerosolized pentamidine prophylaxis.

In the last 15 years we have seen a fall in the prevalence of PJP in the general HIV-positive population. However, those presenting late with CD4 counts $<200 \times 10^6$/l and those who are poorly compliant with HAART have a high incidence of PJP. In these groups the bronchoscopic yield in patients with pulmonary infiltrates is high.

Cases of *Pneumocystis* pneumonia are rising in non-HIV-infected immunosuppressed patients. PJP is noted to be more common in post-transplant patients (particularly following renal, liver and bone marrow transplant) who are all receiving long-term immunosuppressant agents. More recently, patients being treated with monoclonal antibodies for autoimmune and connective tissue disease have been developing various opportunistic infections including PJP. There is most evidence of PJP in patients treated with the anti-tumour necrosis factor alpha drug, infliximab, for rheumatoid arthritis, inflammatory bowel disease and psoriasis. There are also case reports of *Pneumocystis* pneumonia in patients treated with rituximab and alemtuzumab.[8,9]

Treatment

Co-trimoxazole and corticosteroids are the mainstay of treatment. The clinical course of PJP prior to the routine use of adjunctive corticosteroids was often of rapid deterioration into respiratory failure. In the late 1980s evidence was published which showed that systemic corticosteroids reduced the severity and duration of the clinical course of the disease.[10] Patients with HIV-associated PJP who commence HAART during their acute illness may deteriorate at around day 7–10 due to immune reconstitution. For this reason the initiation of HAART is sometimes deliberately delayed. However, there is emerging evidence that in patients with a CD4 count below 200 cells/μl at presentation, mortality is lower if HAART is commenced within the first 14 days.[11] Corticosteroids are often continued during the initiation of HAART.

Conclusion

The diagnosis of PJP should be considered in all hypoxic patients with pulmonary infiltrates on the chest radiograph. In unwell patients with known low CD4 counts, prolonged immunosuppression or suspected undiagnosed HIV infection, it is reasonable to commence treatment on clinical suspicion if invasive diagnostics are not possible.

Further Reading

1 Stringer JR, Beard CB, Miller RF, Wakefield AE. A new name (*Pneumocystis jiroveci*) for *Pneumocystis* from humans. *Emerg Infect Dis* 2002; **8**: 891–6.

2 Poon MC, Landay A, Prasthofer EF, Stagno S. Acquired immunodeficiency syndrome with *Pneumocystis carinii* pneumonia and *Mycobacterium avium-intracellulare* infection in a previously healthy patient with classic hemophilia. Clinical, immunologic, and virologic findings. *Ann Intern Med* 1983; **98**: 287–90.

3 Small CB, Klein RS, Friedland GH, Moll B, Emeson EE, Spigland I. Community-acquired opportunistic infections and defective cellular immunity in heterosexual drug abusers and homosexual men. *Am J Med* 1983; **74**: 433–41.

4 Stover DE, Meduri GU. Pulmonary function tests. *Clin Chest Med* 1988; **9**: 473–9.

5 Broaddus C, Dake MD, Stulbarg MS *et al.* Bronchoalveolar lavage and transbronchial biopsy for the diagnosis of pulmonary infections in the acquired immunodeficiency syndrome. *Ann Intern Med* 1985; **102**: 747–52.

6 Cruciani M, Marcati P, Malena M, Bosco O, Serpelloni G, Mengoli C. Meta-analysis of diagnostic procedures for *Pneumocystis carinii* pneumonia in HIV-1-infected patients. *Eur Respir J* 2002; **20**: 982–9.

7 Cadranel J, Gillet-Juvin K, Antoine M *et al.* Site-directed bronchoalveolar lavage and transbronchial biopsy in HIV-infected patients with pneumonia. *Am J Respir Crit Care Med* 1995; **152**: 1103–6.

8 Kumar D, Gourishankar S, Mueller T *et al. Pneumocystis jirovecii* pneumonia after rituximab therapy for antibody-mediated rejection in a renal transplant recipient. *Transpl Infect Dis* 2009; **11**: 167–70.

9 Kaur N, Mahl TC. *Pneumocystis jiroveci (carinii)* pneumonia after infliximab therapy: a review of 84 cases. *Dig Dis Sci* 2007; **52**: 1481–4.

10 The National Institutes of Health-University of California Expert Panel for Corticosteroids as Adjunctive Therapy for Pneumocystis Pneumonia. Consensus statement on the use of corticosteroids as adjunctive therapy for pneumocystis pneumonia in the acquired immunodeficiency syndrome. *N Engl J Med* 1990; **323**: 1500–4.

11 Lawn SD, Török ME, Wood R. Optimum time to start antiretroviral therapy during HIV-associated opportunistic infections. *Curr Opin Infect Dis* 2011; **24**: 34–42.

PROBLEM

35 Lymphocytic Interstitial Pneumonia

Elizabeth Hadley, Boris Lams, Christopher Kosky

Case History

A 40-year-old male Nigerian builder presents to hospital with a six-month history of increasing dyspnoea and 10 kg weight loss. Four months ago he had an episode of minor haemoptysis. Three months ago he returned from Nigeria having been resident there for a year. Four weeks ago haemoptysis returned and has persisted. He denies fevers, night sweats or rashes. He says he can now only walk 20 metres before being limited by shortness of breath. He was born in Nigeria. He does not smoke. He denies any risk factors for human immunodeficiency virus (HIV) infection. He has not had contact with animals and has not been knowingly exposed to asbestos or other dusts.

On examination he is not clubbed, pulse is 90 beats/min, temperature is 37.8°C, blood pressure is 115/80 mmHg and oxygen saturation (SaO_2) is 94% on air. Cardiovascular examination is normal. Respiratory examination reveals normal breath sounds and no added sounds. A full blood count reveals a low white blood cell count (3.5×10^9) with a normal differential cell count. Haemoglobin is low (9.8 g/dl) with a normal mean corpuscular volume (86 fl). Platelet count is normal (162×10^9). Erythrocyte sedimentation rate (ESR) is elevated at 82 mm/hr. The C-reactive protein (CRP) is in the normal range. Serum sodium is low (128 mmol/l) and renal function is normal. Total serum protein is elevated (96 g/l) with a low serum albumin (24 g/l). A chest radiograph is performed (Figure 35.1).

What is the differential diagnosis and what investigations are required?

What is lymphocytic interstitial pneumonia (LIP)?

What investigations could be performed to confirm LIP?

What is the prognosis of LIP?

Background

The term LIP was introduced by Liebow and Carrington in 1966 to describe a diffuse lymphocytic interstitial infiltrate that was distinct from other patterns of interstitial pneumonia.[1,2] LIP is viewed as a distinct variant of diffuse pulmonary lymphoid hyperplasia. Pathologically there is a polyclonal lymphocytic infiltrate into the pulmonary

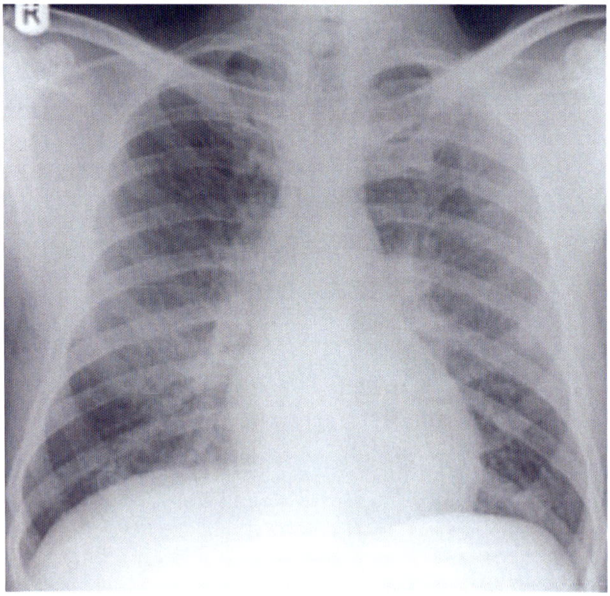

Figure 35.1 Chest radiograph at presentation.

interstitium and alveolar spaces. Modern immunohistochemistry and molecular techniques should allow distinction from lymphoma, although a small number of patients with LIP can undergo malignant transformation.[3]

Clinical features are those of slowly progressive cough and dyspnoea, often over periods of months to years. The patient may experience fatigue, weight loss and mild fevers. There are often inspiratory crackles at the lung bases and there may be finger clubbing. Laboratory features include a mild anaemia, raised ESR and a polyclonal increase in immunoglobulins. The presence of a monoclonal band suggests the presence of an underlying lymphoproliferative malignancy.

Idiopathic LIP is distinctly rare and a pathological diagnosis of LIP should prompt a search for an underlying cause such as autoimmune disorders (rheumatoid arthritis, Sjögren's syndrome, Hashimoto's disease, pernicious anaemia, chronic active hepatitis, or systemic lupus erythematosus), infections (human T cell lymphotrophic virus [HTLV-1], hepatitis B) or immunodeficiency states (HIV infection or severe combined immune deficiency, Castleman's disease).[4] LIP has also been reported with phenytoin therapy.

Differential diagnosis

In this case the chest radiograph shows alveolar shadowing in a perihilar distribution. The patient's blood results reveal hyponatraemia, possibly due to syndrome of inappropriate antidiuretic hormone (SIADH) commonly associated with chest disease. Normocytic anaemia may be due to chronic disease. Leukopenia can be a normal variant in Africans; however, it can also occur in viral infection and sarcoid. Low albumin and a raised total protein are suggestive of high circulating immunoglobulins. The differential diagnosis includes:

- ***Pneumocystis jirovecii* pneumonia.** Nigeria, like many sub-Saharan countries, has a high incidence of HIV infection. The chest radiograph findings of perihilar alveolar shadowing are suggestive of *Pneumocystis jirovecii* pneumonia in the context of undiagnosed HIV infection. The raised immunoglobulins may reflect the polyclonal gammopathy that can occur in HIV infection. However, haemoptysis and the normal serum CRP would be unusual in *Pneumocystis jirovecii* pneumonia.
- **Pulmonary amyloid.** Diffuse alveolar septal amyloid could also cause the combination of perihilar alveolar shadowing and raised immunoglobulins. In amyloidosis, raised immunoglobulins are due to underlying monoclonal gammopathy. Haemoptysis is unusual in alveolar septal amyloid, occurring more commonly in tracheobronchial amyloid.
- **Lymphocytic interstitial pneumonia.** LIP would also account for diffuse alveolar shadowing. LIP is strongly associated with HIV infection. Raised serum protein is due to raised immunoglobulins from polyclonal gammopathy.

Further investigations were performed. Serology for HIV was positive with a CD4 count of 194×10^6/l. Protein electrophoresis revealed a polyclonal increase in gammaglobulins with no underlying monoclonal band. A diagnosis of LIP was suspected.

Investigations

Lymphocytic interstitial pneumonia has a characteristic appearance on high-resolution computed tomography (HRCT) of the chest. In this case a HRCT chest scan was performed (Figure 35.2). There is diffuse ground glass opacity, cysts and interstitial thickening. Ground glass opacity is the diffuse increased attenuation of the lung parenchyma. It can be appreciated better if the lung parenchymal density is compared with that in the air within the airways, which appears comparatively darker (the dark bronchus sign). Ground glass opacity and cystic lesions commonly occur in LIP and *Pneumocystis jirovecii* pneumonia. Interstitial thickening is a feature of LIP.

Lymphocytic interstitial pneumonia can require lung biopsy to confirm the diagnosis. In this case the patient underwent a bronchoscopy, bronchoalveolar lavage (BAL) and transbronchial biopsy. The BAL revealed a lymphocytosis; immunofluorescent staining for *Pneumocystis jirovecii* was negative. The transbronchial biopsy revealed a lymphocytic infiltrate of uncertain aetiology.

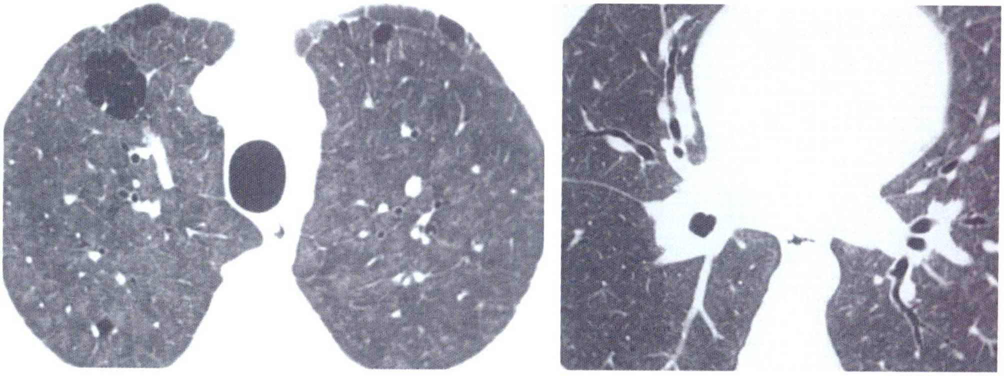

Figure 35.2 HRCT chest scan at presentation.

A video-assisted thoracoscopy was performed. Biopsy specimens revealed a polyclonal infiltrate of B cells characteristic of LIP.

Prognosis

The prognosis of LIP is variable and it can spontaneously regress. A third of cases may progress to pulmonary fibrosis and there are reports of progression to pulmonary lymphoma. Idiopathic and autoimmune LIP may respond to treatment with corticosteroids. LIP associated with HIV usually responds to highly active antiretroviral therapy (HAART).

In this case the patient was started on HAART and showed substantial improvement clinically and radiologically.

Conclusion

All patients with LIP should have access to a multidisciplinary team experienced in interstitial lung disease, and undergo smoking cessation and pulmonary rehabilitation.

Further Reading

1 Carrington BC, Liebow AA. Lymphocytic interstitial pneumonia (abstract). *Am J Pathol* 1966; **48**: 36.

2 American Thoracic Society/European Respiratory Society International Multidisciplinary Consensus Classification of the Idiopathic Interstitial Pneumonias. *Am J Respir Crit Care Med* 2002; **165**: 277–304.

3 Wells AU, Hirani N. Interstitial lung disease guideline. British Thoracic Society in collaboration with Thoracic Society of Australia and New Zealand and the Irish Thoracic Society. *Thorax* 2008; **63**(Suppl 5): v1–v58.

4 Bragg DG, Chor PJ, Murray KA, Kjeldsberg CR. Lymphoproliferative disorders of the lung: histopathology, clinical manifestations, and imaging features. *AJR Am J Roentgenol* 1994; **163**: 273–81.

SECTION NINE

09

Pleural Disease

PROBLEM

36 Parapneumonic Effusion

Liju Ahmed, Richard Leach

Case History

A 38-year-old female clerical worker presented to the emergency department with a five-day history of fever, cough productive of green sputum, progressive breathlessness and gradual-onset pleuritic chest pain. She had no relevant past medical history or previous regular medication. She had smoked ten cigarettes a day for 18 years. Alcohol consumption was minimal.

On examination she was febrile (40°C), dehydrated but well perfused. Her blood pressure was 96/60 mmHg, respiratory rate 28 breaths/min and oxygen saturation (SaO_2) 98% on air. Chest examination found bronchial breathing and crepitation at the right base. The remainder of the examination was unremarkable.

Blood tests revealed a haemoglobin level 13.0 g/dl, white cell count 13.7×10^9/l, platelet count 210×10^9/l, sodium (Na^+) 132 mmol/l, potassium (K^+) 4.4 mmol/l, urea 10.6 mmol/l, creatinine 85 μmol/l and C-reactive protein 482 mg/l. The electrocardiogram was normal. The chest radiograph (CXR) showed right lower lobe consolidation. She was treated for community-acquired pneumonia (CAP) with intravenous cefuroxime and oral doxycycline. Unfortunately, despite initial improvement she continued to spike intermittent fevers and her breathlessness increased. Bilateral pleural effusions were present on a repeat CXR (Figure 36.1). Aspiration of right-sided pleural fluid revealed a pH 7.19, lactate dehydrogenase (LDH) 1200 IU/l, glucose 1.6 mmol/l and a negative Gram stain.

What is the cause of the pleural effusion and could it be an empyema?

How would you investigate this patient and how reliable are the tests?

What are the most likely infective organisms in infected pleural fluid?

How would you manage this patient and would you insert a chest drain?

How would you manage failure to improve despite antibiotics and drainage?

What is the main complication of empyema and how would you deal with it?

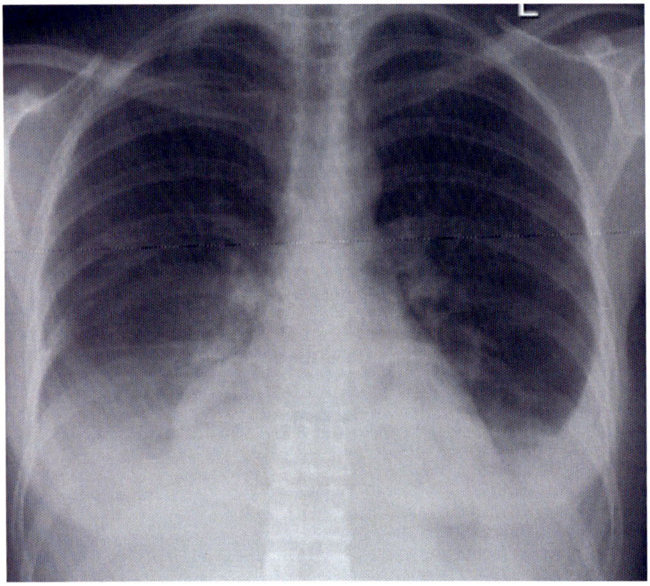

Figure 36.1 Chest radiograph.

Background

Pleural effusions are common and associated with a wide range of diseases, most commonly malignancy, heart failure, pneumonia and pulmonary embolism. Small effusions may be asymptomatic. Larger effusions are associated with chest tightness, dyspnoea and dry cough.

Parapneumonic effusions (PPE) are common following pneumonia, especially in paediatric and elderly populations. Incidence of pleural infection is increasing at 2.8% per year.[1,2] Up to 57% of patients with pneumonia produce additional pleural fluid[3] resulting in about 80 000 cases of pleural infections annually in the UK and USA combined.[3,4] Most PPE follows CAP or hospital-acquired pneumonia (HAP), although iatrogenic and primary pleural infection can occur. Unilateral and bilateral PPE accompanying CAP are associated with a 3.4- and 7-fold increase in mortality and morbidity, respectively.[5] The mortality risk associated with a PPE equates to a partial pressure of oxygen (PaO_2) <60 mmHg in a CAP patient.[6]

Parapneumonic and infected pleural effusions

Normally the pleural space contains about 0.3 ml/kg of fluid. Pleural fluid production and absorption are mainly by parietal pleura, and fluid production is about 0.01 ml/kg/hr or 15 ml/day. Drainage is achieved by contraction of smooth muscles of the lymphatic walls and tissue pressure oscillations related to respiratory movements. The maximum fluid drainage is about 0.2 ml/kg/hr or 300 ml/day. Normal pleural fluid contains a similar concentration of protein (e.g. albumin) to interstitial fluid, small numbers of mesothelial cells, macrophages and lymphocytes, and some larger molecular weight proteins such as LDH. Compared to plasma, it has higher levels of bicarbonate, lower levels of sodium and similar levels of glucose.

Pleural infection is a gradual process that transforms a self-resolving exudative PPE into a complicated multiloculated fibrinopurulent collection leading to organization and scarring which significantly impairs respiratory reserve. The British Thoracic Society (BTS) classification of PPE[3] (Table 36.1) describes:

- **'Simple PPE'**: the initial exudative effusion, with pleural fluid containing an increase in cytokines, LDH less than half that of the serum, pH >7.2 and a normal glucose level. At this stage observation and antibiotic therapy are recommended.
- **'Complicated PPE'**: the early fibrinopurulent stage when the effusion has developed features of infection but is not yet overtly purulent. This occurs as bacteria enter the pleural space through the damaged epithelium with neutrophil chemotaxis and activation of the coagulation cascade. An increase in plasminogen activator inhibitors and decrease in tissue-type plasminogen activator promotes septations. Neutrophil phagocytosis and the inflammatory process increase lactic acid production and decrease pH. The increased metabolic activity reduces glucose levels and LDH is elevated due to leukocyte cell death. Chest tube drainage is recommended for complicated PPE.
- **Empyema**: describes frank pus. It has an estimated mortality of about 20%, which in the UK is higher than that of hospitalized patients with pneumonia. A poor outcome is associated with increased age, hypotension, low serum albumin, renal impairment and hospital-acquired infection. Surgical drainage is required in approximately 20% of empyemas.[3,4]

Table 36.1 BTS classification and characteristics of PPE

Stages	Aspirated fluid appearance	Pleural fluid characteristics	Management
Simple PPE	Clear	pH >7.2 LDH <1000 IU/l Glucose >2.2 mmol/l No organisms on staining/culture	Usually clears spontaneously with antibiotic therapy alone. Chest tube drainage only for symptomatic relief
Complicated PPE	Clear or cloudy	pH <7.2 LDH >1000 IU/l Glucose <2.2 mmol/l May be organisms on staining/culture	Requires chest tube drainage
Empyema	Frank pus	No additional biochemical tests required. May be organisms on staining/culture	Requires chest tube drainage ± surgery/VATS

The American College of Chest Physicians (ACCP) consensus conference classification of PPE uses four categories based on estimated risk of poor outcome.[7] The pleural space anatomy, fluid biochemistry and bacteriology were used to categorize patients into the four groups (Table 36.2). The first two categories were treated with antibiotics and no fluid drainage. The last two categories required drainage either via tube thoracostomy, tube thoracostomy with fibrinolytics and/or video-assisted thoracoscopy (VATS) or surgery.

Table 36.2 ACCP classification and characteristics of PPE

Category	Anatomy	Microbiology	Biochemistry	Risk
1	Minimal Free flowing (<10 mm)	Unknown	Unknown	Very low
2	Small to moderate (>10 mm and <1/2 hemithorax)	Negative Gram stain and culture	pH >7.2	Low
3	Large free flowing, loculations or with pleural thickening	Positive Gram stain/culture	pH <7.2	Moderate
4	As above	Pus		High

Investigation of pleural effusions and empyema

The mortality, morbidity, high incidence of complications and health-care costs associated with empyema necessitate early evaluation and treatment. Figure 36.2 shows a diagnostic algorithm for the diagnosis and management of patients with suspected pleural infection.

The BTS recommends diagnostic pleural fluid sampling in all patients with a pleural effusion associated with sepsis or pneumonia, and the ACCP, BTS and Cochrane guidelines all conclude that clinical outcome is best predicted from pleural fluid characteristics. Meta-analysis of pleural fluid measurements used in the analysis of potential pleural infection indicates that a pleural fluid pH <7.2 has the highest accuracy, followed by glucose <2.2 mmol/l and then LDH >1000 IU/l.[2,6,7] However, even pleural fluid pH is not 100% sensitive and the possibility of pleural infection should be considered despite a pH >7.2 if the patient deteriorates or does not respond to treatment. Care must be taken when sampling pleural fluid, as the local anaesthetic lignocaine is acidic and may interfere with the measured pH value. A blood gas analyser should be used rather than pH litmus paper or a pH meter as these are not reliable. Fluid should also be sent for Gram stain, culture, acid-fast bacilli stain and culture and cytology. About 40% of infections are culture negative. Detection of anaerobes is improved by inoculating blood culture bottles with pleural fluid. Frank pus does not need further pH or biochemical evaluation but microbiology samples should be sent.

A CXR should be performed in every patient with suspected PPE. Small pleural effusions (i.e. maximal thickness <10 mm on ultrasound scan [USS]) should be observed, with pleural fluid sampling only if the effusion enlarges. Pleural USS improves visualization of septations and pleural thickening which occurs in 86%–100% of empyemas and approximately 56% of exudative PPEs. When available, pleural fluid sampling is best

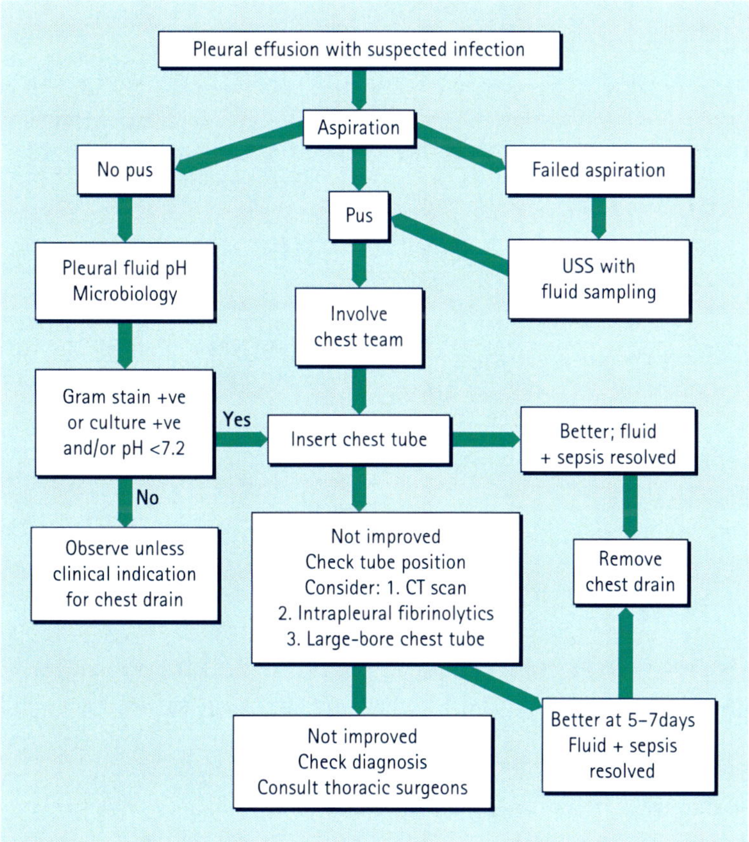

Figure 36.2 Diagnostic algorithm for the management of suspected pleural infection. +ve, positive; CT, computed tomography; USS, ultrasound scan.

performed under USS guidance, especially when effusions are small or loculated. The pH may vary between locules.

Contrast-enhanced chest computed tomography (CT) scans are performed in difficult cases to delineate the size and position of loculated effusions and to guide drainage. Empyema is associated with attenuation of extrapleural subcostal fat and pleural enhancement, which may result in the 'split pleura sign' of enhanced but separated visceral and parietal pleura. CT scans also differentiate between parenchymal and pleural disease (e.g. lung abscess). Bronchoscopy is only indicated if a bronchial lesion is suspected.

If a tuberculous effusion is suspected, pleural biopsy should be performed as this increases diagnostic yield. Pleural fluid adenosine deaminase may be of value in countries where tuberculosis is prevalent. It has a high negative predictive value and may be useful to rule out tuberculosis in countries with low incidence. However, the high sensitivity and low specificity can result in false-positive results in complicated PPE, empyema and neoplasia (especially mesothelioma and some lymphoma).[8]

Causative organisms in infected pleural fluid

In community-acquired infections, aerobic organisms include *Streptococcus milleri* (28%), *Streptococcus pneumoniae* (14%) and *Staphylococcus* (12%), although many other organisms may be implicated. In hospital-acquired infections, methicillin-resistant *Staphylococcus aureus* (MRSA) and other staphylococci account for approximately 50%. Gram-negative organisms, mainly *Escherichia coli*, *Enterobacter* spp. and *Pseudomonas*, are responsible for the majority of the remainder. The Gram-negative organisms (e.g. *E. coli*, *Pseudomonas*, *Haemophilus influenzae*, *Klebsiella*) are usually part of mixed infections with anaerobes and rarely occur in isolation.[3]

In both CAP and HAP, anaerobes occur in 12%–34% but have been reported in up to 76% of cases. They are often associated with aspiration and poor oral hygiene. Anaerobic empyema often presents less acutely with general ill health and weight loss but without fever.

Management of parapneumonic pleural effusions

The diagnosis of PPE and empyema must be considered in patients with 'slow to respond' pneumonia or pleural effusion with fever, or in high-risk patients with non-specific symptoms including weight loss. In this case, the slow response to initial antibiotic therapy, the development of pleural effusions, recurrent fevers and the subsequent finding of a low pH, low glucose and high LDH in pleural fluid biochemistry raise the possibility of an infected PPE or empyema.

- **Antibiotics**. Potentially infected PPE should always be treated with antibiotics. Whenever possible, antibiotic therapy is guided by microbiological results. Initial empirical treatment in community-acquired infections is with a second-generation cephalosporin (e.g. cefuroxime) or a penicillin ± β-lactamase inhibitor (e.g. co-amoxiclav), which have good pleural space penetration and cover most expected organisms. Metronidazole is added if an anaerobic infection is suspected. Alternatively, clindamycin as a single agent or combined with ciprofloxacin may be used. Benzylpenicillin with a quinolone gives the same spectrum with less risk of *Clostridium difficile* diarrhoea. If microbiology is negative, antibiotics should initially cover community-acquired bacterial pathogens and anaerobic organisms.

  In hospital-acquired infections due to HAP, trauma or surgery, antibiotics should cover Gram-positive, Gram-negative and anaerobic organisms. Post-operative and trauma cases should also cover staphylococcal infections. Recommended antibiotics include piperacillin with tazobactam, ticarcillin with clavulanic acid, carbapenems or third-generation cephalosporins. Aminoglycosides are avoided because they have poor pleural space penetration and are less active in acidic pleural fluid. MRSA infection is common and may require vancomycin cover. There is no clear evidence regarding length of treatment, but provided there is adequate pleural drainage, treatment for three weeks is probably appropriate. Once the systemic symptoms and fever resolve, oral antibiotics may be used and co-amoxiclav is a useful single agent with anaerobic cover.
- **Chest tube drainage** is indicated when pleural fluid is frankly purulent or turbid, when organisms are detected on Gram stain or culture, and if pH is <7.2, glucose <2.2 mmol/l or LDH is >1000 IU/l. Early drainage is considered for loculated

effusions and in the elderly or those with comorbid conditions, as these are associated with poor outcome.

The ideal chest tube size is debated. Small-bore (10–14 French) tubes have been shown to be as effective as large drains and are more comfortable, but large-bore drains may be more appropriate for thick, viscid purulent fluid. The position of the drain is important and tube insertion is best carried out under image guidance. Drains should be flushed eight-hourly with 30 ml of normal saline to prevent occlusion. Remove drains when clinical improvement occurs.

- **Intrapleural fibrinolytics** including streptokinase and streptodornase were first reported to be beneficial 50 years ago. Subsequently four small trials and several observational studies suggested potential efficacy. However, a recent, relatively large, UK-based prospective trial showed no benefit in terms of mortality, surgery or hospital stay.[9] Consequently routine use is not recommended although many chest physicians continue to use fibrinolytics in patients unsuitable for surgery.
- **Pleural lavage and intrapleural antiseptics** have been reported to be beneficial in the treatment of pleural infection in several small studies,[10,11] but there are no randomized trial data and this cannot be recommended.
- **Nutritional support.** Hypoalbuminaemia is associated with poor outcome. Supplementary nasogastric feeding and parenteral nutrition should be considered from the time of diagnosis.

Management of patients who 'fail to improve'

Initially review the microbiology and adjust antibiotics. Ensure good tube drainage by flushing with saline and checking for kinks. Consider a repeat CT scan to assess the extent of residual collection. Remove persistently blocked tubes and insert image-guided new small-bore drains into loculated collections. If surgical intervention is not an option, consider large-bore drains, lavage and surgical rib resection under local anaesthetic with subsequent open drainage.

Surgical review is normally recommended if there is clinical deterioration including weight loss, ongoing features of sepsis or a residual pleural collection with loculations and pleural thickening after seven days despite drainage and antibiotics.[11] Surgical options include:

1. VATS to break down adhesions and drain residual collections. This may be unsuccessful in chronic empyema with thickened visceral pleura;
2. Thoracotomy, pleural decortication and removal of pleural debris;
3. Rib resection and open drainage, which can be performed under local anaesthetic.

Long-term complications of empyema

Residual pleural thickening occurs in 13.8% of cases after six months.[12] It does not usually impair lung function. Surgical therapy is considered when there is significant impairment in lung function with reduced total lung capacity (<60% predicted) and >50% reduction of lung perfusion (fibrothorax). Decortication is the definitive treatment but general agreement is to wait for six months before considering surgery as diffuse pleural thickening may resolve spontaneously over a few months.

This patient responded well to tube thoracostomy and antibiotic therapy. She was discharged without any sequelae.

Conclusion

Delayed treatment of, or untreated, pleural infection is associated with high morbidity and mortality. Any patient with prolonged sepsis in the context of pneumonic illness should be investigated for pleural infection. Timely assessment and interventions in these patients can significantly improve the outcome. This patient made a complete recovery with appropriate intervention.

Further Reading

1. Finley C, Clifton J, Fitzgerald JM, Yee J. Empyema: an increasing concern in Canada. *Can Respir J* 2008; **15**: 85–9.
2. Farjah F, Symons RG, Krishnadasan B, Wood DE, Flum DR. Management of pleural space infections: a population-based analysis. *J Thorac Cardiovasc Surg* 2007; **133**: 346–51.
3. Davies HE, Davies RJO, Davies CWH. British Thoracic Society pleural disease guideline 2010. Management of pleural infection in adults. *Thorax* 2010; **65**(Suppl 2): ii41–ii53.
4. Cameron RJ, Davies HRH. Intra-pleural fibrinolytic therapy versus conservative management in the treatment of parapneumonic effusions and empyema. *Cochrane Database Syst Rev* 2011; CD002312.
5. Hasley PB, Albaum MN, Li YH *et al.* Do pulmonary radiographic findings at presentation predict mortality in patients with community-acquired pneumonia? *Arch Intern Med* 1996; **156**: 2206–12.
6. Fine MJ, Smith MA, Carson CA *et al.* Prognosis and outcomes of patients with community-acquired pneumonia. A meta-analysis. *JAMA* 1996; **275**: 134–41.
7. Colice GL, Curtis A, Deslauriers J *et al.* Medical and surgical treatment of parapneumonic effusions: an evidence-based guideline. *Chest* 2000; **118**: 1158–71.
8. Jiménez Castro D, Díaz Nuevo G, Pérez-Rodríguez E, Light RW. Diagnostic value of adenosine deaminase in nontuberculous lymphocytic pleural effusions. *Eur Respir J* 2003; **21**: 220–4.
9. Maskell NA, Davies CW, Nunn AJ *et al.* U.K. Controlled trial of intrapleural streptokinase for pleural infection. *N Engl J Med* 2005; **352**: 865–74.
10. Mennander A, Laurikka J, Kuukasjärvi P, Tarkka M. Continuous pleural lavage may decrease postoperative morbidity in patients undergoing thoracotomy for stage 2 thoracic empyema. *Eur J Cardiothorac Surg* 2005; **27**: 32–4.
11. Rosenfeldt FL, McGibney D, Braimbridge MV, Watson DA. Comparison between irrigation and conventional treatment for empyema and pneumonectomy space infection. *Thorax* 1981; **36**: 272–7.
12. Jiménez Castro D, Díaz G, Pérez-Rodriguez E, Light RW. Prognostic features of residual pleural thickening in parapneumonic pleural effusions. *Eur Respir J* 2003; **21**: 952–5.

PROBLEM

37 Spontaneous Pneumothorax: Langerhans Cell Histiocytosis

Eleanor Giddings, Boris Lams, Elizabeth Hadley

Case History

A 34-year-old male chef presented with acute right pleuritic chest pain and severe breathlessness. He smoked 40 cigarettes a day and had noticed slight dyspnoea for two years. He denied risk factors for human immunodeficiency virus infection. He had no fever, clubbing or cervical lymphadenopathy but the right hemithorax was hyperresonant with reduced expansion and absent breath sounds. Cardiovascular examination was normal with no signs of pulmonary hypertension. Blood results including C-reactive protein were normal. A chest X-ray was performed (Figure 37.1).

What does the chest X-ray show and what is the immediate management?

How should a pneumothorax be managed?

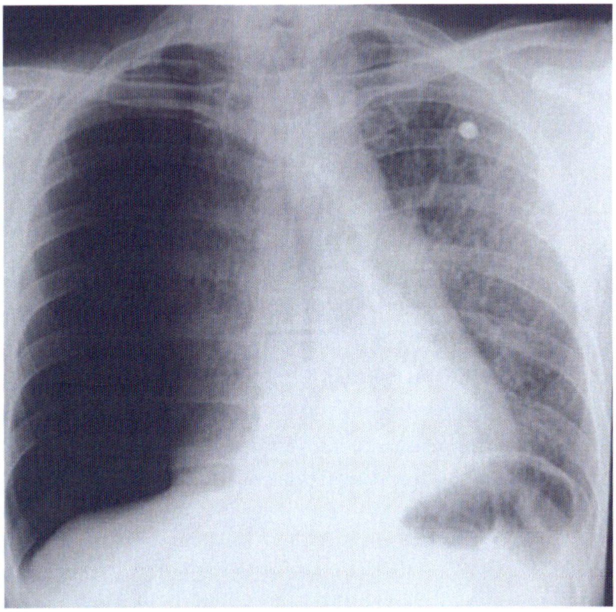

Figure 37.1 Chest X-ray on arrival.

What does the chest computed tomography (CT) scan show and what is the underlying diagnosis?

What is pulmonary Langerhans cell histiocytosis (PLCH)?

What is the management of PLCH?

What is the prognosis of PLCH?

Background

In this case the chest X-ray shows a large right-sided pneumothorax with mediastinal shift. Pneumothoraces are classified into primary spontaneous pneumothorax (PSP) or secondary pneumothorax (SPP).

A PSP is a pneumothorax occurring in a healthy lung. An SPP is a pneumothorax associated with underlying lung disease. An SPP should be suspected in patients over 50 years of age, in those with a significant smoking history or if there is clinical or radiological evidence of underlying lung disease. Causes of a secondary pneumothorax include asthma, chronic obstructive pulmonary disease, *Pneumocystis jirovecii (carinii)* pneumonia, cystic fibrosis, tuberculosis, pulmonary Langerhans cell histiocytosis, lymphangioleiomyomatosis and thoracic endometriosis (catamenial pneumothorax).

Management

In this case the right-sided tension pneumothorax requires immediate treatment by insertion of a cannula through the right second intercostal space in the mid-clavicular line. Then an intercostal chest drain should be placed in the triangle of safety. Written consent is required for elective intercostal drain insertion, but in an emergency verbal consent suffices.[1]

The management of a pneumothorax that is not under tension depends on its type (PSP or SPP), size and the degree of clinical compromise (see Figure 37.2).[2] The size of a pneumothorax is measured from the lung margin to the chest wall. A pneumothorax can be large (>2 cm) or small (<2 cm). Symptoms and degree of clinical compromise are more important than size in determining management. Patients with significant breathlessness and PSP or SPP of any size should have the pneumothorax drained.

A patient with a PSP that is less than 2 cm in size and asymptomatic can be discharged and followed-up in 2–4 weeks. If a PSP is large or symptomatic then it should be aspirated. If aspiration fails then a chest drain should be inserted.

A patient with an SPP should be admitted and treated with oxygen. If the SPP is large or symptomatic a pleural drain should be inserted. If it is between 1 cm and 2 cm and asymptomatic it should be aspirated. An SPP less than 1 cm should be observed.

This patient had a right-sided chest drain inserted. A repeat chest X-ray (Figure 37.3) showed a well-placed intercostal drain with the tip at the apex of the right lung. However, the lung is not fully expanded suggesting a persistent air leak. Diffuse cystic change can be seen in the left lung. The underlying lung disease means that the pneumothorax is secondary. The following day the patient developed increasing breathlessness and a further chest X-ray revealed a new left-sided pneumothorax. A left-sided chest drain was inserted and a high-resolution CT chest scan was performed to look in more detail at the lung parenchyma (Figure 37.4).

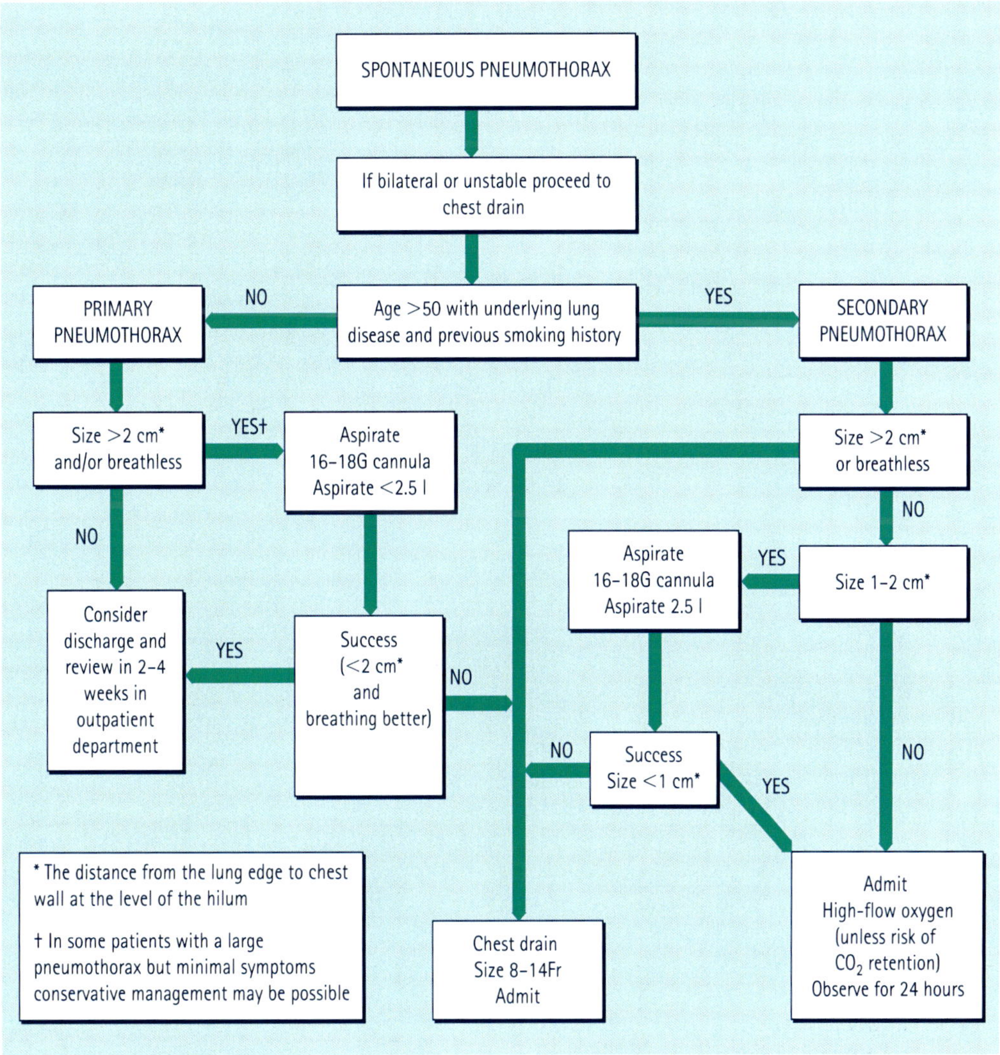

Figure 37.2 Management of a spontaneous pneumothorax. (From the British Thoracic Society Pleural Disease Guideline 2010.[2])

Pulmonary Langerhans cell histiocytosis

Pulmonary Langerhans cell histiocytosis is a rare granulomatous interstitial lung disease that affects young smokers and is associated with significant morbidity. It affects 2–5 per 1 000 000 individuals per year and is diagnosed in <5% of lung biopsies.[3] Those affected are usually Caucasian, smokers and aged between 20 and 40 years although it can present at any age. Men are as often affected as women although women may present later. No geographical, occupational or genetic predisposition has been reported although there have been a few familial cases. The cause is unknown but smoking is thought to be a major risk factor as greater than 90% of those with PLCH smoke, usually more than 20 cigarettes a day.[4,5]

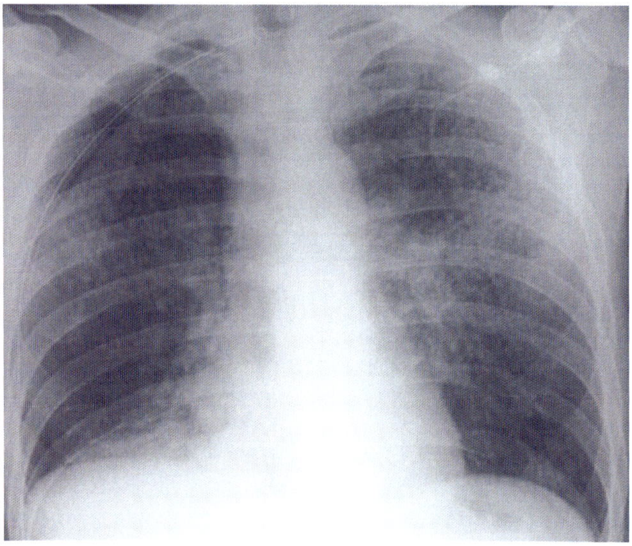

Figure 37.3 Chest X-ray after pleural drain insertion.

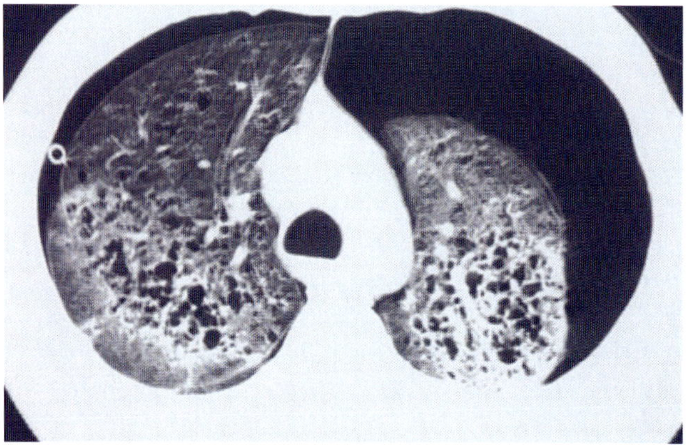

Figure 37.4 High-resolution CT chest scan.

The Langerhans cell (LC) is an antigen-presenting cell of the monocyte–macrophage line, present normally in many tissues including the skin, reticulo-endothelial system and airway epithelium. LCs contain the cytoplasmic Birbeck granule and can be found in association with smoking in normal individuals and in other lung disorders such as idiopathic pulmonary fibrosis.

The LCs of PLCH are characteristically found in clusters and in greater quantities than in other lung diseases. In early cellular PLCH, LCs multiply and accumulate in multiple small bronchiocentric granulomas, forming nodules which frequently extend into the lung parenchyma. The nodules then cavitate to form thick- and then thin-walled cysts and eventually fibrosis. The pulmonary arterioles and venules may also be involved. Older lesions may be relatively acellular and so differentiation may be difficult from end-stage extensive fibrosis, honeycombing and cystic lesions. Pseudo-desquamative interstitial pneumonia, respiratory bronchiolitis and intraluminal fibrosis may occasionally be seen in association with PLCH.

Langerhans cell histiocytosis is confined to the lungs in 85% of patients with the disease. Breathlessness on exertion and a dry cough are the predominant symptoms. Approximately two-thirds of patients with PLCH present with dry cough and breathlessness on exertion, whilst one-third have constitutional features such as fever or weight loss. Less than 25% of patients with PLCH are asymptomatic with incidental findings on chest X-ray. Up to 10% of patients with PLCH present with a spontaneous pneumothorax which may be recurrent or bilateral.[4]

Extrathoracic involvement includes bony lesions, diabetes insipidus from hypothalamic involvement and abdominal pain from hepatic and splenic infiltration. Examination is usually normal although lymphadenopathy and skin lesions may occur. Rarely there is clubbing, or crackles on auscultation. There may be signs of pulmonary hypertension.

Radiological abnormalities depend on the stage of the disease. In one series, less than 10% of chest X-rays of patients with PLCH appeared normal.[4] Initially the nodules are small (<5 mm) and then cavitation occurs into thick- and thin-walled cysts of varying diameter. Some patients with PLCH progress to fibrosis. The chest X-ray may show bilateral, symmetrical, nodular, reticulo-nodular or cystic changes with upper and middle lobe predominance. Classically there is sparing of the costophrenic angles.

A high-resolution CT chest scan in patients with PLCH typically shows nodules and cysts that are uniformly distributed and interspersed by normal lung parenchyma. Nodules may be well or poorly defined, and occasionally large or irregular in shape. Nodules may regress. Cysts usually persist or enlarge. As with chest X-ray, there is sparing of the costophrenic angles. Atypical appearances include single nodules, purely nodular or cystic disease, or enlarged airways.

High-resolution CT has a high sensitivity for PLCH particularly with the following combination: ill-defined nodules of 2–10 mm size, reticulo-nodular infiltrates, upper zone cysts or honeycombing, preservation of lung volume, costophrenic angle sparing. Fibrosis and honeycombing is seen in advanced disease. Increased total lung volumes or hyperinflation is typical although reduced lung volume may occur with fibrosis.

Lung function tests show that approximately half of patients with PLCH have an obstructive picture, particularly those with cystic disease. Restriction can occur late in the disease if fibrosis is present. Most of the patients have reduced diffusion capacity. Reduced diffusion capacity may cause both exertional dyspnoea and exertional hypoxia. Lung volumes are normal or increased, although may be reduced with fibrosis. Arterial blood gases at rest are usually normal early in the disease. Full lung function tests including diffusion capacity are required for disease monitoring.

In the majority of cases the clinical and radiological characteristics are sufficient for the diagnosis of PLCH. Blood tests are usually normal. When presentation is atypical or diagnostic uncertainty remains, an open or video-assisted thoracoscopic lung biopsy should be considered. Biopsy of extrathoracic sites such as bone can also secure the diagnosis. Open lung biopsy gives the highest yield although some focal areas may be missed.

Management of PLCH

Smoking cessation is essential in the management of PLCH. There is limited evidence for other treatments. Corticosteroids may be tried if there are prominent nodular opacities, or if the patient is symptomatic. Respiratory infection is a cause of deteriorating respiratory function and needs prompt treatment.

Chemotherapy such as cladribine, vinblastine, cytarabine, doxorubicin, methotrexate, cyclophosphamide and etoposide has been tried but there is no clear evidence of benefit in isolated PLCH.[6] Radiotherapy can help to palliate bone pain but is not useful for parenchymal involvement.

Lung transplantation should be considered in advanced progressive disease with respiratory failure or severe pulmonary hypertension, although PLCH may recur in transplanted lungs.

Prognosis

Patients with PLCH have a reduced life expectancy compared to a healthy population. However, the disease course is variable; in a half of patients, radiological abnormalities will partially or completely resolve. However, the disease may recur in the future. Pulmonary hypertension is common and independently associated with reduced survival. Patients with PLCH have an increased risk of lung malignancy.

A review of 102 patients showed that those with PLCH had a shorter median survival time than age-matched controls. The estimated five- and ten-year survival rates were 74% and 64%, respectively. Almost half of the deaths were attributed to respiratory failure. The remainder of deaths were due to malignancy.

Prognosis is favourable in patients with either spontaneous improvement or improvement with corticosteroids. Factors associated with a poor prognosis are extremes of age at disease onset, ongoing constitutional symptoms, recurrent pneumothoraces, abnormal lung function, severe pulmonary hypertension and extrathoracic lesions (except bone).

Pregnancy has not been shown to influence the course of PLCH in most patients. Unless the patient has severe respiratory failure, PLCH is not a contraindication to pregnancy. Exacerbations of LC histiocytosis-related diabetes insipidus in pregnancy have been reported.

Conclusion

In this patient the high-resolution CT chest scan showed widespread cystic changes in the upper lobes and bilateral pneumothoraces. In a smoker with bilateral pneumothoraces and this high-resolution CT appearance, the most likely diagnosis would be PLCH. This patient was referred to a thoracic surgeon and underwent a left video-assisted thoracoscopic lung biopsy, pleural abrasion and talc pleurodesis. Histology confirmed PLCH. His right-sided pneumothorax resolved with drainage alone over three days.

Early diagnosis of pulmonary Langerhans cell histiocytosis coupled with strong smoking cessation support is likely to give the best outcomes.

Further Reading

1 National Patient Safety Agency. Chest drains: risks associated with the insertion of chest drains. Rapid Response Report 1065, 2008. www.npsa.nhs.uk/nrls/alerts-and-directives/ (accessed 01 06 11).

2 British Thoracic Society. British Thoracic Society Pleural Disease Guideline 2010. *Thorax* 2010; **65**(Suppl 2): ii1–ii7. www.brit-thoracic.org.uk (accessed 01 06 11).

3 Maskell N, Millar A (eds). *Oxford Desk Reference: Respiratory Medicine*. New York: Oxford University Press, 2009.

4 Tazi A. Adult pulmonary Langerhans' cell histiocytosis. *Eur Respir J* 2006; **27**: 1272–85.

5 Sundar K, Gosselin MV, Chung HL, Cahill BC. Pulmonary Langerhans cell histiocytosis: emerging concepts in pathobiology, radiology, and clinical evoluation of disease. *Chest* 2003; **123**: 1673–83.

6 Lazor R, Etienne-Masroianni B, Khouatra C, Tazi A, Cottin V, Cordier J-F. Progressive diffuse pulmonary Langerhans cell histiocytosis improved by cladribine chemotherapy. *Thorax* 2009; **64**: 274–5.

PROBLEM

38 Mesothelioma and Asbestos-related Pleural Disease

Amina Aitsi-Selmi, Charles Twort

Case History

A 64-year-old carpenter was referred to the chest clinic with a four-week history of increasing breathlessness on exercise, persistent dry cough, weight loss and night sweats. He complained of persistent, right-sided chest ache but denied any wheeze or haemoptysis. Previous antibiotics and inhaler therapy were of no benefit. He had worked in the same joinery factory since he was 23 years old. There was no other significant medical history. He had no previous chest illness or chest radiographs. He had never smoked, had no contact with avian proteins or pets and was not aware of any industrial dust exposure or direct asbestos contact.

On examination he was not dyspnoeic at rest. His saturation was 97% on air and examination of the chest revealed dullness to percussion at the right base with normal breath sounds and no crepitations. Figure 38.1 illustrates (A) his chest radiograph (CXR) and (B) his contrast-enhanced computed tomography (CT) scan. Respiratory function tests showed a restrictive pattern (forced expiratory volume in 1 second [FEV_1] 2.0 l [67% predicted], forced vital capacity [FVC] 2.3 l [66% predicted] and normal gas transfer factor).

What are the possible causes and how is the diagnosis confirmed?

What factors must be considered when planning pleural investigations?

Why is histological diagnosis important in malignant mesothelioma?

What factors influence the risk of malignancy in asbestos exposure?

What is the role of surgery and radiotherapy in mesothelioma management?

Should pleural plaques be followed-up and is it possible to screen for the development of mesothelioma, lung cancer or asbestosis in asbestos-exposed patients?

Will patients be compensated if they have asbestos-related pleural disease?

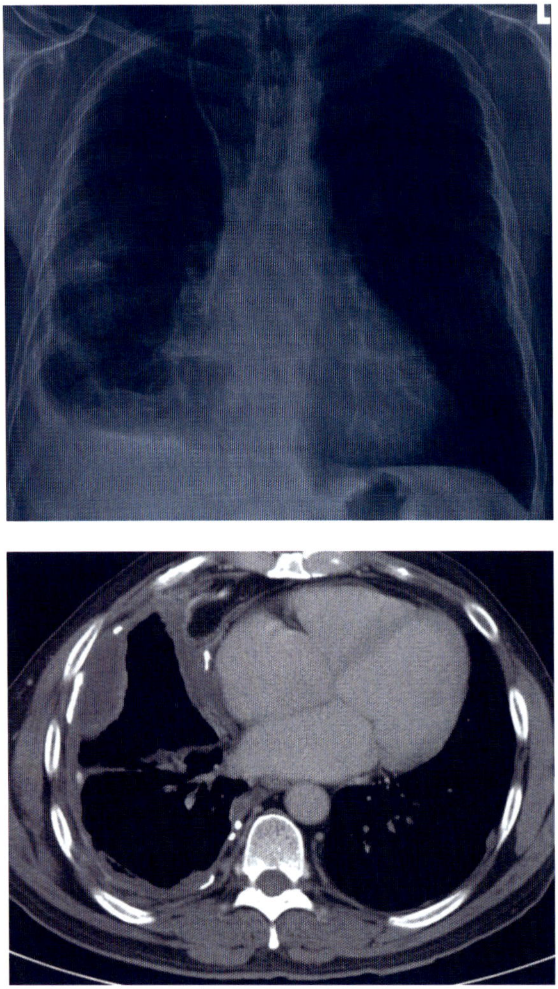

(A)

(B)

Figure 38.1 (A) Chest X-ray and (B) contrast-enhanced CT scan.

Background

Asbestos causes both benign and malignant disease. Exposure is usually occupational and occurs during construction (e.g. fireproofing, insulation), demolition work, manufacturing (e.g. brake linings) or mining. Domestic exposure occurs due to 'carry home' fibres on clothing, geological exposure in some regions (e.g. Corsica) and during domestic refurbishment.

In the UK, industrial asbestos use peaked in the 1970s and asbestos-related disease will be a significant problem for the next 20 years, with the peak incidence of mesothelioma occurring in about 2020. The coroner should be notified of any proven or suspected asbestos-related deaths.

In this case the CXR (Figure 38.1A) reveals right-sided pleural thickening and the CT scan of the chest shows nodular, irregular pleural thickening extending onto the mediastinal surfaces and into the interlobar fissures. The CT scan should include contrast enhancement which helps differentiate benign and malignant pleural disease. Positron emission tomography scans can also be helpful.

Although the patient denied direct asbestos exposure, use of asbestos sheeting for fireproofing was common in 1960–70 in the joinery trade. Consequently, the possibility of asbestos-related disease must be considered.

Benign asbestos-related pleural diseases include:

- **Pleural plaques** (± calcification) which occur bilaterally in the parietal pleura, particularly on the posterolateral chest wall and the dome of the diaphragm, in approximately 50% of asbestos-exposed workers after 20–30 years. They are typically asymptomatic, usually incidental findings on chest radiography and are not premalignant, but the asbestos exposure that caused the plaques carries a risk of malignant disease.
- **Benign asbestos-related pleural effusions** which occur approximately 20 years after exposure and are small and unilateral. They are either asymptomatic or associated with pleurisy, fever and dyspnoea. The effusion is an exudate, often blood stained. It may precede the development of diffuse pleural thickening.
- **Diffuse pleural thickening (DPT)** due to extensive fibrosis of the visceral pleura with areas of adhesion to the parietal pleura and associated obliteration of the pleural space. Unlike pleural plaques, its margins are ill defined and it involves the apices, costophrenic angles and interlobar fissures. Breathlessness, chest pain and occasionally respiratory failure are due to the associated constrictive pulmonary defect. There is no association with the development of mesothelioma, from which it is differentiated by pleural biopsy.

In this case, the clinical symptoms (i.e. pain, breathlessness) and CT scan findings of pleural irregularity with contrast enhancement and mediastinal extension raise the probability of malignant disease (e.g. mesothelioma, metastatic adenocarcinoma). Diagnosis is established by pleural aspiration, biopsy and immunocytochemistry.

- **Pleural fluid aspiration**, with cytological examination, confirms the diagnosis of malignant pleural disease in 40%–87% (mean sensitivity 60%) of subsequently proven malignant cases.[1,2] In 65% the diagnosis is established from the first aspiration, 27% from the second and only 5% from the third. Yield depends on tumour type, with higher diagnostic rates for adenocarcinoma compared to mesothelioma or squamous cell carcinoma. In mesothelioma, cytological examination is positive for malignant cells in one-third of cases but rarely gives a definitive diagnosis.[2]

- **Abrams pleural biopsy** increases histological yield by approximately 7%–27% if combined with pleural fluid cytology in malignant pleural effusions. When cytology is negative, blind needle biopsy has a yield of about 50% for malignant effusions but <50% for mesothelioma.[1] Image-guided (e.g. ultrasound, CT scan) cutting needle biopsies achieve higher yields than blind biopsies and establish the diagnosis in more than 85% of malignant effusions with a sensitivity of 86%–93% for mesothelioma.[1] If the result is negative, as it was in this patient, local anaesthetic thoracoscopy or video-assisted thoracoscopy (VATS) with biopsy under direct vision, or an open pleural biopsy, will help establish the diagnosis.
- **Immunocytochemistry** helps distinguish benign from malignant mesothelial cells and mesothelioma from adenocarcinoma. Epithelial membrane antigen (EMA) is widely used to confirm epithelial malignancy. For the diagnosis of mesothelioma it is recommended to use two markers with positive diagnostic value for mesothelioma (anti-calretinin, anti-WT1 [anti-Wilms tumour 1], anti-EMA or anti-CK5/6 [anti-cytokeratin 5/6]) and two markers with negative diagnostic value to validate the diagnosis (such as anti-Ber-EP4 [human epithelial antigen], anti-TTF-1 [anti-thyroid transcription factor 1] or monoclonal anti-CEA [anti-carcino-embryonic antigen]). In this patient, histological examination confirmed a sarcomatous mesothelioma.

Pleural investigation in potential mesothelioma cases

Prophylactic radiotherapy should be considered when planning diagnostic or drainage procedures in potential mesothelioma cases, as tumour cells may seed in the tracks made by chest instrumentation (e.g. pleural aspiration, biopsy, chest drains, VATS).

In one series of 40 patients, three daily radiotherapy fractions two weeks prior to an intervention reduced the incidence of tumour seeding and local metastases from 40% to zero in untreated and radiotherapy groups, respectively.[3] However, a pooled analysis of three small randomized trials found no significant reduction in the frequency of procedure-tract metastases. Localized post-procedure radiotherapy is more frequently instigated and intervention sites should be marked with India ink to assist subsequent radiotherapy field alignment.[4]

Histological diagnosis in malignant mesothelioma

The diagnosis of malignant mesothelioma should be confirmed histologically except when the patient is too unwell or frail for biopsy. Confirmation strengthens the case for compensation as well as informing individual treatments and prognosis.

Malignant mesothelioma can be epithelioid (approximately 50%), sarcomatoid or mixed (biphasic). Sarcomatoid types have the worst prognosis with an average survival time of 5–10 months and the epithelioid types the best survival time at 8–16 months.[2] Histological confirmation may also be necessary for participation in clinical trials.

Factors that influence the risk of mesothelioma and lung cancer in asbestos exposure

Asbestos is a naturally occurring hydrated silica fibre that can be divided into two groups on the basis of shape, lung clearance kinetics and pathogenic potential:

- **Chrysotile** (white asbestos) is a curly serpentine fibre which represents 80%–90% of commercially used asbestos (mainly in developing countries).
- **Amphiboles** are straight, needle-like fibres including amosite (brown asbestos) and crocidolite (blue). Amphiboles clear more slowly from the lung and are more carcinogenic than chrysotile.

All fibre types of asbestos are lung carcinogens. However, the long latency periods, usual exposure to mixed fibre types and other factors like smoking make it difficult to determine the carcinogenicity of each fibre type.[2,5] There is a dose–response relationship between exposure to friable, inhaled asbestos and the risk of lung cancer. The risk increases with both maximum intensity of exposure and the cumulative dose. Recent studies suggest a sixfold increase in the risk of lung cancer in non-smokers. Smoking increases this risk. In asbestos workers, death from lung cancer increased 16-fold if they smoked more than 20 cigarettes per day and 9-fold if they smoked fewer than 20 per day, compared to non-smokers. Workers with asbestosis are at even greater risk of lung cancer. There has been controversy as to whether this is because asbestosis is a marker for heavier asbestos exposure or if the inflammatory process of asbestosis is important *per se* in promoting carcinogenesis.

The risk of developing a mesothelioma also increases with extent and duration of asbestos exposure. For equal exposure, crocidolite increases this risk by four to ten times compared to chrysotile. However, this increased risk is not sufficient to ascribe total causation to the small percentage of crocidolite fibres in mixed-fibre exposure. Occupation also affects the risk of developing mesothelioma. Asbestos manufacture is associated with a 6.7% increase in lung malignancies per fibre-ml/year compared to crocidolite mining at 0.17% and chrysotile mining at <0.17%. Non-occupational exposure to asbestos including household exposure (e.g. cohabitants of asbestos workers) and residential exposure from pollution in mining areas or from local asbestos factories may cause disease.[6] The risk of developing mesothelioma also increases with increasing duration from the time of first exposure.

The roles of surgery, radiotherapy and chemotherapy in mesothelioma management

Chemotherapy with pemetrexed and cisplatin is currently the mainstay of palliative chemotherapy for mesothelioma.

After careful selection of patients suitable for surgery, the most favourable outcomes are reported with trimodal therapies including extrapleuropneumonectomy (EPP), combinations of pre- and post-operative chemotherapy and radiotherapy.

The overall survival rate for EPP followed by radiation and adjuvant chemotherapy is 36% at two years (52% for patients with epithelial cell-type tumours; and 16% in sarcomatous or mixed histology tumours). A 46% five-year survival rate has been reported for patients with epithelioid mesothelioma, no mediastinal lymph node involvement and negative resection margins at surgery.[7] However, the majority of patients have recurrent disease usually in the ipsilateral hemithorax or abdomen. Unfortunately, these initial encouraging results have not been supported by the preliminary results from the MARS trial.

Other surgical palliative measures, like talc pleurodesis to control pleural effusions, can be combined with biopsy and pleurectomy for those with more extensive mesotheliomas. Radiotherapy relieves pain and reduces chest wall masses in about 50% of cases but rarely palliates breathlessness or superior vena cava obstruction.[2]

Screening in asbestos-exposed patients

There is no consensus about the appropriate follow-up of asbestos-exposed patients including those with pleural plaques. In practice, the majority are seen when symptoms develop. However, the American Thoracic Society guidelines (1986)[8] and Helsinki criteria (1997)[9] suggest that all patients with significant asbestos exposure require a baseline CXR, spirometry and a single-breath diffusion capacity. Patients with a history of exposure more than ten years previously but no manifest disease may reasonably be monitored with CXR and lung function studies every 3–5 years to identify the onset of asbestos-related disease. The positive predictive value of a minimally abnormal CXR in making the diagnosis of asbestosis exceeds 50% when the background population asbestos exposure is high, and falls below 30% when it is infrequent. Use of multiple test criteria to identify abnormal lung function reduces sensitivity without enhancing specificity for asbestos-related disease.[10]

Screening for lung cancer with annual CXR, CT or sputum cytology does not reduce morbidity or mortality in populations of smokers without significant adverse occupational exposure. Newer technologies (e.g. low-dose spiral CT scans) are being evaluated in high-risk groups. There is no definite role for tumour markers (e.g. osteopontin, mesothelin) in the screening of high-risk individuals or those presenting with features suggestive of mesothelioma.

Compensation in asbestos-related pleural disease

The British Thoracic Society issued guidance on compensation for asbestos-related diseases.[2] Identification of asbestos exposure is essential and the legal test is that the diagnosis and causation should be established on the balance of probability. Patients are not eligible for compensation if their exposure occurred whilst they were self-employed. Histological diagnosis is not mandatory but prevents subsequent debate. Compensation can be claimed in two ways in the UK:

- **From the Government**. A claim for Industrial Injuries Disablement Benefit (using form BI 100PD from the Benefits Agency; Tel. 0800 882200 or www.dwp.gov.uk) applies to prescribed diseases including DPT, asbestosis, lung cancer (associated with DPT or asbestosis) and mesothelioma and scheduled occupations (i.e. exposure to asbestos). Alternatively the War Pensions Scheme may provide compensation for disease resulting from asbestos exposure in the armed forces (form WPA 0001). Compensation is not available for pleural plaques alone. The value of the compensation reflects the degree of disability and age at diagnosis. Next of kin may claim within six months posthumously.
- **Common Law**. This allows a claim for compensation from a previous employer. Even when the employer is no longer in existence, a claim is possible through their previous insurer. Patients must be advised to seek legal advice promptly (and this should be documented in the notes) as proceedings for these claims must start within three years of diagnosis or they become 'statute barred' and cannot be pursued in the courts. If neither an employer nor an insurer can be identified, a claim can be made to the Department of Environment, Transport and Regions under the Pneumoconiosis Act 1979. Isolated pleural plaques are no longer considered for compensation. Awards for asbestosis range from £15 000–45 000 depending on disability and these patients may accept higher 'once and for all' awards. Typical awards

for mesothelioma including additional claims for loss of earnings and ongoing care may exceed £50 000–200 000.

Conclusion

This patient presented with a unilateral pleural effusion with radiographic evidence of irregular pleural thickening, and a history of progressive breathlessness, chest wall pain, weight loss and sweats, having probably worked with asbestos starting 41 years previously. These clinical features are characteristic of malignant pleural mesothelioma and this was subsequently confirmed histologically.

Further Reading

1 British Thoracic Society. BTS pleural disease guideline 2010. *Thorax* 2010; **65**(Suppl 2): ii1–ii76.

2 British Thoracic Society Standards of Care Committee. BTS statement on malignant mesothelioma in the United Kingdom, 2007. *Thorax* 2007; **62**(Suppl 2): ii1–ii19.

3 Boutin C, Rey F, Viallat JR. Prevention of malignant seeding after invasive diagnostic procedures in patients with pleural mesothelioma. A randomized trial of local radiotherapy. *Chest* 1995; **108**: 754–8.

4 West SD, Foord T, Davies RJ. Needle-track metastases and prophylactic radiotherapy for mesothelioma. *Respir Med* 2006; **100**: 1037–40.

5 Nicholson WJ. The carcinogenicity of chrysotile asbestos–a review. *Ind Health* 2001; **39**: 57–64.

6 Camus M, Siemiatycki J, Meek B. Nonoccupational exposure to chrysotile asbestos and the risk of lung cancer. *N Engl J Med* 1998; **338**: 1565–71.

7 Sugarbaker DJ, Flores RM, Jaklitsch MT *et al.* Resection margins, extrapleural nodal status, and cell type determine postoperative long-term survival in trimodality therapy of malignant pleural mesothelioma: results in 183 patients. *J Thorac Cardiovasc Surg* 1999; **117**: 54–65.

8 American Thoracic Society. The diagnosis of nonmalignant diseases related to asbestos. *Am Rev Respir Dis* 1986; **134**: 363–8.

9 Tossavainen A. Consensus report. Asbestos, asbestosis, and cancer: the Helsinki criteria for diagnosis and attribution. *Scand J Work Environ Health* 1997; **23**: 311–6.

10 American Thoracic Society. Diagnosis and initial management of nonmalignant diseases related to asbestos. *Am J Respir Crit Care Med* 2004; **170**: 691–715.

Index